"*The Matthews Model of Clinical Reasoning* is a book both for occupational therapy students and seasoned practitioners. It offers a new model for understanding our clients and developing client-centered evaluations and intervention plans. It provides not only a theoretical base from which to build depth but also detailed information in a step-by step approach to assessment and treatment. Students will find this approach instructive while seasoned practitioners will find a new model method to add to their repertoire of client-centered care."

—**Victoria P. Schindler,** *PhD, OTR, BCMH, FAOTA, co-editor*,
Occupational Therapy in Mental Health, *Professor Emeritus, Stockton University*

"*The Matthews Model of Clinical Reasoning* presents a refreshing approach to the field of occupational therapy. It differs from the antiquated ways of past thinking by emphasizing a person's life story rather than diagnosis. As an occupational therapist who switched practice areas after an extended absence from the profession, this model, presented in a user-friendly format, was a great resource that taught me how to be more client-centered and occupation-based throughout the evaluation and intervention process for the people I serve. Dr. Knis-Matthews is an innovative changemaker whose book takes us on an exciting person-centered journey, creating a ripple effect from educator to student to future practitioner."

—**Mary-Jo Zinnie,** *licensed occupational therapist with 25 years of experience*

"As a student in the midst of level II fieldwork, the MMCR model has provided me with a blue-print to strategize a person's evaluation and intervention process. While I learned foundational information in my occupational therapy courses, this book presents, in a visual and friendly manner, *how* to apply this knowledge into practice. By examining the MMCR model case study chapters, I am able to generalize my clinical reasoning skills across various practice settings, evaluation findings, a person's worldviews, and multiple occupational performance issues. I recommend this book to any student wanting to learn more about applying clinical reasoning and ways to approach occupation-based intervention in a clinical setting."

—**Jessica Onorati,** *OTS, occupational therapy student currently in level II fieldwork*

Matthews Model of Clinical Reasoning

The *Matthews Model of Clinical Reasoning* (MMCR) provides occupational therapy practitioners a systematic approach to develop their clinical reasoning skills during the evaluation and intervention process when collaborating with persons served across multiple practice locations.

The three core constructs of person, environment, and occupation lay the foundation for practitioners to compartmentalize information from selected evaluations, determine relevant intervention priorities, implement occupation-based intervention plans, and interpret successful outcomes. This book, influenced by these constructs, the practice framework, and accreditation standards for academic preparedness, provides the reader with the foundational information on how to apply the core constructs using a MMCR systematic approach for evaluation and intervention. Within the chapters are a variety of instructional methods, interviews with practitioners of various levels of experience, and case study examples. Clinical reasoning guidesheets are presented to assist the reader to follow the MMCR clinical reasoning process in terms of evaluation findings, application of frame of reference (FOR)/practice models, intervention strategies, and documentation.

Occupational therapy students and practitioners will be provided with the foundational skills to systematically think about and apply the steps of the clinical reasoning process, starting with a person's evaluation through the completion of the intervention plan.

Laurie Knis-Matthews, PhD, OT, has been an occupational therapist for over thirty years, primarily focused on mental health practice. Laurie has been conceptualizing the MMCR since she began teaching full-time in academia over twenty-five years ago.

Matthews Model of Clinical Reasoning

A Systematic Guide to Occupation-Based Evaluation and Intervention Planning

Edited by Laurie Knis-Matthews

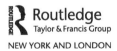

Routledge
Taylor & Francis Group

NEW YORK AND LONDON

Cover image © Getty Images

First published 2024

by Routledge
605 Third Avenue, New York, NY 10158

and by Routledge
4 Park Square, Milton Park, Abingdon, Oxon, OX14 4RN

Routledge is an imprint of the Taylor & Francis Group, an informa business

Library of Congress Cataloging-in-Publication Data
Names: Knis-Matthews, Laurie, editor.
Title: Matthews model of clinical reasoning : a systematic guide to occupation-based evaluation and intervention planning / edited by Laurie Knis-Matthews.
Other titles: Model of clinical reasoning
Description: New York, NY : Routledge, 2024. | Includes bibliographical references and index.
Identifiers: LCCN 2023019597 (print) | LCCN 2023019598 (ebook) | ISBN 9781032491615 (hbk) | ISBN 9781032491608 (pbk) | ISBN 9781003392408 (ebk)
Subjects: MESH: Occupational Therapy—methods | Clinical Reasoning
Classification: LCC RM735.3 (print) | LCC RM735.3 (ebook) | NLM WB 555 | DDC 615.8/515—dc23/eng/20230721
LC record available at https://lccn.loc.gov/2023019597
LC ebook record available at https://lccn.loc.gov/2023019598

ISBN: 978-1-032-49161-5 (hbk)
ISBN: 978-1-032-49160-8 (pbk)
ISBN: 978-1-003-39240-8 (ebk)

DOI: 10.4324/9781003392408

Typeset in Times New Roman
by Apex CoVantage, LLC

To my husband, Scott. Our journey started over twenty-five years ago in the very occupational therapy class this book is based upon. I could not think of a more perfect person to share in all of my life adventures. My sons, Michael and Max. You are the pride and joy of my life. I am so incredibly proud of your accomplishments, and in turn you inspire me every day.

All of the people who helped formulate the MMCR model for this book. It took a village to put this book together, and I am incredibly grateful for your patience, kindness, friendship, perseverance and dedication. Thank you for encouraging me to present this model to a wider audience and infuse different views into our profession.

To my students, mentees, colleagues and friends. My ideas for this model were inspired by all the people I have come into contact with on this journey. Thank you for challenging my worldviews so I can continue to grow and learn.

To the people I worked with as an occupational therapist over my career. I am in constant awe of your strength and courage to keep moving forward in a world that is not always kind to others. You have taught me to be compassionate, more empathetic and a better person.

To my former self. Don't be afraid to step outside of your comfort zone. Change comes with risk taking and sharing ideas with others. Just because something has always been done a certain way does not mean it cannot change or should stay as the status quo.

Contents

About the Author

Dr. Laurie Knis-Matthews has been an occupational therapist for almost thirty years. She graduated from Kean College with a bachelor's of science in 1992 and then earned a master's degree (1996) and doctoral degree (2005) in occupational therapy from New York University.

Laurie's clinical experiences have been primarily focused on the mental health practice area. She has worked with children, adolescents and adults in diverse settings such as psychiatric inpatient units, group homes, day programs, addiction services and shelters.

Laurie is a passionate advocate for the core tenets of authentic occupation for all people and institutions. She weaves these beliefs into her teaching, research and academic service as well as within her own community. Laurie utilizes her lifelong devotion to learning as a highly skilled group leader across all settings, academic and intervention, as she listens intently to each person's perspective, clearly rephrasing and moving the discussion or goal process forward.

Earlier in her academic career, Laurie began as an adjunct professor for both of the occupational therapy programs at Kean University and New York University. In 1999, she accepted a full-time tenure-track position as an assistant professor at Kean University. Soon after earning tenure, Laurie served as chairperson of the department from 2007 to 2017. She was awarded the ranking of professor in 2012. As a professor at Kean University she teaches both the master's- and doctoral-level courses such as psychosocial seminar, theoretical guides to practice, research methods and doctoral proposal courses.

During her experiences in the doctoral program, Laurie established herself as a qualitative researcher. She is most interested in pursuing scholarly work that gives voice to people with different viewpoints and life experiences. Her doctoral work focused on the experiences of parents who were substance dependent and participating in a year-long drug treatment program. In 2010, this research was later published as a special issue in *Occupational Therapy in Mental Health*. In 2017, her first article, relating to the Matthews Model of Clinical Reasoning (MMCR), was published in *Occupational Therapy in Mental Health*.

In collaboration with Kean University occupational therapy students, Laurie has continued focus on her scholarly agenda utilizing qualitative methods to investigate and publish research related to such topics as the cultural lens of mental illness, high school transition for female young adults diagnosed with autism and the meaning of higher education for individuals diagnosed with a mental illness. She has also presented many of these scholarly activities at national, regional and local conferences. Laurie has been an ongoing reviewer for such journals as *Occupational Therapy in Mental Health*, *American Journal of Occupational Therapy*, *International Journal of Occupational Therapy*, and *Canadian Journal of Occupational Therapy*.

Laurie has a loving husband, Scott, who is also an occupational therapist and founder of Intensive Therapeutics pediatric center in West Caldwell, New Jersey. Scott and Laurie have two teenage boys, Michael and Max. Laurie is a proud swim, band, art and volleyball mom. She enjoys gardening, writing, watching Marvel movies and spending time with her friends.

Contributing Authors

Christine A. Bodzioch, MS, OTR/L, CBIS, CSRS
Adjunct Professor
Department of Occupational Therapy
Kean University
Union, New Jersey

Shaniqua Bradley, PhD, LCSW
Assistant Professor
Department of Social Work and Child Advocacy
Montclair State University
Montclair, New Jersey

Nancy R. Dooley, PhD, OTR/L
Associate Professor and Program Director
Occupational Therapy Doctorate Program
Johnson & Wales University
Providence, Rhode Island

Ashley N. Fuentes, OTD, OTR/L
Occupational Therapist
Kessler Institute for Rehabilitation
West Orange, New Jersey
*Doctoral student from Kean University, New Jersey, while working on the book

Paige Garramone, MS, OTR/L
Occupational Therapist
Kean University Occupational Therapy Community Cares Clinic
Hillside, New Jersey

Pauline Gasparro, OTR/L, CHT
Certified Hand Therapist
Ivy Rehab Physical Therapy
Randolph, New Jersey

Maureen Grainger, MS, OTR/L
Occupational Therapist
Centura Health
Denver, Colorado

Valerie Hengemuhle, MS, OTR/L
Occupational Therapist
Holy City Pediatric Therapy
Charleston, South Carolina

Daryll Adrian A. Henson, OTD, OTR/L, CEAS I
Occupational Therapist
Holsman Healthcare
Jersey City, New Jersey
*Doctoral student from Kean University, New Jersey, while working on the book

Erik M. Horn, ATC, OTD
Occupational Therapist
*Doctoral student from Kean University, New Jersey, while working on the book

Allison C. Inserra, OTD, OTR/L
Occupational Therapist
Kean OT Community Cares Clinic
Hillside, New Jersey
Overlook Medical Center
Summit, New Jersey
*Doctoral student from Kean University, New Jersey, while working on the book

Susan E. Kushner, OTD
Occupational Therapist
*Doctoral student from Kean University, New Jersey, while working on the book

Marlee Murphy, MS, OTR/L
Occupational Therapist
The Rehab Center at St. Joseph's Hospital
Savannah, Georgia

Jessica L. Ortiz, OTD, OTR
Occupational Therapist
*Doctoral student from Kean University, New
    Jersey, while working on the book

Geraldine Pagaoa-Cruz, MS OTR/L
Director of Rehabilitation
Dignity Health Rehabilitation Hospital
Henderson, Nevada

Thais K. Petrocelli, OTD, MHA, OTR/L
Assistant Professor/Doctoral Capstone Coordi-
    nator
Department of Occupational Therapy
University of St. Augustine
St. Augustine, Florida

Lynne Richard, PhD, OT/L
Associate Professor
Department of Occupational Therapy
Florida International University
Miami, Florida

**Victoria P. Schindler, PhD, OTR, BCMH,
    FAOTA**
Professor Emeritus
Master of Science in Occupational Therapy
    Program
Stockton University
Galloway, New Jersey
Co-editor, *Occupational Therapy in Mental
    Health*

Margaret Swarbrick, PhD, FAOTA
Professor and Associate Director
Rutgers Center of Alcohol and Substance Use
    Studies, Graduate School of Applied and
    Professional Psychology
Wellness Institute Collaborative Support Pro-
    grams of New Jersey
Freehold, New Jersey

Acknowledgements of Contributions

Teresita Cruz
Henderson, Nevada

Ignacio Cruz
Henderson, Nevada

Sergio DeAlmeida, MS, OTR/L
Professional Therapy Associates, LLC
Brick, New Jersey

Dennis DuBois, BA
High School Athletic Coach
BA in Liberal Studies
Thomas Edison State University
Trenton, New Jersey

Lydia W. Eskander
Member of the Lebanese community

Mary Falzarano, PhD, OT
Kean University, Assistant Professor, Retired
Hillside, New Jersey

Melissa Farkas, OTR/L
Children's Specialized Hospital
Hamilton, New Jersey

C. Shane Flaviano, MD, FAAPMR
Medical Director
Dignity Health Rehabilitation Hospital
Henderson, Nevada

Marline Francois, LCSW
CEO and Clinical Director
Hearts Empowerment Counseling Center
PhD Student

Department of Family Science and Human
    Development
Montclair State University
Montclair, New Jersey

Juana Guglielmino, MS, OTR/L
Kean University, Class of 2020
Hillside, New Jersey

Elvis Gyan, MA, MDiv, PhD Student, Doctoral Assistant
Department of Family Science and Human
    Development
Montclair State University
Montclair, New Jersey

Brielle Hassa, MS, OTR/L
Intensive Therapeutics
West Caldwell, New Jersey

Orah Jooyandeh, MS, OTR/L
Dr. L. Hanes and Associates
Newark, New Jersey

Daniel Kim, RPh, MBA
Director of Pharmacy
Dignity Health Rehabilitation Hospital
Henderson, Nevada

Nicole Kiseli, MS, OTR/L
Kean University OT Community Cares Clinic
Hillside, New Jersey

Meagan Koch, OTR/L
Cranial Technologies
Morristown, New Jersey

Theresa Lapinski
South Plainfield, New Jersey

Tammy L. Lewis, BS
Parent/Special Education Advocate, Youth
    Director, Youth Mentor for Girls Ages 7–13
BS in Early Childhood Education
Kean University
Union, New Jersey

Inti Marazita, MS, OTR/L
Assistant Professor
University of St. Augustine
St. Augustine, Florida

Danielle Minetti, MS, OTR
Occupational Therapist
North Valley Regional School District
Norwood, New Jersey

Randee Myers, MS, OTR/L
Kean University, Class of 2021
Union, New Jersey

Daniella Nath, MS OTR/L
Bayonne Visiting Nurse Association
Bayonne, New Jersey

Cynthia Nead, COTA
Inpatient SCI & TBI
Kessler Institute for Rehabilitation
West Orange, New Jersey

Alivia Nufrio, OTR/L
FOX Rehabilitation
Bridgewater, New Jersey

Adelaida Pagaoa
Jacksonville, Florida

Thomas Pagaoa
Jacksonville, Florida

Noelle Rayment-Cruz
Architecture Student
Bethesda, Maryland

Della Spratt, MOTR/L
MUSC Health Florence
Florence, South Carolina

Emily Thomas, MS, OTR/L
The Children's Hospital of Philadelphia
Philadelphia, Pennsylvania

Katheryne Wall, OTR/L
Holmdel Public Schools
Holmdel, New Jersey

The profession of occupational therapy is the land of the gray so that is why clinical reasoning is so important and hard. I think that Laurie's book could make it easier by using something that is sound and strategic. It is based on the fact that everyone's life story is different, because that's the beauty of clinical reasoning (Jackie).

Preface

In Brief: What Is the Matthews Model of Clinical Reasoning?

The Matthews Model of Clinical Reasoning (MMCR) provides occupational therapy practitioners a systematic approach to develop their clinical reasoning skills during the evaluation and intervention process when collaborating with persons served across multiple practice locations. The three core constructs of person, environment and occupation lay the foundation for practitioners to compartmentalize information from selected evaluations, determine relevant intervention priorities, implement occupation-based intervention plans and interpret successful outcomes.

Stance: How My Personal Experiences as a Student, Occupational Therapist and Academician Contributed to the Reasons for Writing This Book

In 1992, I earned my bachelor's degree in occupational therapy from Kean College in New Jersey. During my education preparation, the medical model was the gold standard of care in the profession, and many practitioners primarily worked in hospital systems. Although it was emphasized in school, the construct of occupation was not fully immersed into the curriculum and often was nonexistent in practice. I recall learning about manual muscle and range of motion testing in class but not fully understanding how this information connected to a person's story. Characteristics of the medical model (practitioner as expert, focus on the diagnosis and separation of the mind/body connection) guided intervention approaches.

During this time, there was increased pressure to fix peoples' problem areas, leading to the selection of preparatory methods and activities during intervention. At this time, practitioners often used predetermined activities for all people on their caseload despite the person's life story, identified goals or suggested discharge plan. Following a one-size-fits-all approach, popular craft activities and therapeutic exercises such as tile trivets, making doormats, cones and resistance band exercises were common.

Early in my career I attended a conference and the main speaker emphasized the importance of client-centeredness and occupation-based treatment. The conference speaker told a story of a practitioner hiding the "cones" from the closet in a rehabilitation unit for one week. Throughout the week, practitioners had different reactions to the missing, cones as some searched for the cones, others were visibly upset the cones were misplaced and some colleagues tried to immediately purchase new ones. Toward the end of the week, some of the practitioners started to become less reliant on those cones and more interested in other activities that a person might actually find meaningful. This "experiment" served as the catalyst to begin talking about occupation. Ah, success!

This one short but powerful story told during a conference ignited my earliest ideas for the MMCR. Creating a ripple effect, this and similar stories took me on a twenty-year journey to create a systematic approach to clinical reasoning when developing an evaluation and intervention plan for each person served. I soon returned to school to earn both an advanced master's and doctoral degree in occupational therapy at New York University. This positive experience solidified my interest in lifelong learning and mentoring others in the profession.

Eventually the culmination of these experiences and skills became stepping stones to enter into the field of academia. As a professor in the occupational therapy program at Kean University, I have taught a specific psychosocial seminar course twice a year for over the last twenty years. During this course, my students use clinical reasoning skills to think deeply about the constructs of person-environment-occupation factors to create occupation-based intervention plans applicable to any practice setting.

As part of this seminar course, my students also actively participate in level one fieldwork experiences. Students often come back from their clinical fieldwork experiences very frustrated and confused as they may ask a seasoned practitioner questions about the reasons for selecting an evaluation or creating goals related to a person's story. At times, the seasoned practitioner may not be able to answer that question directly, but hints that clinical reasoning emerges from experiences or is more just second nature. From a student perspective, it often appears this process naturally develops with time and experience. I propose that clinical reasoning is a much more complicated process. Occupational therapy practitioners must strategically think about each person's evaluation and intervention plan in a systematic way to ensure measured success. There are no cookie-cutter approaches, as intervention plans differ depending on the person served, the constraints of the practice location and numerous other factors.

As an educator, my questions became: How do I teach clinical reasoning skills? How do novice practitioners learn to think in a systematic way, emphasizing client-centered principles and occupation-based treatment applicable to multiple populations and settings? To address these ongoing student frustrations related to clinical reasoning, I began developing a systematic *approach on how to think* about evaluation and intervention. Over my teaching career, I had numerous opportunities to formulate and evolve my thoughts about how clinical reasoning is integrated within the occupational therapy profession. I have been able to deconstruct the clinical reasoning process and "try out" various learning activities to help students apply this process for multiple settings. This book is intended to create a "spark" and subsequent ripple effect to the readers of this book. Perhaps it is time to "hide the cones" in your practice location and embrace the true client-centered journey.

Style and Unique Features of This Book

Following the MMCR, several unique features are incorporated throughout this book to assist practitioners to learn how this potentially abstract clinically reasoning model can be applied to daily practice over any practice location.

Progression of Learning and Tone of the Book

From my experiences as an occupational therapy educator, my priority is to teach the next generation of practitioners at a level that is understandable, non-threatening, interesting and dare I say . . . fun? The progression of learning and tone of this book will often mirror how I introduce new learning concepts to my students in the classroom. Each chapter builds on the next to solidify those foundation skills with more complexity and depth over time.

Utilizing Information From Other Works to Build Upon a Systematic Approach to Clinical Reasoning

Undeniably, the connection among the three constructs of person, environment and occupation in relation to a person's story has always been central to our profession. While the emphasis of these core constructs distinguishes occupational therapy from other professions, it also unifies our distinct values and areas of expertise. This book, influenced by numerous occupation-based practice models, the practice framework and accreditation standards for academic preparedness, provides the reader with the foundational information on how to apply these core constructs using an MMCR systematic approach for evaluation and intervention. Refer to Table 0.1 to view a sampling for Accreditation Council for Occupational Therapy Education (ACOTE) standards that are related to this model.

Table 0.1 Sampling of ACOTE Standards Relating to the Clinical Reasoning Process Addressed in the MMCR (ACOTE, 2018)

ACOTE Standard	*Associate's (OTA)* *Bachelor's (OTA)*	*Master's (OT)* *Doctoral (OT)*
B.2.1	Apply, analyze, and evaluate scientific evidence, theories, models of practice, and frames of reference that underlie the practice of occupational therapy to guide and inform interventions for persons, groups, and populations in a variety of practice contexts and environments.	
B.3.2	Apply, analyze, and evaluate the interaction of occupation and activity, including areas of occupation, performance skills, performance patterns, context(s) and environments, and client factors.	
B.3.6	Demonstrate activity analysis in areas of occupation, performance skills, performance patterns, context(s) and environments, and client factors to formulate the intervention plan	
B.4.1	Demonstrate therapeutic use of self, including one's personality, insights, perceptions, and judgments, as part of the therapeutic process in both individual and group interaction	
B.4.2	Demonstrate clinical reasoning to address occupation-based interventions, client factors, performance patterns, and performance skills.	Demonstrate clinical reasoning to evaluate, analyze, diagnose, and provide occupation-based interventions to address client factors, performance patterns, and performance skills.
B.4.3	Utilize clinical reasoning to facilitate occupation-based interventions that address client factors. This must include interventions focused on promotion, compensation, adaptation, and prevention.	
B.4.4	Contribute to the evaluation process of client(s)' occupational performance, including an occupational profile, by administering standardized and nonstandardized screenings and assessment tools and collaborating in the development of occupation-based intervention plans and strategies. Explain the importance of using psychometrically sound assessment tools when considering client needs, and cultural and contextual factors to deliver evidence-based intervention plans and strategies. Intervention plans and strategies must be client centered, culturally relevant, reflective of current occupational therapy practice, and based on available evidence	Evaluate client(s)' occupational performance, including occupational profile, by analyzing and selecting standardized and non-standardized screenings and assessment tools to determine the need for occupational therapy intervention(s). Assessment methods must take into consideration cultural and contextual factors of the client. Interpret evaluation findings of occupational performance and participation deficits to develop occupation-based intervention plans and strategies. Intervention plans and strategies must be client centered, culturally relevant, reflective of current occupational therapy practice, and based on available evidence.

(Continued)

Table 0.1 (Continued)

ACOTE Standard	Associate's (OTA) Bachelor's (OTA)	Master's (OT) Doctoral (OT)
B.4.6	Under the direction of an occupational therapist, collect, organize, and report on data for evaluation of client outcomes.	Collect, analyze, and report data in a systematic manner for evaluation of client and practice outcomes. Report evaluation results and modify practice as needed.
B.4.9	Demonstrate an understanding of the intervention strategies that remediate and/or compensate for functional cognitive deficits, visual deficits, and psychosocial and behavioral health deficits that affect occupational performance.	Design and implement intervention strategies to remediate and/or compensate for functional cognitive deficits, visual deficits, and psychosocial and behavioral health deficits that affect occupational performance.
B.4.10	Provide direct interventions and procedures to persons, groups, and populations to enhance safety, health and wellness, and performance in occupations. This must include the ability to select and deliver occupations and activities, preparatory methods and tasks (including therapeutic exercise), education and training, and advocacy.	Recommend and provide direct interventions and procedures to persons, groups, and populations to enhance safety, health and wellness, and performance in occupations. This must include the ability to select and deliver occupations and activities, preparatory methods and tasks (including therapeutic exercise), education and training, and advocacy.
B.4.18	Assess, grade, and modify the way persons, groups, and populations perform occupations and activities by adapting processes, modifying environments, and applying ergonomic principles to reflect the changing needs of the client, sociocultural context, and technological advances.	
B.4.21	Demonstrate the principles of the teaching–learning process using educational methods and health literacy education approaches: To design activities and clinical training for persons, groups, and populations. To instruct and train the client, caregiver, family, significant others, and communities at the level of the audience.	Demonstrate, evaluate, and utilize the principles of the teaching–learning process using educational methods and health literacy education approaches: To design activities and clinical training for persons, groups, and populations. To instruct and train the client, caregiver, family, significant others, and communities at the level of the audience.

Utilizes Various Instructional Methods

The clinical reasoning process is unique, strategic and fluid for each person served. Students often begin this process by memorizing chunks of information without understanding how it all relates together. This process becomes more challenging to transfer this basic knowledge originally introduced during academic preparation and apply it across practice settings. The goal of this book is to provide practitioners with the foundational skills to systematically think about and apply the steps of the clinical reasoning process, starting with a person's evaluation through the completion of the intervention plan. To make these complex and abstract ideas more manageable, a variety of instructional methods are presented throughout the book.

Multiple Perspectives of the Clinical Reasoning Process

While this model was developed primarily by one author, numerous colleagues and current and former students have participated in the creation of this book. The authors are a mixture of experts, scholars, practitioners and students with multiple perspectives and provide unique ways to incorporate the MMCR and help the reader think outside of the traditional therapy box.

Try It

Within the Try It sections of each chapter, readers are encouraged to practice parts of the clinical reasoning process after explanations are provided by the author.

A-HA Moments

Within the A-HA Moments sections of each chapter, certain parts of the clinical reasoning process are highlighted to alert the reader to pause and reflect more deeply.

Voices of the Practitioners

Ten practitioners working in different practice locations with various years of experience and academic degrees were interviewed to more fully explore the clinical reasoning process. Their unique perspectives are presented throughout the book. Please review Table 0.2 presented at the end of this section for more information about the practitioners interviewed.

Participant Chart

Table 0.2 Voices of the Practitioner Information

Participant	Age	Self-Identified Gender	Degree Obtained	# of Years Practicing as an OT	Current Practice Setting	# of Total Practice Settings the OT Has Been Employed In
Jackie	28	F	MS OT	4	Pediatric, outpatient services	2
Casey	30	F	MS OT	5.5	Pediatric, outpatient services	3
Rebecca	44	F	BS OT	21.5	Pediatric, outpatient services	3
Kristen	45	F	MS OT	22	Pediatric, outpatient services	3
Julie	26	F	MS OT	0.5	Adult mental health, inpatient and outpatient services	2
Abigail	48	F	BS OT	23	Academia	8
Pam	27	F	MS OT	2	Adult rehab, outpatient services	1
Louise	64	F	COTA	44	Adult rehab, outpatient services	4

(Continued)

Table 0.2 (Continued)

Participant	Age	Self-Identified Gender	Degree Obtained	# of Years Practicing as an OT	Current Practice Setting	# of Total Practice Settings the OT Has Been Employed In
Rose	27	F	MS OT	4.5	Adult rehab, inpatient services	1
Morgan	27	F	MS OT	2.5	Adult rehab, inpatient services	2

*Note: Participants chose pseudonyms to maintain confidentiality

Clinical Reasoning Guidesheets

Six specific clinical reasoning guidesheets are presented to assist the reader to follow the MMCR clinical reasoning process in terms of evaluation findings, application of frame of reference (FOR)/ practice models, intervention strategies and documentation. Each of the six clinical reasoning guidesheets will help readers organize their thoughts about a person's story and intervention.

Each guidesheet is presented twice in the appendices: the first guidesheet is presented so the reader can use it to clinically reason during the evaluation or intervention process. The second guidesheet has pre-filled notes (like a cheat sheet) to help remember key points until it becomes more second nature.

Case Study Examples

Mini case examples are provided in every chapter to help the reader apply potentially abstract ideas to practice. The last four chapters of this book present additional case studies to demonstrate how the MMCR and all of the clinical reasoning guidesheets are used together to support the clinical reasoning process for a person served.

What This Textbook Does Not Cover

While guided by theoretical perspectives and evidence-based practice, the specific approach to evaluation and intervention varies by person based on complex issues such as the facets of environment, occupations and the person's unique characteristics. With few exceptions, this complexity results in many of our decisions falling into the dreaded "gray area".

As previously stated, this book is not intended to be a cookbook to clinical reasoning, as no such thing really exists in occupational therapy. Rather, the MMCR provides a systematic approach for practitioners to become more aware of their clinical reasoning development during the evaluation and intervention process.

This book offers an alternative way of thinking about how to conceptualize the occupational therapy process and begin moving the needle to change the status quo of traditional services. Practitioners may choose to follow the entire model or use certain parts of the model that seem most applicable to their practice location, philosophy toward intervention, etc.

While practitioners do emphasize intervention with individuals, groups and populations, the scope of this book will primarily focus on the clinical reasoning process related to a person's life story and change process.

The constructs of person, environment and occupation are a part of our occupational therapy fabric and discussed extensively in our profession. While the American Occupational Therapy Association (AOTA) practice framework and other occupation-based practice models have influenced the MMCR, at times information is presented that may diverge from these other works. This book describes one clinical reasoning model: the MMCR.

The Organization of This Book

Section 1 (Chapters 1–6) provides the reader with background information to develop a deeper understanding on how clinical reasoning is defined, the evolution of clinical reasoning in occupational therapy and how it is related to our profession's domain of concern. Once the practitioner has a greater understanding of clinical reasoning, the MMCR will be introduced, emphasizing an in-depth understanding of the person, environment and occupation constructs. The evaluation process will be described in terms of the MMCR. This will help the practitioner to select evaluations related to both occupational profiles and analysis of performance and analyze evaluation data surrounding the constructs of person, environment and occupation to determine treatment priorities that are client centered and occupation based.

Section 2 (Chapters 7–12) provides in-depth information for practitioners to develop intervention plans that address issues identified during the occupational profile and analysis of performance evaluations. Using a systematic approach, these chapters explain why intervention is implemented in a specific way and how practitioners actually promote change that is occupation based.

Section 3 (Chapters 13 and 14) explains how practitioners create a documentation system, including evaluation summaries, goals, progress notes and discharge summaries, following the MMCR model.

Section 4 (Chapters 15–18) provides case examples for a deeper understanding of how this model can be applied with various types of people and practice settings.

Appendices contain reproducible clinical reasoning guidesheets to provide practitioners with opportunities to practice these skills. As these skills become more automatic and secondary in nature, practitioners will be able to "think on their feet" to make quicker decisions about a person's plan.

Reference

Accreditation Council for Occupational Therapy Education. (2018). *2018 ACOTE standards and interpretive guide*. https://acoteonline.org/accreditation-explained/standards/

Acknowledgements

The creation of this book has been a work in progress for over twenty years. For a long time, I kept these ideas to myself or slowly proposed a few ideas to students in my classroom to gauge their reactions to this way of thinking. Many of my ideas emerged based on the types of questions students asked in the classroom, so I began writing down information on sticky notes and taking pictures of the classroom white board when we were having A-HA Moments together while working through a case example. Over the years, students periodically pitched different versions of the model for me to consider or wrote lyrics to songs about the top-middle-bottom occupational performance issues for fun. I want to thank all of the Kean University students for sharing their viewpoints, stories and questions with me. There have been so many impactful moments in my teaching career and specifically for the evolution of this model. As you are the next generation of future leaders, our profession is in good hands. I would also like to thank the administration of Kean University, who provided me with release time and support to pursue this project to completion.

After I stepped down as the department chairperson, I had more time to pursue my scholarly agenda. Over the years, I had quite an accumulation of pieces of paper, pictures and sticky notes identifying potential ideas for this model. Now it was time to begin putting these thoughts together, take ownership of this model and give it a proper name: the Matthews Model of Clinical Reasoning (MMCR). I want to thank my earliest support system for this model: Dr. Lynne Richard, Dr. Clarie Mulry, Dr. Mary Falzarano and Katheryne Wall. They listened to my scattered ideas and helped to shape these abstract thoughts into something more sustainable.

I want to thank Brien Cummings for providing support and encouragement during the initial stages of the publication process. As I continued searching for a publisher to share my ideas, I found a perfect match with the Routledge/Taylor & Francis Publishing family. I want to thank editor Amanda Savage for taking a chance on me to share this model to a larger audience and Katya Porta for guiding me in this detailed and often complicated process.

I could not have written this book alone, as it was important to include other scholarly viewpoints, experts in various practice areas and people I knew would be critical yet supportive of my ideas. Dr. Lynne Richard, Dr. Margaret Swarbrick, Dr. Nancy R. Dooley and Dr. Victoria P. Schindler are a perfect combination of scholars to move this model to the next level. This group of women are well respected, smart, scholarly and experts in their fields. Thank you for providing your time, thoughts and dedication to this project.

Every once in a while, there is a standout student who is on a different career path. A student who is truly fascinated by scholarly pursuits, creating new ideas and hard work. Ashley N. Fuentes contributed to almost every part of this book in such ways as co-author, technical support, data gathering, editor and MMCR reviewer from a student perspective. She continuously helped me to think and write for new practitioners and students in the field.

Next, a talented group of academicians and practitioners accepted the challenge of following the MMCR guidelines to develop case studies that varied in practice areas, duration of intervention time, evaluation selection and guidelines for practice. It is not easy to shift your clinical reasoning into a new way of thinking and then have it published in a book. Thank you to Christine A. Bodzioch, Dr. Shaniqua Bradley, Ashley N. Fuentes, Paige Garramone, Pauline Gasparro, Valerie Hengemuhle, Allison C. Inserra, Danielle Minetti, Marlee Murphy, Geraldine Pagaoa-Cruz, Dr. Thais K. Petrocelli and Katheryne Wall.

While juggling their academic coursework, doctoral students Ashley N. Fuentes, Daryll Adrian A. Henson, Erik M. Horn, Susan E. Kushner and Jessica L. Ortiz worked together for over a year to present the review of literature chapter and also conduct multiple interviews with practitioners and academicians to learn about their clinical reasoning process to present the powerful Voices of the Practitioners sections of this book. They are simply the best.

I would also like to thank Diana Cruz, Erik M. Horn, Randee Myers and Tamar Stern for assisting with much appreciated technical support, literature searches and the clinical reasoning guidesheet creation ideas. A final thank you to the many clinicians, consultants and academicians who helped create these detailed case study chapters and Voices of the Participants sections.

Section 1

Clinical Reasoning and Evaluation

1 Exploring the Literature Related to Clinical Reasoning

Ashley N. Fuentes, Erik M. Horn, Susan E. Kushner, Daryll Adrian A. Henson, Jessica L. Ortiz, Lynne Richard, and Laurie Knis-Matthews

Note: It is not within the scope of this textbook to provide comprehensive information about clinical reasoning for content mastery. Please refer to the numerous publications written about clinical reasoning that are rich in depth and breadth.

History of Clinical Reasoning

Clinical reasoning, in some form, has been around since the dawn of medicine when early physicians were in the practice of explaining illnesses and symptoms as moral failings or imbalances within the body. Clinical reasoning itself as a skill or practice tool was initially studied in the 1950s (Custers, 2018). As the healthcare industry became increasingly complex with a growth in professions, there was a realization that the training and teaching of clinical reasoning was an important skill needed to improve client outcomes (Brailovsky et al., 2001; Norman, 2005; Yazdani & Abardeh, 2019; Yazdani et al., 2017).

Moving into the 1970s, research focused primarily on understanding clinical problem-solving (Norman, 2005). In the 1980s and 1990s, the medical field investigated the role of memory and mental representation as a person recalls previous knowledge when addressing new problem situations (Norman, 2005). By the 1990s, other health professions began to recognize that the medical model perspective of knowing and teaching clinical reasoning was not sufficient, and other specific models of clinical reasoning began to emerge (Edwards & Richardson, 2008). As reported by Yazdani and Abardeh (2019), the 20th century contributed the most to the theoretical work of clinical reasoning, but this research must continue well into the 21st century.

How Clinical Reasoning Is Described

In the literature, the term clinical reasoning in the health professions is often used interchangeably with other terms such as professional reasoning, medical problem-solving, decision-making and/or clinical judgment (Angus et al., 2018; Márquez-Álvarez et al., 2019; Norman, 2005). The variety of terms used to describe clinical reasoning suggests that it is a complex construct, and this can lead to difficulty communicating exactly what it entails (Young et al., 2020). However, researchers, clinicians and educators agree that clinical reasoning is a core clinical skill required by healthcare practitioners (Enslein & Wiles, 2020; Lateef, 2018; Simpkins et al., 2019; Yazdani & Abardeh, 2019).

DOI: 10.4324/9781003392408-2

Voices of the Practitioners: What Is Clinical Reasoning?

Clinical reasoning is that internal dialogue you have with yourself to decide what you need to do with that person in that moment, the next day or in the long term. The clinical reasoning skills as an OT are very different from any other professional in the medical field. We understand so many different things: the person, environment, occupation. (Morgan)

Clinical reasoning is a combination of thinking and experience that you have to guide what kind of intervention you are going to provide the client. (Kristen)

I describe clinical reasoning as a therapist's approach to working with someone. This approach is apparent through the continuum of care to ultimately meet their needs as occupational beings. (Jackie)

While health professions describe clinical reasoning skills as essential to clinical practice, profession-specific definitions can differ based on particular domains of practice. For example, physicians Epstein and Hundert (2002) report that clinical reasoning involves cognitive processes that lead clinicians to a diagnosis and treatment plan. Within the nursing field, Banning (2008) identifies the term as an essential competence that focuses on useful and efficient healthcare evidence to direct patient management. In physical therapy, Huhn et al. (2018) describe clinical reasoning as the integration of thinking and decision-making when encountering clinical scenarios. Occupational therapists Unsworth and Baker (2016) define clinical reasoning as the thinking processes practitioners utilize throughout their therapeutic relationship and interventions with persons served.

Characteristics Often Associated With Clinical Reasoning

A growing body of literature (Bissessur et al., 2009; Gonzalez, 2018; Konopasek et al., 2014; Liao et al., 2018; Marcum, 2012; Yazdani & Abardeh, 2019; Yazdani et al., 2017; Vanstone et al., 2019) suggests that clinical reasoning consists of both analytic and non-analytic processes. *Analytic processes* consist of cognitive elements and are based on objective analysis when a practitioner's expertise alone is insufficient, requiring more evidence. *Non-analytic processes* rely on the affective domain and are more prone to error because those processes are based on subjective experiences, prior knowledge and the practitioner's expertise. In practice, both processes are often used in tandem to determine assessment and intervention choices (Bissessur et al., 2009; Lateef, 2018; Marcum, 2012; Monteiro et al., 2018).

Key characteristics utilizing analytic and non-analytic processes of clinical reasoning have been identified across the literature (Banning, 2008; Cerullo & Monteiro da Cruz, 2010; Goodin et al., 2019; Kuipers & Grice, 2009; Marcum, 2012; Norman, 2005; Vanstone et al., 2019; Victor-Chmil, 2013) and include critical thinking, problem-solving, therapeutic use of self and ethical considerations (refer to Table 1.1).

Critical thinking is often highlighted in the literature as a key component that forms clinical reasoning (Banning, 2008; Cerullo & Monteiro da Cruz, 2010; Victor-Chmil, 2013). Critical thinking differs from clinical reasoning, as it is based solely on knowledge, evidence and science, rather than intuition (Cerullo & Monteiro da Cruz, 2010; Marcum, 2012; Vanstone et al., 2019; Victor-Chmil, 2013).

Problem-solving involves practitioners utilizing information that is available to them to generate a solution to an existing problem. It has been noted that experts, or more experienced practitioners, have encountered multiple similar problems over time and are able to utilize their prior

Table 1.1 Characteristics Often Associated With the Clinical Reasoning Process

Characteristic	Definition	Citation
Critical thinking	A process that relies on objective analysis and evaluation of a clinical situation. It is based on knowledge, evidence and science and not dependent on the current situation or assumptions.	Banning, 2008 Cerullo & Monteiro da Cruz, 2010 Victor-Chmil, 2013
Problem-solving	The practitioner uses information that is available to them to generate a solution to an existing problem. Experts, or more experienced practitioners, have encountered multiple similar problems over time and are able to utilize prior knowledge and familiarity to formulate decisions with more efficiency.	Goodin et al., 2019 Kuipers & Grice, 2009 Norman, 2005
Therapeutic use of self	Therapeutic use of self is a conscious use of one's knowledge, personality and actions to enhance a therapeutic collaboration. It is often vital for the practitioner to understand a person's unique story in a way that provides safety, empathy and trust for the story to unfold.	AOTA, 2020a Mosey, 1986 Patnaude, 2021 Solman & Clouston, 2016
Ethical considerations	The ability to reason through a dilemma or conflict by collecting the facts of the situation and creating a resolution based on values, best interests and a moral outcome. Encompasses such concepts as beneficence, autonomy and justice.	AOTA, 2020b

knowledge and familiarity to formulate decisions with more efficiency (Goodin et al., 2019; Kuipers & Grice, 2009; Norman, 2005).

Therapeutic use of self is a conscious use of one's knowledge, personality and actions to enhance a therapeutic collaboration (Mosey, 1986; Patnaude, 2021; Solma & Clouston, 2016). It is vital for the practitioner to understand a person's unique story in a way that provides safety, empathy, and trust for the story to unfold (AOTA, 2020a).

Practitioners must consider *ethical considerations* when engaging in the clinical reasoning process. This involves the ability to reason through a dilemma or conflict by collecting the facts of the situation and progress to a morally sound decision. Ethics encompasses such concepts as beneficence, autonomy and justice (AOTA, 2020b). It is a practitioner's responsibility to provide services that are of high quality, ethical and effective.

Clinical Reasoning Explored Within the Occupational Therapy Profession

Clinical reasoning is a multifaceted, abstract set of professional skills that are utilized within the field of occupational therapy (Murphy & Stav, 2018). Clinical reasoning involves a dynamic, complex thought process that is exercised by practitioners throughout the occupational therapy process, as well as longitudinally throughout their careers. Occupational therapy practitioners use clinical reasoning to evaluate an individual's strengths and challenges and consider an individual's occupational needs prior to executing a plan of intervention (Baird et al., 2015). When used successfully, this form of thinking is effective in directing intervention to adhere to the specific needs of each person (Márquez-Álvarez et al., 2019).

Evolution of Clinical Reasoning Throughout Occupational Therapy

In occupational therapy, there was a recognition of the need to develop specific studies of clinical reasoning for the profession. In 1989, the American Occupational Therapy Association (AOTA) and the American Occupational Therapy Foundation (AOTF) funded the Clinical Reasoning Study to investigate and better understand reasoning processes unique to occupational therapy. A special issue of the *American Journal of Occupational Therapy* (AJOT) on clinical reasoning published in November 1991 included many of the seminal works on clinical reasoning from this initiative. Mattingly (1991a) and Fleming (1991), along with others, created a foundational work that continues to be used in occupational therapy today.

Márquez-Álvarez et al. (2019) conducted a scoping review of the literature to examine the evolution of clinical reasoning within occupational therapy and to explore the purpose and implementation of clinical reasoning in the profession. They broke down clinical reasoning in occupational therapy into three phases: (1) exploratory phase (1982–1993) in which clinical reasoning was first being defined, described, and explored; (2) transition phase (1994–2003) in which the number of studies about clinical reasoning increased to support occupational therapy with more rigorous scientific research; and (3) consolidation phase (2005–present) (Márquez-Álvarez et al., 2019).

The exploratory phase shows an investigative perspective primarily using the qualitative approaches of ethnography and phenomenological methods. In the transition phase, new research perspectives on clinical reasoning were developing through empirical studies, although qualitative studies continued to be the primary approach of study (Márquez-Álvarez et al., 2019). The consolidation phase shows that a variety of both qualitative and quantitative approaches are being utilized for research on professional reasoning in occupational therapy (Márquez-Álvarez et al., 2019).

How Clinical Reasoning Is Presented in the Occupational Therapy Practice Framework

In more recent years, the occupational therapy profession has become increasingly client-centered and has expanded beyond the medical model. These changes are reflected in the new *Occupational Therapy Practice Framework* (OTPF) 4th edition, as it replaced the term "clinical reasoning" with "professional reasoning" (AOTA, 2020a). The term professional reasoning is purposefully broad to encompass all practice settings and describe how practitioners utilize knowledge and skills throughout the occupational therapy process in a variety of settings outside of the medical model. The OTPF goes on to define professional reasoning as the "process that practitioners use to plan, direct, perform, and reflect on client care" (Schell, 2019).

A client-centered approach implies that the person's perspective and occupations directly affect the planning and reevaluation of intervention sessions and considers the person's context and environments, performance patterns, performance skills and client factors (AOTA, 2020a). The exponential expansion of knowledge and necessary skills required to engage in the occupational therapy process necessitates more sophisticated thinking and reasoning by practitioners. For our purposes here, the term clinical reasoning will be used throughout this book but recognize that the reasoning process happens broadly across all settings—not just in the "clinic."

Voices of the Practitioners: How I Developed My Clinical Reasoning Skills

Clinical reasoning just unfolds pulling from my understanding, education and own experiences. There is physical clinical reasoning and cognitive clinical reasoning. I pull from research articles, models of practice and things about what has worked in the past. (Jackie)

Clinical reasoning comes with experience, intuitiveness and it is learned. It is what helps us decide how to work with people from the evaluation process, through the treatment and then reevaluation. Thank goodness I have mentorship because my supervisor is also an OT, so he helps me with that OT lens. His feedback has been very helpful in thinking about and planning my sessions. (Julie)

Clinical reasoning happens on the spot because there is a problem that you need to troubleshoot. You have to be able to critically think in order to be able to clinically reason a problem. This goes hand in hand but is not the same thing. Each one complements one another. The only way you are going to get better at reasoning is with more reflection. (Abigail)

Types of Clinical Reasoning in Occupational Therapy

In occupational therapy, different types of clinical reasoning have been identified and proposed. Mattingly (1991b) wrote about narrative reasoning, and Fleming (1991), building on this work, identified three other types of clinical reasoning: procedural, interactive and conditional. Please see Table 1.2 for an overview.

Mattingly (1991b) proposed a *narrative model* of reasoning rather than focusing solely on scientific reasoning commonly followed in the medical profession. This type of clinical reasoning emphasizes storytelling from the person's perspective. This helps the practitioner to understand the totality of the person's unique story beyond the diagnosis, disease or illness. This information assists the practitioner to form a collaborative relationship to assist the person in creating a future story.

Building on Mattingly's work, Fleming identified three types of clinical reasoning (procedural, interactive and conditional) that occupational therapy practitioners often use to shift from one strategy to another. *Procedural reasoning* emphasizes the use of science and evidence as the practitioner identifies occupational problems related to disease and disability to implement an intervention plan (Fleming, 1991; Neistadt, 1996). Using problem-solving strategies, practitioners identified problems, set goals and developed treatment plans (Fleming, 1991).

At times, practitioners use *interactive reasoning* to learn more about the illness perspective from the vantage point of the person served. Practitioners may use this style of clinical reasoning to determine the success of the intervention plan, engage the person as an active participant in the plan or develop a deeper sense of trust. This reasoning emphasizes the interpersonal relationships such as the collaboration between the person and the practitioner (Fleming, 1991).

Conditional reasoning takes on a broader understanding of the person's contexts by considering the social and temporal concerns (Fleming, 1991). This type of reasoning takes into consideration what the *best* approach is for this specific person and considers current and future outcomes.

Building on the previous clinical reasoning models, *pragmatic reasoning* considers therapists' knowledge and experiences when determining an intervention plan within a given practice location (Neistadt, 1996; Schell & Schell, 2018). Pragmatic reasoning emphasizes what is possible in the setting. This can include the practitioner's level of experience, organizational policies, time and available physical resources (Schell & Schell, 2018).

Table 1.2 Types of Clinical Reasoning in Occupational Therapy

Types of Reasoning	Definition	Focus	Citation
Narrative reasoning	Understanding and engaging with the person's occupational story. Provides a personalized understanding of the person and what is important to them. Mattingly referred to this as "thinking in stories."	Person	Mattingly, 1991a, 1991b
Procedural or scientific reasoning	Use of science and evidence as the practitioner identifies occupational problems in relationship to the diagnosis and/or disability to problem-solve.	Diagnosis and its effect on the individual	Fleming, 1991 Neistadt, 1996
Interactive reasoning	Interactive reasoning happens in the context of the person and their relationship to others—including the practitioner. It is a shared understanding of someone as a social person.	Person and interpersonal relationships	Fleming, 1991
Conditional reasoning	An iterative or ongoing process of revision to treatment based on the situational context. This type of reasoning takes into consideration what the *best* approach for this specific person is considering current and potential future outcomes.	Provisional on the person's response and participation in the therapeutic process	Fleming, 1991 Mattingly & Fleming, 1994
Pragmatic reasoning	Considers practitioners' knowledge and experiences when determining an intervention plan in each environment or practice setting. Emphasizes what is possible in the setting—including what skills the OT does or does not have, organizational policies, time and physical resources.	Person and environment	Neistadt, 1996; Schell & Schell, 2018

Clinical Reasoning in Occupational Therapy Education

Voices of the Practitioners: My Earliest Recollections of the Clinical Reasoning Process

I learned about clinical reasoning for the first time in my fieldwork experiences. My supervisor asked why I chose this exercise, and I had to start explaining why I made that decision. (Louise)

As a student, clinical reasoning was a much longer process and it took a lot more time. I relied more on the experience of others. I would watch others work and then pull from their clinical reasoning to support mine. I learned a lot about clinical reasoning from the certified occupational therapy assistants (COTAs) that I work with. (Rebecca)

During one of my level two experiences, clinical reasoning seemed to be missing because every patient had the same exact goals and the same exact activities that other people were doing. In that experience, I was encouraged to look at the pieces instead of looking at the whole person. (Rebecca)

The use of theories and models, knowledge about the effects of conditions on participation and available evidence on interventions all aid the practitioner's clinical or professional reasoning (AOTA, 2020a). Competent practitioners use clinical reasoning skills to understand the unique considerations for each person served and apply this information to the evaluation and intervention plan. Therefore, it's important to explore how these skills are introduced and reinforced in the classroom, which will shape the future practitioner's clinical competency.

Occupational therapy educators are tasked with using the most effective teaching approaches for students to develop and transfer their clinical reasoning skills as future practitioners (Neistadt, 1996). However, specific teaching instructions highlighting all of these clinical reasoning models are not always found in occupational therapy curriculum. Occupational therapy faculty use a limited number of instructional methods to specifically develop clinical reasoning in students (Henderson et al., 2017). There are specific strategies that occupational therapy educators gravitate toward while teaching, formulating and exercising clinical reasoning in the classroom and in clinical practice.

Neistadt (1996) proposed that much of the curriculum emphasizes *procedural reasoning*, utilizing such teaching-learning activities as case study exams, guest speakers, videotaping, incorporating why questions and level one experiences. There is research (deBeer & Martensson, 2015; Murphy & Radloff, 2019; Murphy & Stav, 2018) demonstrating the effectiveness of using a variety of procedural reasoning types of teaching-learning activities. For example, deBeer and Martensson (2015) used a mixed-methods approach to examine the impact a fieldwork supervisor's feedback has on a student's clinical reasoning abilities. The researchers found that the students' clinical reasoning skills improved when corrective feedback was given with suggestions on how to improve.

Case-based learning is another type of procedural reasoning method that is commonly used to teach clinical reasoning skills by using authentic, or real-world cases, to guide students through the problem-solving process. Murphy and Stav (2018) conducted a study to examine clinical reasoning skills of entry-level occupational therapy students using a case-based format. The researchers compared two groups of students using the instructional method of video case-based studies presented in an online format with additional learning activities as compared with students who were instructed by the use of text-based case studies. They proposed that the video case study format facilitated stronger inductive reasoning skills than the text-based instructional format as the students utilized observations and decision-making skills to draw upon their conclusions.

The research of Murphy and Radloff (2019) supports continued and/or increased use of case-based learning opportunities in occupational therapy programs. A curriculum that is carefully implemented to connect theory to practice through the use of case studies can benefit the occupational therapy student. Murphy and Radloff (2019) also report that building on the concepts of each case and determining an optimal format for presentation (i.e., video simulation, standardized patients, written cases) ultimately increase student competency in their preparation for clinical practice.

More Models Are Needed to Guide the Use of Clinical Reasoning in Practice

While there is a growing body of knowledge on clinical reasoning in occupational therapy, there are still many gaps (Araujo et al., 2022; Hooper, 2008). The unique characteristics of the occupational therapy profession call for a discipline-specific, shared understanding of the clinical reasoning process (Maruyama et al., 2021). Occupational therapy scholars have called for a clinical reasoning process that is methodical, immersed in theory and backed up by data. There is a need for occupational therapy practitioners to align their practices with the best evidence and instructional methods (Bondoc, 2005; Knis-Matthews et al., 2017; Rochmawati & Wiechula, 2010; Schaaf, 2015).

This call to action is prompted by concerns that there appears to be a continuing disconnect between education and practice and that the increasing demands require practitioners to use their clinical reasoning processes to implement occupation-based interventions across practice settings (Colaianni & Provident, 2010; Craig, 2012; Gillen, 2015; Knis-Matthews et al., 2021; Kreider et al., 2014; Krishnagiri et al., 2017). Decades after occupational therapy's paradigm shift from impairments to participation and occupation, practitioners continue to be challenged in using their clinical reasoning skills to implement occupation-based care (Andonian, 2017; Colaianni & Provident, 2010; Craig, 2012; Knis-Matthews et al., 2021).

Introducing the MMCR to Guide the Clinical Reasoning Process

Because the occupational therapy profession is rooted in the use of models to guide practice, highlight the distinct value of occupations and demonstrate the benefits of occupational therapy to society, there is an ongoing need to integrate more models to direct the teaching and learning of clinical reasoning into the profession. It is essential to support occupational therapy educators and students in the development of clinical reasoning skills and create more clarity around this process.

The Matthews Model of Clinical Reasoning (MMCR) structures how an occupational therapy practitioner reasons about all aspects of the person to create an effective occupation-based, holistic, client-centered plan of assessment and intervention across populations and practice settings (Knis-Matthews et al., 2017). Additionally, the MMCR has the potential to inform future research that supports efficacious educational practices in clinical reasoning. The next chapters of this book will methodically prepare the reader for this clinical reasoning process suitable across all populations and practice settings.

References

American Occupational Therapy Association. (2020a). Occupational therapy practice framework: Domain and process (4th ed.). *American Journal of Occupational Therapy*, *74*(Suppl. 2), 7412410010. https://doi.org/10.5014/ajot.2020.74S2001

American Occupational Therapy Association. (2020b). AOTA 2020 occupational therapy code of ethics. *American Journal of Occupational Therapy*, *74*, 7413410005. https://doi.org/10.5014/ajot.2020.74S3006

Andonian, L. (2017). Occupational therapy students' self-efficacy, experience of supervision, and perception of meaningfulness of Level II fieldwork. *Open Journal of Occupational Therapy*, *5*(2), 1–12. https://doi.org/10.15453/21686408.1220

Angus, L., Chur-Hansen, A., & Duggan, P. (2018). A qualitative study of experienced clinical teachers' conceptualisation of clinical reasoning in medicine: Implications for medical education. *Focus on Health Professional Education: A Multi-Disciplinary Journal*, *19*(1), 52–64. https://doi.org/10.11157/fohpe.v19i1.197

Araujo, A. D. S., Kinsella, E. A., Thomas, A., Gomes, L. D., & Marcolino, T. Q. (2022). Clinical reasoning in occupational therapy practice: A scoping review of qualitative and conceptual peer-reviewed literature. *American Journal of Occupational Therapy*, *76*, 7603205070. https://doi.org/10.5014/ajot.2022.048074

Baird, J. M., Raina, K. D., Rogers, J. C., O'Donnell, J., & Holm, M. B. (2015). Wheelchair transfer simulations to enhance procedural skills and clinical reasoning. *American Journal of Occupational Therapy*, *69*(Suppl. 2), 6912185020. https://doi.org/10.5014/ajot.2015.018697

Banning, M. (2008). Clinical reasoning and its application to nursing: Concepts and research studies. *Nurse Education in Practice*, *8*(3), 177–183. https://doi.org/10.1016/j.nepr.2007.06.004

Bissessur, S. W., Geijteman, E. C. T., Al-Dulaimy, M., Teunissen, P. W., Richir, M. C., Arnold, A. E. R., & De Vries, T. P. G. M. (2009). Therapeutic reasoning: From hiatus to hypothetical model. *Journal of Evaluation in Clinical Practice*, *15*(6), 985–989. https://doi.org/10.1111/j.1365-2753.2009.01136.x

Bondoc, S. (2005). Occupational therapy and evidence-based education. *Education Special Interest Section Quarterly*, *15*(4), 1–4.

Brailovsky, C., Charlin, B., Beausoleil, S., Coté, S., & Van der Vleuten, C. (2001). Measurement of clinical reflective capacity early in training as a predictor of clinical reasoning performance at the end of residency: An experimental study on the script concordance test. *Medical Education*, *35*(5), 430–436. https://doi.org/10.1046/j.1365-2923.2001.00911.x

Cerullo, J. A. S. B., & Monteiro da Cruz, D. A. L. (2010). Clinical reasoning and critical thinking. *Revista Latin-Americana de Enfermagem*, *18*(1), 124–129. https://doi.org/10.1590/S0104-11692010000100019

Colaianni, D., & Provident, I. (2010). The benefits of and challenges to the use of occupation in hand therapy. *Occupational Therapy in Health Care*, *24*(2), 130–146. https://doi.org/10.3109/07380570903349378

Craig, D. G. (2012). Current occupational therapy publications in home health: A scoping review. *American Journal of Occupational Therapy*, *66*(3), 338–347. https://doi.org/10.5014/ajot.2012.003566

Custers, E. J. F. M. (2018). Training clinical reasoning: Historical and theoretical background. In E. J. F. M. Custers, O. ten Cate., & S. J. Durning (Eds.), *Principles and practice of case based clinical reasoning education: A method for preclinical students* (pp. 21–34). Springer.

deBeer, M., & Martensson, L. (2015). Feedback on students' clinical reasoning skills during fieldwork education. *Australian Occupational Therapy Journal*, *62*(4), 255–264. https://doi.org/10.1111/1440-1630.12208

Edwards, I., & Richardson, B. (2008). Clinical reasoning and population health: Decision making for an emerging paradigm of health care. *Physiotherapy: Theory and Practice*, *24*(3), 183–193. https://doi.org/10.1080/09593980701593797

Enslein, T. W., & Wiles, B. (2020). Impact and reasoning: Applying community service learning in a non-traditional field. *Journal of Experiential Education*, *43*(2), 136–155. https://doi.org/10.1177/1053825920902797

Epstein, R. M., & Hundert, E. M. (2002). Defining and assessing professional competence. *JAMA*, *287*(2), 226–235. https://doi.org/10.1001/jama.287.2.226

Fleming, M. H. (1991). The therapist with the three-track mind. *American Journal of Occupational Therapy*, *45*(11), 1007–1014. http://doi.org/10.5014/ajot.45.11.1007

Gillen, G. (2015). What is the evidence for the effectiveness of interventions to improve occupational performance after stroke? *American Journal of Occupational Therapy*, *69*, 1–3. https://doi.org/10.5014/ajot.2015.013409

Gonzalez, L. (2018). Teaching clinical reasoning piece by piece: A clinical reasoning concept-based learning method. *Journal of Nursing Education*, *57*(12), 727–735. https://doi.org/10.3928/01484834-20181119-05

Goodin, T. L., Caukin, N. G., & Dillard, H. K. (2019). Developing clinical reasoning skills in teacher candidates using a problem-based learning approach. *Interdisciplinary Journal of Problem-Based Learning*, *13*(1). https://doi.org/10.7771/1541-5015.1707

Henderson, W., Coppard, B. M., & Qi, Y. (2017). Identifying instructional methods for development of clinical reasoning in entry-level occupational therapy education: A mixed methods design. *Journal of Occupational Therapy Education*, *1*(2). https://doi.org/10.26681/jote.2017.010201

Hooper, B. (2008). Therapists' assumptions as a dimension of professional reasoning. In B. A. Schell & J. W. Schell (Eds.), *Clinical and professional reasoning in occupational therapy* (pp. 13–35). Lippincott, Williams & Wilkins.

Huhn, K., Gilliland, S. J., Black, L. L., Wainwright, S. F., & Christensen, N. (2018). Clinical reasoning in physical therapy: A concept analysis. *Physical Therapy*, *99*(4), 440–456. https://doi.org/10.1093/ptj/pzy148

Knis-Matthews, L., Koch, M., Nufrio, A., Neustein Gorman, M., Zaki, F., & Wall, K. H. (2021). The perceptions of four novice occupational therapists' preparedness and ability to perform occupation-based practice in pediatric practice. *Journal of Occupational Therapy Education*, *5*(4). https://doi.org/10.26681/jote.2021.050416

Knis-Matthews, L., Mulry, C. M., & Richard, L. (2017). Matthews model of clinical reasoning: A systematic approach to conceptualize evaluation and intervention. *Occupational Therapy in Mental Health*, *33*(4), 360–373. https://doi.org/10.1080/0164212X.2017.1303658

Konopasek, L., Kelly, K. V., Bylund, C. L., Wenderoth, S., & Storey-Johnson, C. (2014). The group objective structured clinical experience: Building communication skills in the clinical reasoning context. *Patient Education and Counseling*, *96*(1), 79–85. https://doi.org/10.1016/j.pec.2014.04.003

Kreider, C. M., Bendixen, R. M., Huang, Y. Y., & Lim, Y. (2014). Review of occupational therapy intervention research in the practice area of children and youth 2009–2013. *American Journal of Occupational Therapy*, *68*(2), e61–e73. https://doi.org/10.5014/ajot.2014.011114

Krishnagiri, S., Hooper, B., Price, P., Taff, S. D., & Bilics, A. (2017). Explicit or hidden? Exploring how occupation is taught in occupational therapy curricula in the United States. *American Journal of Occupational Therapy*, *71*, 1–9. https://doi.org/10.5014/ajot.2017.024174

Kuipers, K., & Grice, J. W. (2009). Clinical reasoning in neurology: Use of the repertory grid technique to investigate the reasoning of an experienced occupational therapist. *Australian Occupational Therapy Journal*, *56*(4), 275–284. https://doi.org/10.1111/j.1440-1630.2008.00737.x

Lateef, F. (2018). Clinical reasoning: The core of medical education and practice. *International Journal of Internal and Emergency Medicine*, *1*(2), 1015.

Liao, H.-C., Yang, Y.-M., Li, T.-C., Cheng, J.-F., & Huang, L.-C. (2018). The effectiveness of a clinical reasoning teaching workshop on clinical teaching ability in nurse preceptors. *Journal of Nursing Management*, *27*, 1047–1054. https://doi.org/10.1111/jonm.12773

Marcum, J. A. (2012). An integrated model of clinical reasoning: Dual-process theory of cognition and metacognition. *Journal of Evaluation in Clinical Practice*, *18*(5), 954–961. https://doi.org/10.1111/j.1365-2753.2012.01900.x

Márquez-Álvarez, L.-J., Calvo-Arenillas, J.-I., Talavera-Valverde, M.-Á., & Moruno-Millares, P. (2019). Professional reasoning in occupational therapy: A scoping review. *Occupational Therapy International*, *2019*, Article ID 6238245. https://doi.org/10.1155/2019/6238245

Maruyama, S., Sasada, S., Jinbo, Y., & Bontje, P. (2021). A concept analysis of clinical reasoning in occupational therapy. *Asian Journal of Occupational Therapy*, *17*(1), 17–25. https://doi.org/10.11596/asiajot.16.119

Mattingly, C. (1991a). What is clinical reasoning? *American Journal of Occupational Therapy*, *45*, 979–986. https://doi.org/10.5014/ajot.45.11.979

Mattingly, C. (1991b). The narrative nature of clinical reasoning. *American Journal of Occupational Therapy*, *45*(11), 998–1005. https://doi.org/10.5014/ajot.45.11.998

Mattingly, C., & Fleming, M. H. (1994). *Clinical reasoning: Forms of inquiry in a therapeutic practice*. F. A. Davis.

Monteiro, S., Norman, G., & Sherbino, J. (2018). The three faces of clinical reasoning: Epistemological explorations of disparate error reduction strategies. *Journal of Evaluation in Clinical Practice*, *24*(3), 666–673. https://doi.org/10.1111/jep.12907

Mosey, A. C. (1986). *Psychosocial components of occupational therapy*. Raven Press.

Murphy, L. F., & Radloff, J. C. (2019). Using case-based learning to facilitate clinical reasoning across practice courses in an occupational therapy curriculum. *Journal of Occupational Therapy Education*, *3*(4). https://doi.og/10.26681/jote.2019.030403

Murphy, L. F., & Stav, W. B. (2018). The impact of online video cases on clinical reasoning in occupational therapy education: A quantitative analysis. *The Open Journal of Occupational Therapy*, *6*(3). https://doi.org/10.15453/2168-6408.1494

Neistadt, M. E. (1996). Teaching strategies for the development of clinical reasoning. *American Journal of Occupational Therapy*, *50*(8), 676–684. https://doi.org/10.5014/ajot.50.8.676

Norman, G. (2005). Research in clinical reasoning: Past history and current trends. *Medical Education*, *39*(4), 418–427. https://doi.org/10.1111/j.1365-2929.2005.02127.x

Patnaude, M. E. (2021). Student success: Therapeutic reasoning process. In J. C. O'Brien, M. E. Patnaude, & T. G. Reidy (Eds.), *Therapeutic reasoning in occupational therapy* (pp. 1–17). Elsevier.

Rochmawati, E., & Wiechula, R. (2010). Education strategies to foster health professional students' clinical reasoning skills. *Nursing and Health Sciences*, *12*, 244–250. https://doi.org/10.1111/j.1442-2018.2009.00512.x

Schaaf, R. C. (2015). Creating evidence for practice using data-driven decision making. *American Journal of Occupational Therapy*, *69*, 6902360010. https://doi.org/10.5014/ajot.2015.010561

Schell, B. (2019). Professional reasoning in practice. In B. Schell & G. Gillen (Eds.), *Willard and Spackman's occupational therapy* (13th ed., pp. 384–397). Wolters Kluwer.

Schell, B. A. B., & Schell, J. W. (2018). *Clinical and professional reasoning in occupational therapy*. Wolters Kluwer.

Simpkins, A. A. M., Koch, B., Spear-Ellinwood, K., & Paul St, J. (2019). A developmental assessment of clinical reasoning in preclinical medical education. *Medical Education Online*, *24*(1). https://doi.org/10.1080/10872981.2019.1591257

Solman, B., & Clouston, T. (2016). Occupational therapy and the therapeutic use of self. *British Journal of Occupational Therapy*, *79*(8), 514–516. https://doi.org/10.1177/0308022616638675

Unsworth, C., & Baker, A. (2016). A systematic review of professional reasoning literature in occupational therapy. *British Journal of Occupational Therapy*, *79*(1), 5–16. https://doi.org/10.1177/0308022615599994

Vanstone, M., Monteiro, S., Colvin, E., Norman, G., Sherbino, J., Sibbald, M., Dore, K., & Peters, A. (2019). Experienced physician descriptions of intuition in clinical reasoning: A typology. *Diagnosis*, *6*(3), 259–268. https://doi.org/10.1515/dx-2018-0069

Victor-Chmil, J. (2013). Critical thinking versus clinical reasoning versus clinical judgment: Differential diagnosis. *Nurse Education*, *38*(1), 34–36. https://doi.org/10.1097/NNE.0b013e318276dfbe

Yazdani, S., & Abardeh, H. M. (2019). Five decades of research and theorization on clinical reasoning: A critical review. *Advances in Medical Education and Practice*, *10*, 703–716. https://doi.org/10.2147/AMEP.S213492

Yazdani, S., Hosseinzadeh, M., & Hosseini, F. (2017). Models of clinical reasoning with a focus on general practice: A critical review. *Journal of Advances in Medical Education & Professionalism*, *5*(4), 177–184.

Young, M. E., Thomas, A., Lubarsky, S., Gordon, D., Gruppen, L. D., Rencic, J., Ballard, T., Holmboe, E., Da Silva, A., Ratcliffe, T., Schuwirth, L., Dory, V., & Durning, S. J. (2020). Mapping clinical reasoning literature across the health professions: A scoping review. *BMC Medical Education*, *20*, 1–11. https://doi.org/10.1186/s12909-020-02012-9

2 The MMCR Approach to Evaluation Guided by the Profession's Domain of Concern

Laurie Knis-Matthews and Nancy R. Dooley

Occupational Therapy and Our Domain of Concern

In 1981, Anne Cronin Mosey published *Occupational Therapy: Configuration of a Profession* in which she began laying out the framework for our profession and subsequently influenced the creation for the Matthews Model of Clinical Reasoning (MMCR). Mosey described a model as the way a profession looks at itself, the connection to the other professions and its relationship with society. Mosey described the six facets of a profession's model as philosophical assumptions, ethical code, theoretical foundations, domain of concern, legitimate tools and the nature of and principles for sequencing the various aspects of practice (Mosey, 1981).

Practitioners are encouraged to read this seminal work in its entirety, but the domain of concern will be described in more detail. The domain of concern represents our areas of expertise, what makes our profession unique, and details our body of knowledge (Mosey, 1981). It is written in such a way that laypeople are often able to distinguish our areas of expertise and role delineation between professions. For example, most people in our society are able to articulate the differences between a dentist and a physician, while it may be more difficult to articulate the expertise of other professions such as a recreational therapist and a music therapist.

TRY IT: Explaining Our Domain of Concern to Others. What Is Occupational Therapy?

To make deliberate decisions about a person's evaluation and intervention plan, practitioners should be able to articulate their areas of expertise and role delineation to others such as the person served and interprofessional partners. To explain our domain of concern in layman terms, try answering the following:

Provide a clear and succinct explanation of your expertise as a practitioner.

Adjust your explanations of occupational therapy to a variety of audiences such as the person served, interprofessional team members or during a presentation at a health fair.

Identify one or two other professions and articulate the similarities and differences with occupational therapy.

Domain of Concern: The Occupational Therapy Practice Framework

The *Occupational Therapy Practice Framework (OTPF): Domain and Process* is one example of a document that illustrates our current domain of concern. Replacing *Uniform Terminology*

DOI: 10.4324/9781003392408-3

for Occupational Therapy in 2002, there have been four revisions of this official document of the American Occupational Therapy Association (AOTA), with the most recent fourth edition published in 2020. The second edition of the *Uniform Terminology Occupational Therapy* document defined and explained the constructs of occupational performance areas and performance components for the practitioner to use this information to guide intervention (AOTA, 1989). However, this document barely mentioned the process for conducting evaluations and providing occupation-based treatment, leaving readers to potentially misinterpret the steps for intervention.

Beginning with the first edition of the *Occupational Therapy Practice Framework: Domain and Process* (AOTA, 2002), the document finally included a process section and supplied the missing link for practitioners. This document is divided into two parts: domain and process. The domain section of the practice framework outlines our profession's scope and the areas in which practitioners have established expertise (AOTA, 2020). The process section of the practice framework outlines the action steps taken by practitioners while engaging in the delivery of occupational therapy services, including evaluation, intervention and outcomes (AOTA, 2020). Grounded in clinical reasoning, this section provides practitioners with a framework *of how to think* about evaluation, interventions and outcomes. This distinction, connected with the pillars of client centeredness and occupation-based intervention, further solidified the occupational therapy profession's domain of concern. This connection further served as the foundation to shape the MMCR.

The Occupational Therapy Practice Framework *Explains the Evaluation Process*

The fourth edition of *The Occupational Therapy Practice Framework: Domain and Process* describes the parts of the evaluation process in considerable detail (AOTA, 2020), and the reader should review this important document. The occupational therapy process typically begins with a referral for services. These referrals can come from a variety of sources, such as a person seeking services, family members, educators, other professionals such as physical therapists, physicians and nurses. A practitioner's clinical reasoning process begins when a referral is generated for a person seeking occupational therapy services.

Once a referral is initiated, the practitioner may conduct a screening process to determine if an evaluation is warranted and/or directly begin the evaluation process. The practitioner collects data during the evaluation period to create a baseline measure of the person's strengths and challenges to direct the eventual course of intervention.

The process section of the practice framework describes equally important but differentiating parts of the evaluation process: the occupational profile and the analysis of performance. Following guidance from the practice framework (AOTA, 2020), a practitioner should conduct *both* types of evaluations: an occupational profile and analysis of performance. Practitioners use various occupational profiles during the evaluation period to create opportunities to more fully understand the person's life story and goals. Each decision made in terms of the number and types of evaluations selected are guided by the practitioner's clinical reasoning.

Voices of the Practitioners: Using the Occupational Profile as Part of the Evaluation

There are so many little pieces to the puzzle and valuable information. I will ask them questions about things as they are talking. Towards the end, I go back over everything and repeat the things they mentioned were getting in the way. Then I will continue with more follow-up questions. (Casey)

I get the most information from my first interview when I learn about the person, environment and occupation and any struggles they are having. (Morgan)

I use active listening to understand people's stories. I want to understand their perspective of what it is like for them to live with an illness. (Kristen)

I always push the importance of the occupational profile. We have kids working on things like archery, drumming, accordions, tying their shoelaces and braiding their hair. We had a little boy come from Mexico, and his goal was to hit a pinata with two hands for his birthday. There was another little boy from Spain, who needed to work on archery because it was an important part of the curriculum there. (Casey)

Occupational Profiles or Top Evaluations

How the Occupational Profile Helps a Practitioner to Understand a Person's Story

An occupational profile is a *type* of evaluation used to facilitate a practitioner's understanding of a person's story related to their occupations, activities, interests and goals (AOTA, 2020; Knis-Matthews et al., 2017). There is not one specific occupational profile to use during the evaluation process, nor is there a standardized format when completing the profile. An occupational profile is typically completed in an interview-style format so the practitioner can ask numerous open-ended types of questions with probing, clarifying and restatements of ideas. The practitioner can generate the profile-type questions or can use specific evaluations designed to understand a person's story. In the MMCR, occupational profiles are categorized as the "top" type of evaluations.

These top evaluations, utilizing an occupational profile format, examine a person's life story centered in the constructs of person, environment and occupation.

Some areas of inquiry for a top type of evaluation are:

- Explore the unique characteristics of the person (especially beyond labels such as diagnosis, gender or age).
- What lifestyle change(s) does this person want to make?
- How do the various facets of the environment impact a person's story?
- Identify and describe the person's long-term and short-term personal goals.
- Explore a person's perception of strengths and challenges.
- Uncover details of the person's interests, values, activities and occupations.

The occupational profile sets the tone for an occupation-based intervention approach. Without an understanding of the person's unique life story and what goals are to be accomplished, the intervention plans cannot be individualized or meaningful to the person served. Please refer to Table 2.1, which highlights some common occupational therapy evaluations in the top-oriented category.

As the overarching purpose of a top evaluation is to understand a person's story more fully, a practitioner may be expecting these types of evaluations to use an interview format such as the Canadian Occupational Performance Measure (COPM) (Law et al., 2019) or the Occupational Circumstances Assessment Interview Rating Scale (OCAIRS) (Forsyth et al., 2005). This is not always the case, as it is the practitioner, using the art of practice, who conducts these top evaluations in various ways to learn about the person's story. For example, while the Role Checklist requires the person to identify past, present and future roles by checking off boxes, the evaluation rarely ends there (Scott, 2019). After the checklist is completed, the practitioner typically asks the person to identify the most meaningful roles and then utilize the skills of probing, restating and clarifying statements surrounding these selected roles to more fully understand the story.

Table 2.1 Top-Oriented Evaluations With a Focus on Occupational Profiles: Sampling of Occupational Profiles or Top-Oriented Evaluations

Title of Evaluation	Brief Description	Applicable populations	Reference
Canadian Occupational Performance Measure (COPM)	A measure designed to assess a person's perceived occupational performance and satisfaction within the areas of self-care, productivity and leisure.	Designed for use with all persons regardless of diagnosis as young as 8 years old. Cannot be used directly with very young children or individuals with severe cognitive deficits.	Law, M., Baptiste, S., Carswell, A., McColl, M. A., Polatajko, H., & Pollock, N. (2019). *Canadian occupational performance measure (COPM)* (5th ed. rev.). COPM Inc.
Child Occupational Self-Assessment (COSA)	An outcome measure used to gather a person's perceptions of their occupational competence and the importance for everyday activities.	Children between the ages of 8 to 13, have adequate cognitive abilities and have a desire to collaborate in the development of therapy goals.	Keller, J., Kafkes, A., Basu, S., Federico, J., & Kielhofner, G. (2005). *A user's manual for child occupational self-assessment (COSA) (version 2.1).* Model of Human Occupation Clearinghouse.
Goal Attainment Scaling (GAS)	A method of scoring the extent to which a person's goals have been met throughout the course of treatment.	Individuals within the mental health area and rehabilitation health area.	Research Utilization Laboratory. (1976). *Goal attainment scaling manual.* Jewish Vocational Service.
Kawa Model	A metaphoric tool that symbolizes a person's perceived life journey through the creation of a river.	Persons who are able to share their story using the metaphor of a river.	Iwama, M. K., Thomson, N. A., & Macdonald, R. M. (2009). The Kawa Model: The power of culturally responsive occupational therapy. *Disability and Rehabilitation, 31*(14), 1125–1135. http://doi.org/10.1080/09638280902773711
Modified Interest Checklist	A checklist used to gather information related to a person's interests and engagement in activities in the past, present and future.	Adolescents and adults.	Model of Human Occupation Clearinghouse. (2020). *Modified interest checklist.* Department of Occupational Therapy, University of Illinois at Chicago.
Occupational Circumstances Assessment Interview Rating Scale (OCAIRS) Version 4	A semi-structured interview used to gather, analyze and report data regarding a person's occupational participation.	Adolescents or adults with the cognitive and emotional ability to participate in an interview.	Forsyth, K., Deshpande, S., Kielhofner, G., Henriksson, C., Haglund, L., Olson, L., Skinner, S., & Kulkarni, S. (2005). *A user's manual for the occupational circumstances assessment interview and rating scale (OCAIRS) (version 4.0).* Model of Human Occupation Clearinghouse.
Occupational Performance History II (OPHI-II)	A semi-structured interview with the purpose of exploring the person's life history within the areas of work, play and self-care performance.	Persons over the age of 12 who are cognitively aware, are emotionally stable and can participate in an interview.	Kielhofner, G., Mallinson, T., Crawford, C., Nowak, M., Rigby, M., Henry, A., & Walens, D. (2004). *A user's manual for the occupational performance history interview (OPHI-II) (version 2.1).* Model of Human Occupation Clearinghouse.
Pediatric Volitional Questionnaire (PVQ)	An observational tool used to learn about the child's motivations based on their daily behaviors within their environment.	Children between the ages of 2 and 12.	Basu, S., Kafkes, A., Schatz, R., Kiraly, A., & Kielhofner, G. (2008). *A user's manual for the pediatric volitional questionnaire (version 2.1).* Model of Human Occupation Clearinghouse.

(Continued)

Table 2.1 (Continued)

Title of Evaluation	Brief Description	Applicable populations	Reference
Perceived Efficacy and Goal Setting System (PEGS)	A tool that facilitates children to self-report their perceived competence in everyday activities and to set goals for their intervention.	Children between the ages of 5 and 9.	Missiuna, C., Pollock, N., & Law, M. C. (2004). *PEGS: The perceived efficacy and goal setting system: Manual*. Harcourt Assessment.
Role Checklist Version 3: Participation and Satisfaction	A short screening tool that assesses a person's participation levels, satisfaction and reasons for non-participation.	Persons aged 18 and older.	Scott, P. J. (2019). *Role Checklist Version 3 participation and satisfaction (RCv3)*. Model of Human Occupation Clearinghouse, Department of Occupational Therapy, University of Illinois at Chicago.
Wellness in Eight Dimensions	A method for persons to reflect on their strengths and areas for improvement within the eight dimensions of wellness (emotional, financial, social, spiritual, occupational, physical, intellectual, and environmental).	Persons who are able to reflect on their own life experiences and complete a self-assessment.	Swarbrick, P., & Yudof, J. (2014). *Wellness in eight dimensions*. Collaborative Support Programs of NJ, Inc.

Deciding on How Many and Which Occupational Profiles to Select for Each Person Served

Each type of occupational profile or top evaluation is unique and highlights the person's story from a slightly different vantage point. For example, the Role Checklist (Oakley et al., 1986; Scott, 2019) and Interest Checklist (Matsutsuyu, 1969; Model of Human Occupation Clearinghouse, 2020) are both top types of evaluations, but practitioners determine if they want to understand the person's story from the vantage point of role identification and/or leisure interests.

While there are many different types of top-oriented evaluations, one or possibly two evaluations should be selected if the practitioner is inquiring about the person's lived experiences, personal goals and occupational preference. The essence of a person's life experiences or goals will not change based on the selected top evaluation. In other words, the person served will find a way to discuss what is most important regardless of the evaluation selected. It is the practitioner, using an evaluation tool, who creates a safe environment for people to tell their story and determine intervention priorities. No matter which top evaluation is selected, practitioners should utilize their art of practice to probe, clarify and restate certain aspects of the story from these specific vantage points.

Analysis of Performance or Bottom Evaluations

Analysis of Performance Evaluations Guides a Practitioner to Understand Potential Challenges of a Person's Story

While occupational profiles are tools used to gather data about a person's life story, this information alone is not enough to evaluate a person's baseline measure of performance. People typically seek services because they want assistance to make a change or reach a goal. While people are experts in their life experiences, practitioners are masterful in problem solving the obstacles that might interfere with goal attainment. For example, while using the Role Checklist, a practitioner learns about a person's valued roles. If the person expresses dissatisfaction with a specific role and wants to create change, the practitioner then investigates potential reasons for this issue. Is it due to memory loss? Motor planning? Emotional regulation? Difficulties in specific social skills? To identify what might be getting in the way, practitioners may need to administer numerous bottom evaluations due to their narrow scope and specific criteria.

Equally important, but distinctive from an occupational profile, are evaluations that focus on analysis of performance, referred to in the MMCR as "bottom" type evaluations. These types of evaluations measure potential client factors and/or performance skills that may facilitate or hinder occupational performance (AOTA, 2020; Knis-Matthews et al., 2017).

As we will explore in future chapters, practitioners, using their clinical reasoning skills, select the most relevant bottom evaluations specifically connected to a person's life story and goal achievement. This selection can be complicated, as bottom evaluations range in style from standardized, non-standardized, rating scales only; a battery of isolated evaluations pulled together under one umbrella evaluation; or specific parts of different evaluations pulled together. The combinations are endless. For example, manual muscle testing (Daniels & Worthingham, 1980) directly evaluates the strength of a person's muscles. Based on the score, practitioners begin to predict how people may be able to participate in their occupations or if compensatory strategies are needed. Manual muscle testing is considered one bottom-oriented evaluation. It is not uncommon for a practitioner to combine additional evaluations together such as manual muscle testing with range-of-motion testing (Dirette & Gutman, 2021; Hellebrandt et al., 1949) during the evaluation process.

Some bottom evaluations only provide the scoring criteria but not the actual evaluation, such as the Comprehensive Occupational Therapy Evaluation (COTE) scale (Brayman et al., 1976). This rating scale provides direction and parameters for the practitioners to observe specific behaviors divided into three sections (general, interpersonal and task) to observe and evaluate. However, practitioners using the COTE scale must create their own activities or situations to observe these skills. Please refer to Table 2.2, which highlights some common occupational therapy evaluations that fall into the bottom-oriented category.

Quick Recap of the Evaluation Process: A-HA Moment

According to the practice framework, there are two parts of the evaluation process:
Occupational profile or top-oriented evaluations—these evaluations are typically conducted with an interview format to learn more about the person's story, goals, valued occupations or environmental context. As most top evaluation results all eventually lead to the person's goals, a practitioner does not typically need to conduct more than one or two.

Analysis of performance or bottom-oriented evaluations—these evaluations typically focus on investigation of a person's client factors and/or performance skills. These evaluations are useful to determine what may be hindering the progress toward a person's goal. These types of evaluations tend to be narrower in domain, so numerous evaluations might be needed to identify those challenges

Table 2.2 Bottom-Oriented Evaluations With a Focus on Analysis of Performance: Sampling of Analysis of Performance or Bottom-Oriented Evaluations

Title of Evaluation	Brief Description	Applicable Populations	Reference
Allen Cognitive Level Screen (ACLS)	A standardized screening tool to assess functional cognition through the use of visual motor tasks.	Persons ages 6 with psychiatric problems or disruptions in global cognitive processing capacities such as having experienced a TBI or CVA.	Allen, C. K., Austin, S. L., David, S. K., Earhart, C. A., McCraith, D. B., & Riska-Williams, L. (2007). *Manual for the Allen cognitive level screen-5 (ACLS-5) and large Allen cognitive level screen-5 (LACLS-5).* ACLS and LACLS Committee. Allison, J., & Shotwell, M. (2020). The comprehensive occupational therapy evaluation. In B. J. Hemphill & C. K. Urish (Eds.), *Assessments in occupational therapy mental health: An integrative approach* (pp. 632–653). Slack Incorporated.
Beery Visual Motor Integration (Beery VMI) 6th Edition	A tool used to assess a person's ability to integrate their visual and motor abilities through the use of developmental sequencing of geometric figures.	Can be used with persons as early as 2 years old and up. The sixth edition has normed this assessment for ages 2 to 18.	Beery, K. E., Buktenica, N. A., & Beery, N. A. (2010). *The Beery-Buktenica developmental test of visual-motor integration.* Pearson, Inc.
Bruininks-Oseretsky Test of Motor Proficiency 2nd Edition (BOT-2)	An assessment to evaluate gross and fine motor skills in children with the use of eight total subtests, including fine motor precision, fine motor integration, manual dexterity, upper-limb coordination, bilateral coordination, balance, running speed and agility and strength.	Used with children from ages 4 to 21.	Bruininks, R. H., & Bruininks, B. D. (2005). *BOT 2: Bruininks-Oseretsky Test of motor proficiency* (2nd ed.). Pearson, Inc.
Executive Function Performance Test	An evaluation used to examine basic tasks essential for self-maintenance and independent living. The tasks include simple cooking, telephone use, medication management and bill payment.	Can be used for ages 13 and up.	Baum, C. M., & Wolf, T. J. (2013). *Executive function performance test (EFPT).* Washington University.

Assessment	Description	Population/Use	Reference
Kohlman Evaluation of Living Skills (KELS)	A tool used to assess a person's ability to function in basic living skills: (1) self-care, (2) safety and health, (3) money management, (4) community mobility and telephone and (5) employment and leisure participation. Also identifies the areas in which they need further assistance. The evaluation can be used to make recommendations for safe living situations based on the life skills assessed.	Appropriate to use with older adults in inpatient psychiatric units and acute care hospitals. Also, with those with cognitive conditions.	Kohlman Thomson, L., & Robnett, R. (2016). *KELS Kohlman evaluation of living skills* (4th ed.). AOTA Press.
Manual Muscle Testing (MMT)	A standardized assessment used to evaluate muscle strength and function through the use of positioning, applied motion and applied resistance.	Appropriate to use with persons of any age who do not have pain in the area to be tested, a dislocated or unhealed fracture, recent surgery, myositis ossification or any fragile bone condition.	Kendall, F. P., McCreary, E. K., & Provance, P. G. (1993). *Muscles, testing and function* (4th ed.) Williams & Wilkins. Dirette, D. P., & Gutman, S. A. (2021). *Occupational therapy for physical dysfunction* (8th ed.). Wolters Kluwer.
Modified Ashworth Scale	A tool utilized to measure the degree of spasticity.	Persons who present with lesions of the central nervous system ages 6 and up.	Bohanan, R., & Smith, M. (1987). Interrater reliability of a modified Ashworth scale of muscle spasticity. *Physical Therapy, 67*(2), 206–207. http://doi.org/10.1093/ptj/67.2.206
Motor-Free Visual Perception Test (MVPT-4)	An assessment utilized to measure a person's visual perceptual skills that are commonly used in everyday activities. It focuses on five types of visual perceptual abilities, including spatial relationships, visual discrimination, figure-ground, visual closure and visual memory.	Used with people ages 4 to 80.	Colarusso, R. P., & Hammil, D. D. (2015). *MVPT-4: Motor-free visual perception test-4.* ATP Assessments Academic Therapy Publications.
Peabody Developmental Motor Scales 2nd Edition (PDMS-2)	An assessment containing six subtests utilized to evaluate a child's gross and fine motor skills that develop early in life. Subtests include reflexes, stationary, locomotion, object manipulation, grasping and visual-motor integration.	Children from birth to age 5.	Folio, M. R., & Fewell, R. R. (2000). *Examiner's manual Peabody developmental motor scales* (2nd ed.). PRO-ED, Inc.
Range of Motion (ROM) Testing	A measure of flexibility in various functional movement patterns. This may include the use of a goniometer to test the angle of joints.	Can be used with persons of any age who do not have heart and respiratory diseases, connective tissue disorders, pain or an acute injury.	Reese, N., & Brandy, W. (2016). *Joint range of motion and muscle length testing* (3rd ed.). Elsevier. Dirette, D. P., & Gutman, S. A. (2021). *Occupational therapy for physical dysfunction* (8th ed.). Wolters Kluwer.
Sensory Profile 2	A standardized assessment designed to evaluate a child's sensory processing preferences within their home, school and community-based activities.	Children up to the age of 14 years and 11 months.	Dunn, W. (2014). *Sensory profile 2.* Pearson, Inc.

There Are Many Choices of Evaluations for the Practitioner to Select

Similar to top-type evaluations, there are many bottom types of evaluations to choose from in occupational therapy. Although analysis of performance or bottom type of evaluations appear more popular in the occupational therapy profession, selection is more complicated. Many bottom evaluations are narrower in scope and measure specific client factors and/or performance patterns. At times, practitioners utilize numerous bottom-type evaluations together or may use just one bottom evaluation.

Occupational therapy practitioners determine how many evaluations are needed, and it often varies depending on numerous factors such as the person served, intervention locations and what evaluations are available. There is no cookbook recipe for this determination, but it is based on a practitioner's clinical reasoning skills. However, an important point is to remember that some combination of both top and bottom evaluations is required to understand the totality of the person's story and what client factors or performance patterns are considered. If practitioners only conduct a top evaluation, then it may lead to guessing what skills should be addressed during intervention. In contrast, only conducting a series of bottom evaluations does not put these foundation skills into context to eventually conduct occupation-based intervention approaches.

Voices of the Practitioners: How to Use Top- and Bottom-Type Evaluations Together

During my evaluations, I follow a bottom-up approach. I initially get information from observations and standardized assessments. I always use at least some sort of a top evaluation like a modified Role Checklist. (Pam)

Using a top-down approach, it is natural for me to get to know the person using an occupational profile. I often use the COPM as the semi-structured interview for the occupational profile. I always use an evaluation that is more standardized and objective along with the occupational profile. I feel like that really helps me to paint a good picture of the person and what gets in the way. (Casey)

Top-Down and Bottom-Up Approaches to the Evaluation Process

An occupational therapy practitioner, guided by clinical reasoning, determines the sequence of top- or bottom-oriented evaluations administered during the evaluation process. Should the practitioner initially focus on gathering detailed information about the person's story and goals to eventually uncover what might be a barrier? Should the practitioner focus on evaluating specific client factors and performance skills to align with the person's story or goals? The answer is yes to both questions.

Two approaches (top-down, bottom-up) described by Weinstock-Zlotnick and Hinojosa (2004) provide a strategy when creating evaluation and intervention plans. Pay attention to the words "down" and "up" as the evaluation process might initially start with the top or bottom approach but must balance both sides to ensure it is client centered and demonstrates measured evidence of skills related to analysis of performance.

Influenced by Weinstock-Zlotnick and Hinojosa, in the MMCR, a top-down approach starts with an occupational profile (top) and provides the practitioner with detailed information about the person's story, interests, occupations and goals. While this specific information is necessary to learn about the individual person, it does not always emphasize the strengths and challenges of the person's client factors or performance skills. Following this line of clinical reasoning, practitioners begin with the top information and then go down to evaluate a person's client factors or performance skills.

In contrast, a practitioner using a bottom-up approach emphasizes evaluating analysis of performance measures first to determine how those skills are relevant to a person's occupations. The strengths and challenges to a person's client factors and performance skills can be uncovered with numerous bottom-oriented evaluations. Following this line of clinical reasoning, the practitioner begins with understanding the bottom-oriented information and then places it in the context of the person's story.

Influenced by earlier versions of *Uniform Terminology* suggesting performance areas, performance components and performance had equal importance, there appeared to be more familiarity with bottom-up approaches (Weinstock-Zlotnick & Hinojosa, 2004). However, at times, practitioners emphasized bottom evaluations but did not connect them with a person's occupation, leaving the door open for more preparatory types of interventions (i.e., cones or collages!). In other words, the practitioners conducted bottom evaluations but did not go "up" to align these skills with the person's unique life story or assumed these skills would just generalize over to other contexts at a later time.

While our profession has consistently embraced the meaning of occupation, the profession experienced a gradual paradigm shift toward occupation-based treatment and client-centered principles when *Uniform Terminology* was replaced with the first edition of the *Practice Framework* (AOTA, 2002). Weinstock-Zlotnick and Hinojosa (2004) proposed that neither approach should dominate our profession, but should be determined specifically for each person served. There are emergency situations requiring immediate attention by the practitioner, for example, a person who has sustained third-degree burns and requires a strategic range-of-motion protocol to prevent contractures or a person who is at risk for falls and preparing to return home alone. In these situations, there is not sufficient time to conduct an initial occupational profile. In this case, a bottom-up approach might be more beneficial to begin the evaluation process.

Other times, the person's client factors and performance skills need to be understood within a person's life story, so it is not assumed these skills will automatically generalize. For example, Angel wants to improve his endurance to continue making his famous empanadas. The context is important here. How much endurance does Angel require if making empanadas is part of his full-time job in a restaurant? Is the amount of endurance different if making empanadas at home with his brothers? A practitioner can decide to begin with either approach if information about the person's unique story and potential challenges are both addressed throughout the evaluation and intervention process.

TRY IT: Distinguishing the Types of Evaluations in Occupational Therapy

A practitioner's clinical reasoning is part of the evaluation selection for the person served. This process begins with strategically using a balance of top and bottom types of evaluations.

Reflect on common evaluations typically used in occupational therapy.

Identify which are top evaluations emphasizing occupational profile information or are bottom evaluations emphasizing client factors and performance skills. Justify your answers.

Describe the ways these evaluations would be (or are) typically administered.

Strategically create a plan to balance both types of evaluations during the evaluation process.

When Selecting Evaluations, Pay Careful Attention to Initial Publication Dates, Document Revisions and Societal Influences

When creating each person's specific evaluation protocols and timelines, there are four guiding areas to be considered:

- OTPF
- Available top and bottom evaluations to select for the person served
- Possible practice model and/or frames of reference to use as a guideline for action
- Best evidence available

While these four areas are equally important for practitioners to consider when beginning the evaluation process, there can be a misalignment between the updated evaluations available, content discrepancy based on the newest editions of the practice framework and adequate practice models and/or frames of references to guide these evaluations.

There are many reasons for this misalignment. It takes years to develop evaluations, expand practice models and conduct the research guiding these changes. For example, it takes an extraordinary amount of time, effort and research to develop a standardized evaluation. Some of the evaluations commonly used in practice have not been updated for some time. In 1985 the Barth Time Construction (BTC) (Barth, 1985) was created when the profession's domain of concern followed the first edition of *Uniform Terminology* (AOTA, 1979). Practitioners still continue to use this evaluation but no longer follow the standardized format, as it is difficult to purchase the exact materials on the market. In 2007, the Volitional Questionnaire (VQ) was published (de las Heras et al., 2007) during the third edition of the *Model of Human Occupation* (Kielhofner, 2002). Since that time, the *Model of Human Occupation* has evolved, with the fifth edition published in 2017 (Taylor, 2017), while VQ has not been updated to reflect these changes in the guiding practice model. When deciding which evaluations to use for the person served, reflect on the publication dates and what factors may have been an influence during this time.

Factors to Consider When Selecting Evaluations for the Person Served: A-HA Moment

As described in this chapter, there are many factors to consider during the initial stages of data gathering. Next time you are selecting a combination of evaluations for a specific person, ask yourself the following questions:

Am I incorporating both an occupational profile (top) and analysis of performance type (bottom) of evaluation?

Are the bottom evaluations standardized or non-standardized? What are the benefits and challenges of each type? Is my reason for conducting these evaluations for this person based on sound clinical reasoning?

Am I using the most current evaluations? Does this evaluation connect with the most current information identified in our practice framework? What evidence supports my decisions?

How do these evaluation selections align with a frame of reference, practice model and/or the practice framework?

Summary

As part of Mosey's model (1981), the domain of concern delineates our profession's area of expertise. The OTPF is one example of an official document that illustrates our most current domain of concern. The process section of the practice framework describes differentiating parts of the evaluation process: the occupational profile and the analysis of performance. An occupational profile is a type of evaluation used by practitioners to more fully understand the person's life story and goals. In the MMCR, occupational profiles are categorized as a "top" type of evaluations. Equally important is analysis of performance-type evaluations that measure client factors and/or performance skills, referred to in the MMCR as "bottom" type evaluations. It is recommended that practitioners conduct both types of evaluations to understand a person's story and what might be getting in the way of their goal attainment. The MMCR provides a framework to guide practitioners through the evaluation process, leading to eventual intervention plans.

References

American Occupational Therapy Association. (1979). *Occupational therapy product output reporting system and uniform terminology for reporting occupational therapy services.* pracdept@aota.org

American Occupational Therapy Association. (1989). Uniform terminology for occupational therapy—second edition. *American Journal of Occupational Therapy, 43,* 808–815. https://doi.org/10.5014/ajot.4312.808

American Occupational Therapy Association. (2002). Occupational therapy practice framework: Domain and process. *American Journal of Occupational Therapy, 56,* 609–639. https://doi.org/10.5014/ajot.56.6.609

American Occupational Therapy Association. (2020). Occupational therapy practice framework: Domain and process (4th ed.). *American Journal of Occupational Therapy, 74*(Suppl. 2), 7412410010. https://doi.org/10.5014/ajot.2020.74S2001

Barth, T. (1985). *Barth time construction.* Health Related Consulting Services.

Brayman, S. J., Kirby, T. F., Misenheimer, A. M., & Short, M. J. (1976). Comprehensive occupational therapy evaluation scale. *American Journal of Occupational Therapy, 30*(2), 94–100.

Daniels, L., & Worthingham, C. (1980). *Muscle testing: Techniques of manual examination* (4th ed.). W. B. Saunders Company.

de las Heras, C. G., Geist, R., Kielhofner, G., & Li, Y. (2007). *A user's manual for the volitional questionnaire (VQ), version 4.1.* MOHO Clearinghouse.

Dirette, D. P., & Gutman, S. A. (2021). *Occupational therapy for physical dysfunction* (8th ed.). Wolters Kluwer.

Forsyth, K., Deshpande, S., Kielhofner, G., Henriksson, C., Haglund, L., Olson, L., Skinner, S., & Kulkarni, S. (2005). *A user's manual for the occupational circumstances assessment interview and rating scale (OCAIRS) (version 4.0).* Model of Human Occupation Clearinghouse.

Hellebrandt, F. A., Duvall, E. N., & Moore, M. L. (1949). The measurement of joint motion: Part III: Reliability of goniometry. *Physical Therapy Review, 29,* 302–307.

Kielhofner, G. (2002). *Model of human occupation* (3rd ed.). Lippincott Williams & Wilkins.

Knis-Matthews, L., Mulry, C. M., & Richard, L. (2017). Matthews Model of clinical reasoning: A systematic approach to conceptualize evaluation and intervention. *Occupational Therapy in Mental Health, 33*(4), 360–373. http://doi.org/10.1080/0164212X.2017.1303658

Kohlman, L., & Robnett, R. (2016). *KELS: Kohlman evaluation of living skills.* AOTA Press.

Law, M., Baptiste, S., Carswell, A., McColl, M. A., Polatajko, H., & Pollock, N. (2019). *Canadian occupational performance measure (COPM)* (5th ed. rev.). COPM.

Matsutsuyu, J. S. (1969). The interest checklist. *American Journal of Occupational Therapy, 23*(4), 323–328.

Model of Human Occupation Clearinghouse. (2020). *Modified Interest Checklist.* Department of Occupational Therapy, University of Illinois at Chicago.

Mosey, A. C. (1981). *Occupational therapy: Configuration of a profession.* Raven Press.

Oakley, F., Kielhofner, G., Barris, R., & Reichler, R. K. (1986). The role checklist: Development and empirical assessment of reliability. *Occupational Therapy Journal of Research*, *6*(3), 157–170. http://doi.org/10.1177/153944928600600303

Scott, P. J. (2019). *Role checklist version 3: Participation and satisfaction (RCv3)*. Model of Human Occupation Clearinghouse.

Taylor, R. R. (2017). *Kielhofner's model of human occupation* (5th ed.). Wolters Kluwer.

Weinstock-Zlotnick, G., & Hinojosa, J. (2004). Bottom-up or top-down evaluation: Is one better than the other? *American Journal of Occupational Therapy*, *58*, 594–599. https://doi.org/10.5014/ajot.58.5.594

3 Compartmentalizing Evaluation Information and Understanding the Person Served

Laurie Knis-Matthews and Lynne Richard

Creating a System to Compartmentalize the Incoming Evaluation Information

Now that all of the evaluations are completed, the practitioner has a vast amount of information about the person served. To organize this information, it is necessary to begin compartmentalizing it. Students and new practitioners may find this moment stressful and overwhelming, while it appears second nature to seasoned practitioners. Remember, in the clinical reasoning process, expert or more experienced practitioners have multiple representations and patterns to assist them. Often, because of experience, the reasoning can appear automatic or effortless to the novice. This process begins with reflecting on the constructs of person, environment, and occupation (PEO). As practitioners are conducting the evaluations in real time, they are mentally shifting and sorting the incoming information around these constructs in such a way as to understand the person's story, occupations, and eventual goals. This is commonly referred to as "reflection-in-action" (Schon, 1983). It is a process of thinking about what you are doing as you do it. The benefits are that practitioners immediately start to frame the data and begin to identify and transform information into usable pieces.

Do not be alarmed if this process initially appears difficult and confusing. Trust the process! As mentioned earlier in this book, the author has created reproducible clinical reasoning guidesheets to navigate this process until the practitioners are able to do it with more efficiency and effectiveness. In other words, until it becomes second nature.

Voices of the Practitioners: Compartmentalizing Evaluation Information

I'm not writing down the triangle anymore but keeping that [triangle] in the back of my head. I do think that comes with time and experience otherwise. As a student I can't tell you the amount of times I have drawn that [triangle] and applied that [triangle] to so many different types of case studies. That's the way of making it become natural and it evolved into becoming more second nature. (Pam)

I compartmentalize it first in my mind and then I always have a folder for each person. I get it in my head, but I also feel I have to put it down on paper, so that if someone else is going to treat the person, and get to my folder, it's all there. I may first write a little note but after a while I have a lot of information. (Louise)

DOI: 10.4324/9781003392408-4

Let's begin with an introduction of the first MMCR clinical reasoning guidesheet. See Figure 3.1 (also found in Appendix 1): Clinical Reasoning Guidesheet: MMCR Guide to Understanding a Person's Story (Triangle). Take a few moments and examine this guidesheet before moving on with the next sections of this book. There are two clinical reasoning worksheets listed in the appendices. One is a blank guidesheet to be completed by the practitioner, while the other one is like a cheat sheet that emphasizes specific information discussed in these book chapters.

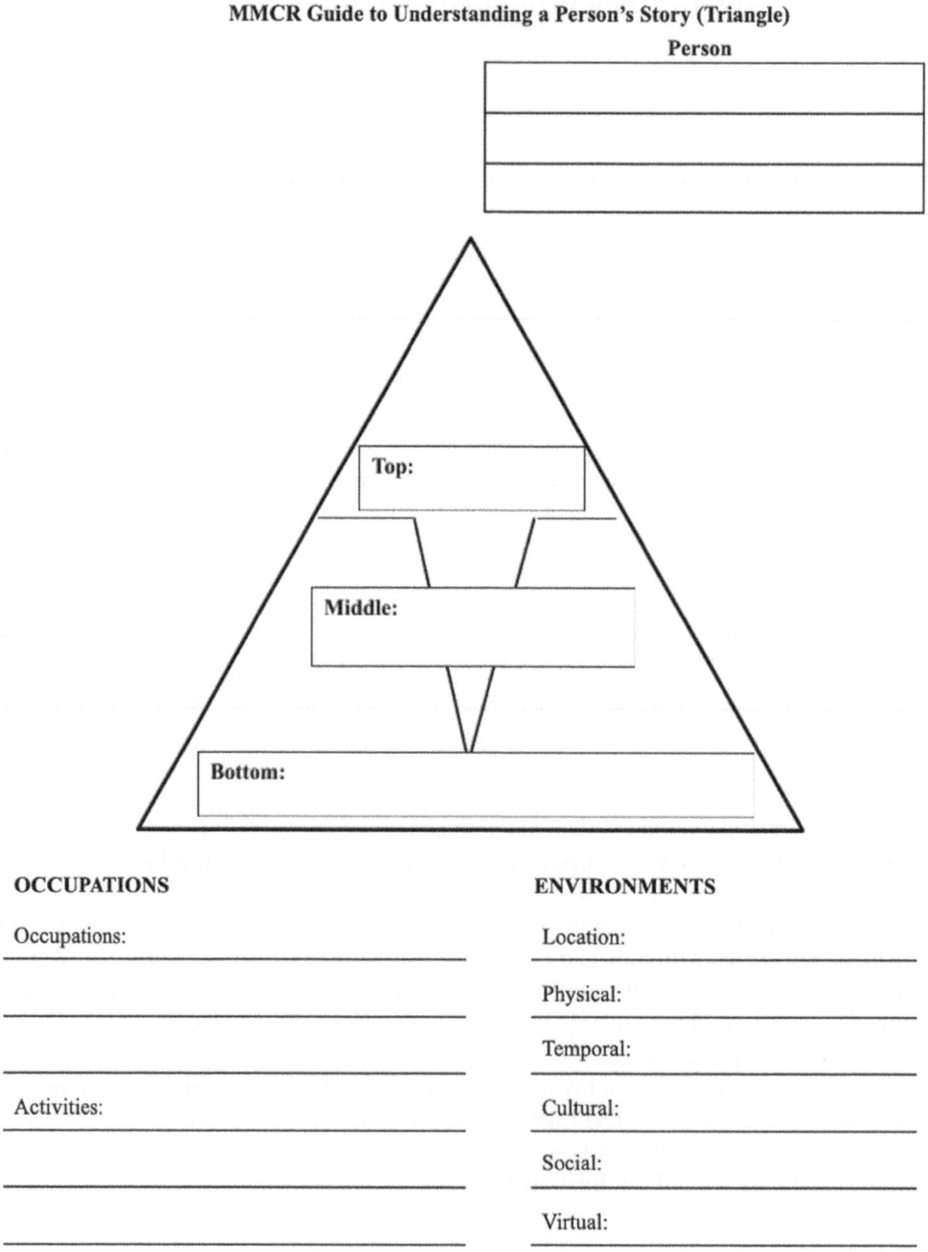

MMCR Guide to Understanding a Person's Story (Triangle)

Person

Top:

Middle:

Bottom:

OCCUPATIONS

Occupations:

Activities:

ENVIRONMENTS

Location:

Physical:

Temporal:

Cultural:

Social:

Virtual:

Figure 3.1 Clinical Reasoning Guidesheet: MMCR Guide to Understanding a Person's Story (Triangle).

Each part of the MMCR triangle will be discussed in detail, but this guideline will assist the practitioner in beginning to understand the overall conceptual map and how to compartmentalize the person's unique story into useful pieces of information. Now remember these clinical reasoning guidesheets are meant to assist in understanding the process and represent how a practitioner may be compartmentalizing the evaluation information in real time. These clinical reasoning guidesheets are not part of the formal evaluation findings or summary, but are designed to gain competency in this process. The practitioner is encouraged to write phrases, questions, or comments onto the MMCR triangle guidesheet as needed. When the triangle guidesheet is filled out, then practitioners can do what Schon (1983) referred to as "reflection-on-action". This is the time where practitioners can reflect back on the process and review, analyze, and evaluate to determine what might be missing or further explored.

How to Conceptualize Incoming Evaluation Data: A-HA Moment

Occupational therapist practitioners collect information about a person using a combination of evaluations gathered from the occupational profile (tops) and the analysis of performance (bottoms). During the evaluation administration, the practitioners are mentally forming, reflecting, and compartmentalizing interpretations of the evaluation data around the constructs of person-environment-occupation. These interpretations are solidified (in wet sand) once the practitioner has a chance to analyze all the relevant evaluation information within the context of the person's life story. A seasoned practitioner automatically begins the process of reflecting and compartmentalizing this information in real time during the data gathering process of the evaluation.

Why Use a Triangle to Represent the Matthews Model of Clinical Reasoning?

Person

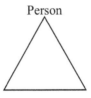

Figure 3.2

A triangle is one of the best shapes in geometry; an equilateral triangle has all three sides of the same length (Merriam-Webster, n.d.) suggesting equality. Similar to the MMCR, the PEO constructs are equally important and work together to make up an understanding of the whole person. Neither the symbolism of a triangle nor the emphasis on the PEO constructs is unique to this model. Earlier influences of the PEO model (Law et al., 1996) and person-environment-occupation-performance (PEOP) model (Baum et al., 2015; Christiansen & Baum, 2005; Cole & Tufano, 2008) provided the foundation to begin creating a systematic approach to evaluation and intervention steeped in client-centered principles and occupation-based interventions (Knis-Matthews et al., 2017). The MMCR provides the framework to put the PEO(P) information into a usable format and support the development of clinical reasoning skills.

Using the MMCR as a Guide, Take a Deeper Look at the *Person* Construct

Person

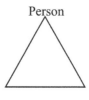

Figure 3.3

Person

The Person section of the triangle identifies some of the basic, but not limited to, specific information about the individual such as age, education, ethnic identity, cultural identity, diagnosis, gender identity, health considerations, medications and side effects, preferred pronouns, pronunciation of name, race, religion, sexual orientation, spirituality, and socioeconomic status. As each person is unique, there is not a cookbook description of how to conceptualize this section. Each time a new person is evaluated, the practitioner will highlight different characteristics that are specific and relevant to the person's story.

It is also important to have some understanding of the current sociocultural environment of disability studies (Kielhofner, 2005). Asking a person how they want to be identified can be the first step in a collaboration. For years, the common nomenclature was to use person-first language— a person with autism vs. an autistic person. Some disability study scholars and activists have challenged this idea, and some promote the use of "identity-first language" (e.g., autistic person) (Dunn & Andrews, 2015). There will be contexts and communities of people who have a preference for how they want to be addressed. Being aware of and sensitive to those preferences will enhance the therapeutic relationship.

Gathering Information About the Person Served

Voices of the Practitioners: How Important Is a Diagnosis to the Person's Story and What Else Needs to Be Learned?

I don't think that diagnosis should guide you, I think it's important to know what the person's diagnosis is just sometimes because of insurance. The families can go to one doctor and get diagnosed and another doctor and not get diagnosed based on the doctor's feelings about them. I don't care that that's their diagnosis. . . . It's not going to tell me anything about the treatment, but I need to know that diagnosis. I think it holds the clinician down from really looking at the child. (Rebecca)

Just left with a script, with or without a diagnosis and that can be misleading. Other times you're only left with a diagnosis like dementia but you really don't get that total understanding until you're actually with the person. That's why I really do rely heavily on that occupational profile both with the person and the family. (Pam)

There is a lot of social unrest in our country right now and we can strengthen our profession by talking about diversity, inclusion, and equity. Understanding these influences can [dampen] or enhance someone's clinical reasoning and relationships. We need to think more about people who are diverse within the culture of health care and professionals. Looking at the diversity side of it will only enhance our clinical reasoning skills. (Abigail)

The occupational therapy process typically begins with gathering initial information about the person who may be participating in services. Traditionally, practitioners are told to approach the evaluation process with an unbiased and neutral stance of the person being served, but in reality, this is more complicated than it sounds.

In order to begin the evaluation process, the practitioner immediately begins connecting labels to the person in order to begin understanding the person more generally. The practitioner begins to formulate a quick but detailed snapshot of the person served. This initial information is often gathered before the formal occupational profile even begins from various sources such as discussion in daily rounds, entry of a school report, what is written in the referral request, discussion with a family member or significant other, etc. For the most part, our initial information gathering about a person is partly based on someone else's interpretation of the person requesting services.

These labels often emphasize the characteristics of the person, so practitioners have a place to begin reflecting on the occupational therapy process in terms of age, gender, religion, race, languages spoken, living situation, and/or diagnosis as applicable. This can be helpful information to begin formulating an evaluation strategy in terms of what potential evaluations are available to use, how to approach the person to begin the evaluation, and relevant safety precautions. For example, the practitioner is going to approach the situation differently when evaluating a young child vs. an older adult.

They will alter their approach to the evaluation process if meeting someone who is actively hallucinating vs. someone who is no longer hearing voices. For example, a nurse may describe a new patient admitted to the hospital as a high-functioning, elderly, white female with a broken hip who lives home alone. A practitioner might immediately begin thinking about hip precautions protocols and how independent she has been and can be after the hip replacement in her living situation. In the clinical reasoning literature, this is referred to as hypothesis generating reasoning—practitioners begin to develop hypotheses about what to expect (i.e., the need for hip precaution instructions based on the diagnosis) and then use these as a stepping-off point to begin the therapeutic process.

While the initial use of labels to begin defining a person can be helpful, it can also be negative or simply untrue without further context. A practitioner may begin formulating a view of the person before the occupational profile even begins, based on the perceptions of others. Common labels such as lower socioeconomic class, poor insight, lower functioning, history of noncompliance with treatment, or aggressive tendencies can create a negative bias before the evaluation even begins.

Our profession has just recently begun to examine bias, discrimination, and stigma within it. All practitioners hold conscious and/or unconscious beliefs about certain people or groups. Increasing an awareness of and the impact of these beliefs on practice and the people served can help practitioners address clients as individuals and not a label. The American Occupational Therapy Association (2020) published a "Guide to Acknowledging the Impact of Discrimination, Stigma, and Implicit Bias on Provision of Services", and there are an increasing number of resources to help you.

Be cautious of these labels, as it can lead to different perceptions, definitions, and judgements of the person. For example, what does homelessness actually mean? Does it mean the person is living under a bridge, in a tent, on a friend's couch, or temporarily staying in a shelter? These are all different "homeless" situations that will alter the evaluation process. Upon admission, a person is labeled as aggressive, and staff are to be cautious upon approach. However, what are the reasons for the aggression? Was the person unexpectedly arrested by the police and without opportunity to call an employer about missing work?

Is the person experiencing withdrawal from a pain medication used to treat a back injury? Noncompliance with medications often creates a negative image of a person—that they are defiant, uncooperative, do not follow through, or are lazy or unmotivated. Before coming to this conclusion ask yourself, "Does the person have a history of noncompliance with medication because the side effects outweighed the benefits of the drug? Can the person afford to purchase these medications? What level of health literacy do they have about their condition and the need for the medication?"

TRY IT: Reflecting on Initial Labels and Information to Describe the Person Served

Reflect on the initial images that came to mind when you read the example earlier describing a woman named June. She is a new person admitted to the hospital as a high-functioning, elderly, white female with a broken hip who lives home alone. Do you assume the person lived in an apartment or a house? What does high functioning mean to you? Did you assume she might be easier to educate and then follow hip precautions?

Now what images come to mind when the description is changed a little more. A new client is admitted to the hospital described as a lower-functioning, elderly, black female with a broken hip who temporarily lives in a shelter.

Let me alter the description one more time with slightly different labels. A new patient admitted to the hospital described as a combative, elderly, male with a broken hip who lives in a psychiatric group home.

Reflect on your life experiences and worldviews. What may have contributed to these initial images and perceptions? How may these characteristics influence your approach to the evaluation and intervention process? How do the labels of person, client, and patient influence your view of the description?

Another resource to explore your implicit biases is the Harvard *Project Implicit*. Go here: *https://implicit.harvard.edu/implicit/takeatest.html* and you can take one or more Implicit Association Tests in categories of disability, age, and skin tone. The results can help you think about your own beliefs.

How Information Gathered Using Top Evaluations Can Help Understand the Person's Story: Looking Beyond the Labels

Oftentimes, initial information about a person is based on someone else's interpretation of the person served. The person's interpretation of events, including biases and worldviews, is captured in these initial documents. This is why it is so necessary for the practitioner to conduct a top evaluation. This provides an opportunity to learn more about the person's story, occupations, and goals on a deeper level. The person's story can facilitate narrative reasoning (Mattingly, 1991).

This type of reasoning goes beyond the facts of the person's story, and the practitioner develops a story to make sense of and explain the clients' experiences. For example, reflect on an initial chart entry identifying a person as not having any children although the person repeatedly reported having two sons. The different versions of this story created conflict between the person and staff, with eventual chart entries describing the person as delusional, aggressive, and paranoid. Upon digging deeper into the interview, the person described a strong connection with a neighbor's children and referred to them as her sons. Some professionals described this as lying or being untruthful. The person was neither—she was expressing her version of what a family means to her. However, this conflicted with the more traditional worldview of family that was held by others. It is important to use this information as a jumping-off point to ask questions for more context of the story.

To be clear, the practitioner should use this section as a loose guide for planning purposes and not definitive for understanding a person's unique life experiences based on a few labels. This might provide some ideas of questions or topics to explore about the person's story during the occupational profile and to be aware of the potential for bias. Be cautious of perceiving all information listed in these initial documents as the absolute truth and carrying more weight than the person's perception of these experiences.

Summary

Once practitioners complete multiple evaluations to gather an abundance of information about the person, it is necessary to analyze this data to determine how it aligns with the person's story, goals, and eventual intervention plan. The MMCR clinical reasoning guidesheet MMCR Guide to Understanding a Person's Story (Triangle) was created to assist practitioners to strategically compartmentalize this incoming information around the constructs of PEO.

The Person section of the triangle identifies some of the basic information about the person served such as age, education, ethnic identity, cultural identity, diagnosis, gender identity, health considerations, medications and side effects, race, religion, sexual orientation, spirituality, and socioeconomic status. While these labels are meant to assist practitioners to broadly begin organizing the evaluation data, they should also be cognizant of biases and safeguard against preconceptions of people.

References

Baum, C. M., Christiansen, C. H., & Bass, J. D. (2015). The person-environment-occupation performance (PEOP) model. In C. M. Baum, C. H. Christiansen, & J. Bass-Haugen (Eds.), *Occupational therapy: Performance, participation and well-being* (4th ed., pp. 49–55). Slack Incorporated.

Christiansen, C., & Baum, C. M. (2005). Person-environment-occupation performance: An occupation-based framework for practice. In C. Christiansen, C. M. Baum, & J. Bass-Haugen (Eds.), *Occupational therapy: Performance, participation, well-being* (pp. 242–267). Slack Incorporated.

Cole, M. B., & Tufano, R. (2008). The person-environment-occupation-performance model. In M. B. Cole & R. Tufano (Eds.), *Applied theories in occupational therapy: A practical approach* (pp. 127–133). Slack Incorporated.

Dunn, D. S., & Andrews, E. E. (2015). Person-first and identity-first language: Developing psychologists' cultural competence using disability language. *American Psychologist*, *70*(3), 255–264. https://doi.org/10.1037/a0038636

Kielhofner, G. (2005). Rethinking disability and what to do about it: Disability studies and its implications for occupational therapy. *American Journal of Occupational Therapy*, *59*, 487–496. https://doi.org/10.5014/ajot.59.5.487

Knis-Matthews, L., Mulry, C. M., & Richard, L. (2017). Matthews model of clinical reasoning: A systematic approach to conceptualize evaluation and intervention. *Occupational Therapy in Mental Health*, *33*(4), 360–373. http://doi.org/10.1080/0164212X.2017.1303658

Law, M., Cooper, B., Strong, S., Stewart, D., Rigby, P., & Letts, L. (1996). The person-environment-occupation model: A transactive approach to occupational performance. *Canadian Journal of Occupational Therapy*, *63*, 9–23. http://doi.org/10.1177/000841749606300103

Mattingly, C. (1991). The narrative nature of clinical reasoning? *American Journal of Occupational Therapy*, *45*(11), 998–1005. https://doi.org/10.5014/ajot.45.11.998

Merriam-Webster. (n.d.). *Merrian-Webster.com dictionary*. Retrieved February 21, 2021, from www.merriam-webster.com/dictionary/equilateral%20triangle

Schon, D. A. (1983). *The reflective practitioner*. Basic Books.

4 Compartmentalizing Evaluation Information and Understanding the Six Facets of the Environment

Laurie Knis-Matthews and Nancy R. Dooley

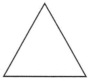

DOI: 10.4324/9781003392408-5

Figure 4.1

Environment:

Location
Physical
Temporal
Social
Cultural
Virtual

How the Environment Has Been Discussed in Occupational Therapy

Within the occupational therapy profession, there has been a steady and growing attention toward the environment construct first appearing in the American Occupational Therapy Association (AOTA) official document in the third version of *Uniform Terminology* (AOTA, 1994), labeled performance context, and then subsequently included in each edition of the *Practice Framework* beginning in the early 2000s (AOTA, 2002). There are many occupational therapy practice models and/or frames of reference to guide practitioners to seek information about various environmental factors. A sampling of these includes the Cognitive Disabilities Model (Allen, 1985), Kawa Model (Iwama, 2006), Model of Human Occupation (MOHO) (Taylor, 2017), Occupational Adaptation (OA) (Schkade & McClung, 2001), and Person-Environment-Occupation Performance (PEOP) Model (Baum et al., 2015).

MMCR and the Six Facets of the Environment

The MMCR addresses six facets of the environmental context (location, physical, temporal, social, cultural, and virtual) during data gathering of the evaluation process. Within this construct, the location facet is the highest categorical level that subsumes the other five environmental facets (physical, temporal, social, cultural, and virtual). Each facet by this context addresses specific parts of the environment for an overall understanding of the person's life story. At times, certain environmental facets may be more dominant when reflecting on the person's story and eventual intervention plan, but all five facets have the potential for equal importance.

Voices of the Practitioners: Learning About the Environment Helps to Understand a Person's Story

The foundation of occupational therapy is understanding the context of the environment, then your clinical reasoning will be supported. (Kristen)

I pay attention to any information about the home environment. I might be working with an older kid and they say, "I live with my mom." However, in the chart it says they live with dad. I need to go back to the team to figure out this mixed information. We need to make sure we are planning to discharge in the right location. (Jackie)

During the evaluation, a parent said that her child was having tantrums at home and he was falling off the seat. He was having a really hard time getting dressed and falling off the seat, especially during dinner. I asked if the child does any of this in school? And she said, no. I went back with more clarifying questions so I can get a broader picture of what's actually going on. I didn't know where the breakdown was happening. Is it happening in every environment or just one environment? Is it a certain time of day? There's so many different pieces that are important to understand what is going on. (Casey)

Reflecting on Each Specific Facet of the Environment

While all environmental facets are interconnected and nearly impossible to separate into a neat package, each one emphasizes a unique perspective of the environment to determine how these facets work together to understand a person's story.

Describing the Six Facets of a Person's Environment, in the Simplest of Terms, While Using an Example of the Sport of Competitive Swimming: A-HA Moment

There are six facets of environment highlighted in the MMCR:

Location: viewed as the highest conceptual level of environment, refers to the sites and places where occupations occur (e.g., riding the bus to a swim meet, the pool facility, eating dinner with other swimmers at a restaurant after the meet).

Each location has specific dimensions of the following five facets. Each of these five facets may have equal importance to a person's story, or specific ones may be more dominant at times.

Physical Environment: non-human or non-living objects present in various locations that are relevant to a person's life story (e.g., swim goggles, swim cap, bathing suit, towel, apples as a snack).

Temporal Environment: understanding a person's story from the perspective of time (e.g., age grouping for swim competitions, length of time as a swimmer, length of time in swim lessons, aging out of the sport, number of and duration of practices per week).

Social Environment: people, groups, communities, organizations, and populations that people feel a sense of belonging to, identify with, or have frequent contact with (e.g., other swimmers on the team, swim coach, relay team members, swim competitors, Olympic swim team members).

Cultural Environment: the expectations of customs, ideals, values, and thoughts of a social group (e.g., following the rules of each stroke so not disqualified, wearing team bathing suits for swim meets, expected sportsmanship behavior while on the pool deck).

Virtual Environment: using technology as a means to carry out occupations or communicate with others (e.g., calling or texting coach when late for practice, watching video of swim meets to model others, using underwater cameras to monitor a swimmer's exact stroke patterns for improvement).

Location: The Specific Sites and Places Where Occupations Occur

Location refers to the sites and places where occupations occur (Knis-Matthews et al., 2017). Within their lifestyles, people move in and out of various places on an hourly, daily, weekly, or yearly basis. Think about the different locations that you are a part of for just one day. At a minimum, this may include the location of school, work, and home. If you think about this more deeply, it may include multiple locations within a one-hour time such as a place in a room where you meditate, the inside of your car while driving, the bagel store you stopped in for breakfast, and then attending your child's school during a teacher's conferences, etc.

Depending on the number and types of locations, these other five facets are necessary to understand the complexity and uniqueness of each person's story. For example, each location has specific non-human objects associated with it (physical), a unique set of norms (cultural), groups of people (social), time spent to create habits and role identification (temporal), and technological capabilities (virtual).

Reflect on the example of a young child going to camp (location). What immediate questions about the facets of the environment come to mind? What is available at the camp in terms of toys, games, books, tables, or chairs (physical environment)? Are there computers and capability for additional online learning activities (virtual environment)? Whom does the camper hang out with during lunch or the day? Does he or she have many groups of friends or one close friend (social environment)? What are the expectations regarding such issues as attendance? How much participation is required during camp activities? Is there a specific dress code (cultural environment)? Is the child brand new to the camp or a returning camper (temporal environment)?

A person's story differs from the occupational therapists' worldviews, so it is important to understand these environmental facets more fully, or not assume everyone shares the same experiences or perceptions. One of the most fascinating roles of a practitioner is to learn how others make meaning of their world based on life experience. Let's explore another example of a person's story that you may be less familiar with.

Riley identifies as a man who is thirty years old and describes one of his occupations as a sex worker during the occupational profile. When reflecting on Riley's lived experience of sex work, some questions that come to mind include: Where are these sexual acts performed? Does Riley work from certain street corners and alleys, in cars, in specific hotels, or the airport (potential locations)? What does Riley use to prevent dangerous situations with aggressive customers (i.e., knife or iron pipe) or contracting a sexually transmitted disease (i.e., using a condom) (physical environment)? How does he collect money for these services? How much does he charge for services, and how much does he keep for himself or split with a pimp or support person (cultural environment)? Does he work alone or with other sex workers (social environment)? How long and how often has he been doing this job, and does he have long-standing customers (temporal environment)? How does he know where and when to meet a customer? Is there a phone number or website? Is there a special phone number to call or a panic button to press if problems are encountered (virtual environment)?

TRY IT: How Does a Practitioner Ask Questions About a Person's Environment During the Occupational Profile?

Learning more about the various facets of a person's environment is based on observations and/or asking questions during the occupational profile. Be mindful of your verbal and non-verbal communication while asking these questions.

Review Riley's situation more closely.

What information do you need to be more familiar with prior to the occupational profile (e.g., clarification of commonly used sex worker labels, research on the lived experiences of sex workers)?

What questions would you specifically ask Riley to learn more about each specific environmental facet of his life story?

How do you incorporate therapeutic use of self to ask these questions in a safe, non-judgmental way using language that is understandable to Riley?

Physical Environment: The Most Important Non-Human Objects Relevant to a Person's Life Story

Physical environment refers to any non-human objects present in a specific location (Knis-Matthews et al., 2017). To demonstrate this point, consider all the non-human objects that are present in a location such as the stadium of a football game, during a museum tour, or while sitting on a bench in the park. While there are hundreds and thousands of objects in a person's non-human environment, the job of the practitioner is to uncover the most significant human or non-living objects related to each person's story. Some examples include a car, child's toy, a piece of adaptive equipment, pots and pans, or a dollar bill.

It is necessary to observe a person's physical environment because these objects can be manipulated for more complexity or simplification in a person's lifestyle. For example, a practitioner can remove a small rug in the kitchen to prevent a person from falling while cooking a meal or simplify steps by reorganizing a person's medication from multiple individual bottles into a larger pill box organizer.

An object in the physical environment may be a dominating factor that contributes to a person's independence or dependence. For example, the number of stairs leading into a person's apartment can determine how much assistance is needed in terms of recommended adaptive equipment or even the addition of a new structure such as a ramp. Fortunately, practitioners are masterful at adapting the non-human environment.

While the previous examples might be more familiar to illustrate a person's physical environment, now I encourage you to reimagine the idea of this facet of the environment. For example, what supplies does a person need to sterilize their contaminated community water? What specific items does a person who travels 10 miles to the nearest grocery store carry while moving through the community? How do you adapt a surfboard for a person who has been surfing for twenty years but recently experienced a bilateral knee amputation?

In our earlier example, Reilly, who was working as a sex worker, might be concerned with items such as a cell phone, condoms, or a knife as part of his necessary non-human environment. Upon closer analysis, most of the items in his physical environment are necessary to keep him safe. These items are central to his life story and must be understood in proper context.

Temporal Environment: How the Person's Story Is Set in Time

Time. What an interesting, deep, and influential construct to our daily lives. Can you relate to any of these following statements or questions? There are just not enough hours in the day. I have too much time on my hands, and I am bored. Just let me sleep five more minutes. Are we there yet? Are you the oldest child in the family? How many more days until the semester ends? How long will this drought last? Is this your first hospitalization? How old are you? I have been a practitioner for the last thirty years. This is my first job and I feel very unsure of myself. There are popular slogans related to this construct such as time is money, absence makes the heart grow fonder, time flies when you are having fun, and a watched pot never boils. All of these statements relate to some aspect of a person's temporal environment.

Temporal information offers insights into the person's unique life story in terms of time (Knis-Matthews et al., 2017). During the data gathering process, practitioners use information obtained about the person in connection to the time construct. For example, the age of the person helps to determine what evaluations should be selected or how to approach the person during the initial meeting. Look for temporal clues in specific words used to describe a person served such as *recently* discharged, *first* hospitalization, *multiple* overdoses, *chronic* arthritis, *newly* diagnosed, *long*-term goal and/or *short*-term goal. A person who is *recently participating or admitted* to a treatment program or hospital is often not aware of the norms or social groups. While transitioning into new locations and situations may be a positive experience, such as starting a new job or the birth of a child, it can still create increased stress levels. As a result, stress (positive or negative) may occur that impacts a person's learning, active participation, and comfort level.

From a healthcare perspective, people who remain in a location for longer time periods tend to be more comfortable with forming social groups and the predictability of rules and expectations. In contrast, people who remain in a location over a shorter time tend to be in a heightened state of anxiety and chaos until the surroundings become more familiar. Reflect on how this aspect of time may influence occupational therapy services with an example of a long-term or short-term hospitalization.

It is important for practitioners to strategically plan a different approach if they are working with a person for only two days before discharge as opposed to one year. People served in short-term hospitalizations are learning about the current location and preparing for discharge to the next location at the same time. Practitioners in both types of locations begin with explaining the meaning of services and more details about the evaluation process to the person served.

However, the practitioner working with a person served in a long-term program has more time to slow down this process with repeated explanations and demonstrations. Meanwhile the practitioner working with a person served in a short-term stay explains the expectations of the current and future locations to the person served. The practitioner quickly begins preparing the person for the next placement or location upon discharge such as a Veterans Administration (VA) hospital, returning to work/employment, skilled nursing facility, outpatient clinic, home alone, etc.

Case Example: Fatima

Fatima was recently released from prison after serving five years for aggravated assault and robbery. The practitioner's task was to prepare her for an upcoming job interview as a gas station attendant. During the initial meetings, the practitioner noticed that she did not make any eye contact or smile. After much rapport building and trust, Fatima stated that making eye contact felt unnatural to her because it was safer to look down or avoid a person's eyes while in prison. Direct eye contact was viewed as a potential challenge or sign of aggression toward other inmates or prison guards.

During her time in prison, Fatima received inadequate dental care and one front tooth was missing while others appeared blackened. She learned to compensate when talking by not showing her teeth to others but was not comfortable smiling confidently. From a temporal perspective, it appeared that over the five years in jail, Fatima created habits consistent with the role of a prisoner. While Fatima was planning to be released from jail and reenter the workforce, it was not easy to demonstrate the roles and habits expected from one location to the next. As a gas station attendant, she was expected to demonstrate such skills as smiling at customers, making eye contact during transactions, and engaging in small talk with co-workers during break periods. Reinforcing these skills in the context of the gas station became the cornerstone of services relevant to Fatima's story.

Social Environment: The People, Groups, or Organizations a Person Feels More Connected To

---

Voices of the Practitioners: Considering the Environmental Factors During Evaluation and Intervention

During the evaluation I want to know more about the social environment. Who is the support system? Where do they live? All of these factors play a role in the plan. (Pam)

I work with families from many different cultural and socioeconomic backgrounds. Our clinical reasoning has to be flexible because it's not always going to fit with my perspective of the family structure. (Rebecca)

I remember during my fieldwork in an outpatient setting, this man had many children from different relationships and we'd always talk about them. It brought him so much joy so I asked him to bring in his kids. I did a session with him and the kids. They got to see what dad was doing and help us out. (Casey)

The social environment consists of people, groups, communities, organizations, and populations that people feel a sense of belonging to, identify with, or have frequent contact with (Knis-Matthews et al., 2017). Think about the numerous social groups to which a person might feel connected. Perhaps it is immediate family members? A sense of security as part of a support group for children diagnosed with special needs? A person identifies with the values and goals of a political party? A connectedness to a larger cause such as the Black Lives Matter movement? Perhaps it is an organization such as people in a religious association?

Social groups are vast and constantly changing. For example, OT students might say that their social groups are currently in transition. They might be identifying with and spending most of their time with peers in the occupational therapy academic program. There may be smaller social groups such as carpools and study groups that ultimately connect to a larger social group such as the occupational therapy profession. Due to current circumstances the social group may be changing since school began, as they spend less time with non-OT friends and family.

At times, a person's choice of social groups may not align with our society's accepted norms and values, creating further stigma. However, it is a complicated process to leave a social group that has created a sense of belonging and security, even if this group is viewed negatively in our society. For example, a friend who was trying to quit smoking felt that she had to stop going outside to the smoking area during breaks at work. On the other hand, she was sad to stop seeing the friends she had created over time who also smoked during breaks.

Social groups can also support or detract from a person's goal achievement. Knis-Matthews (2010) conducted a qualitative study exploring the experiences of parents who were substance dependent and seeking treatment in a long-term drug treatment program. Upon investigation, these parents identified more comfortably with social groups such as drug dealers and friends who were actively using drugs rather than with their children or other adults who were sober. While some of the parents who were sober wanted to change their social groups, they describe much discomfort in the change process due to lack of knowledge and skills.

As practitioners, it is not our place to judge, but to understand the person's story. Social groups change as a person's locations change. For example, consider two people, Colin and Juan, who are in treatment for an opioid addiction and have not actively used drugs for the past few months. Both are getting ready to leave the drug addiction program where most of their social group were peers who were trying to remain drug free. There is unity in larger numbers of people who identify toward a common goal.

Upon discharge, Juan changes location and now attends a Narcotics Anonymous (NA) support group on a daily basis. He has a sponsor and begins spending more time with other people in recovery by participating in activities such as bowling, watching movies, or going out to eat. Juan is surrounding himself with groups of people in sobriety who participate in activities to promote this.

Meanwhile Colin also leaves the location of the addiction program, returns home, and chooses not to participate in additional programming. He begins seeing old friends from the days that he actively used opioids. At first, he is cautious when spending time with his old friends who are still using drugs and consistently declines opioids offered to him. This group of friends do not go to NA meetings, but instead frequent a local bar where drugs are easily accessible. Over time, Colin relapses and begins using opioids with his group of friends.

Cultural Environment: The Rules and Expectations of the Social Groups

Many social groups unify around the expectations of customs, ideals, values, and thoughts. These expectations form the foundations of their worldviews that shape subsequent beliefs and behaviors (Knis-Matthews et al., 2017). Broader organizational systems can influence the cultural expectations. For example, patients in a hospital setting are often told the time to eat meals, attend therapy, or how many people can visit in one day.

Social groups formed within different locations have specific formal and/or informal rules and expectations. For example, think more deeply about the cultural environment of a classroom in the Western world. Students are expected to raise their hands rather than call out an answer to a question or remain seated at a desk until the teacher grants permission to move around the classroom. Meanwhile these school rules differ when the location changes such as moving from the classroom into outdoor recess. Students are now able to physically run and play together; rather than raising their hands, students may shout out a greeting to a peer without consequence. Report cards typically have a section regarding behaviors that formally signal the child's ability to follow school expectations and cultural norms.

Other times a smaller group of individuals set the cultural expectations for the larger social group to follow. For example, a gang, characterized as a social group of street-oriented children, adolescents, or young adults engaging in illegal activities, has very specific cultural expectations for membership (Tonks & Stephenson, 2019). These rules vary depending on the gang, membership, and status of each member. New members follow street code by demonstrating violence toward others or wearing certain types of clothes with gang-related symbols (Lenzi et al., 2014; Macfarlane, 2019; Pyrooz & Sweeten, 2015; Tonks & Stephenson, 2019).

When entering a new location or situation, people often initially inquire about the cultural environment and expectations. Think about a person starting a new job. What are some commonly asked questions? What are the hours? How long is the lunch break? What is the chain of command? What are the paperwork procedures and timelines? The answers to these questions provide information about the rules and expectations of this new location.

People tend to feel more comfortable entering a new location or situation when they are more familiar with the expectations. However, understanding the cultural environment of a new location or situation is often assumed and not fully explained to others, which may lead to confusion, anxiety, and frustration. For example, Cecelia experienced a rocky transition when she was recently admitted into a temporary shelter. The staff described Cecelia as malodorous and disorganized with her personal belongings. During the occupational profile, it was learned that Cecelia felt safer carrying all of her belongings with her at all times for fear of people stealing her stuff. Cecelia also stated that she only took showers when it appeared safe. Meanwhile the group home staff expected all members to shower daily, wear clean clothes, and keep extra personal belongings in their room shared with a roommate. These cultural expectations were not explicitly discussed upon acceptance into the shelter, but Cecelia was "just expected" to know this and have the skill set to do so.

Virtual Environment: Technologies Used to Enhance a Person's Occupations

The virtual environment highlights the opportunities for productive communication with others using such technology as email, telehealth, and computers (Knis-Matthews et al., 2017). From an occupational therapy perspective, the use of technology creates opportunities for individuals to participate in their occupations. While the use of technology has advanced tremendously in our society, the consequences of the 2020 COVID-19 pandemic placed a new spotlight on the virtual environment. Now people are using technology to connect with family and/or friends, attend school, go on dates, communicate with co-workers, pay bills, or buy groceries.

During the 2020 pandemic many occupational therapy practitioners educated clients, family members, and support staff in the use of virtual technologies like video call and conferencing applications for smartphones or computers. In skilled nursing facilities and other residential settings for older adults, virtual technology became the only way to keep residents in touch with their family and friends when visitation was eliminated to stop the spread of infection. Occupational therapy practitioners helped clients learn to use the technology and educated paraprofessional staff in adaptations that could help people overcome cognitive, perceptual, or physical conditions to successfully use the virtual technology. Students from many OT programs met clients individually and in groups over the Internet.

Another important way in which people use virtual environments is gaming. Children and adults play a wide variety of games on different virtual platforms. Many teens stayed connected with their friends by playing together, whether they were across the street or across the country from people sharing the game. Families got together over thousands of miles to experience new holiday activities like Zoom Hanukkah Bingo. Mainstream gaming companies are now adapting programs and controllers for people with disabilities, recognizing the social and emotional benefits of video games for people of all ages (Bailey, 2019; Oculus, 2020).

How Does the Environment Contribute to a Person's Perception of Self?
A-HA Moment

James P. Spradley (1970) conducted an ethnographic study in the late 1960s to uncover the lived experiences of men jailed for public drunkenness. Due to multiple arrests and extended jail time, these men eventually perceived themselves with a negative stereotype of being a bum or reject, because they were unable to follow society's cultural norms and expectations. Once the men began perceiving themselves in this negative way, their actions followed. Spradley described this transformation process as an identity vacuum as the men began shedding their acceptable roles for newly acquired, nonacceptable societal roles (Knis-Matthews, 2010).

Upon reflecting on this study from the MMCR perspective, it appears the environment plays an influential role in the formation of identity vacuums. For example, during this transformation the prolonged (temporal) time spent in jail (location) created new subgroups for these men to feel a sense of connectedness (social) while beginning to follow the rules and norms of jail (culture).

How many people served are in an identity vacuum to varying degrees? A person who is chronically ill and spends most time with doctor appointments. A child who is labeled with special needs and told they cannot join certain activities. A person receiving disability benefits and no longer is able to work to sustain these benefits.

Summary

Considering a person's environment has always been an important part of the occupational therapy framework, the MMCR highlights six specific facets (location, physical, temporal, social, cultural, and virtual) of a person's environment to consider during the evaluation and intervention process. This deeper understanding of a person's environment first begins with identification of the sites and places where the occupations occur (locations). Each location has specific non-human or non-living objects (physical); perspectives related to time (temporal); groups of people, communities, organizations, and populations (social); expectations of customs, ideals, and values (cultural); and technology to carry out those occupations (virtual). Each of these five facets may have equal importance to a person's story, or specific ones may be more dominant at times. However, all six environmental facets together provide a deeper understanding of the person's story.

References

Allen, C. K. (1985). Cognitive levels. In C. K. Allen (Ed.), *Occupational therapy for psychiatric diseases: Measurement and management of cognitive disabilities* (pp. 31–78). Brown & Company.

American Occupational Therapy Association. (1994). Uniform terminology for occupational therapy—third edition. *American Journal of Occupational Therapy, 48,* 1047–1054. https://doi.org/10.5014/ajot.48.11.1047

American Occupational Therapy Association. (2002). Occupational therapy practice framework: Domain and process. *American Journal of Occupational Therapy, 56,* 609–639. https://doi.org/10.5014/ajot.56.6.609

Bailey, J. M. (2019, February 20). Adaptive video game controllers open worlds for gamers with disabilities. *New York Times.* www.nytimes.com/2019/02/20/business/video-game-controllers-disabilities.html

Baum, C. M., Christiansen, C. H., & Bass, J. D. (2015). The person-environment-occupation performance (PEOP) model. In C. M. Baum, C. H. Christiansen, & J. Bass-Haugen (Eds.), *Occupational therapy: Performance, participation and well-being* (4th ed., pp. 49–55). Slack.

Iwama, M. (2006). *The Kawa model: Culturally relevant occupational therapy.* Elsevier.

Knis-Matthews, L. (2010). The destructive path of addiction: Experiences of six parents who are substance dependent. *Occupational Therapy in Mental Health, 26*(3), 201–340. https://doi.org/10.1080/0164212X.2010.498728

Knis-Matthews, L., Mulry, C. M., & Richards, L. (2017). Matthews model of clinical reasoning: A systematic approach to conceptualize evaluation and intervention. *Occupational Therapy in Mental Health, 33*(4), 360–373. https://doi.org/10.1080/0164212X.2017.1303658

Lenzi, M., Sharkey, J., Vieno, A., Mayworm, A., Dougherty, D., & Nylund-Gibson, K. (2014). Adolescent gang involvement: The role of individual, family, peer, and school factors in a multilevel perspective. *Aggressive Behavior, 41*(4). https://doi.org/10.1002/ab.21562

Macfarlane, A. (2019). Gangs and adolescent mental health: A narrative review. *Journal of Child & Adolescent Trauma, 12*(3), 411–420. https://doi.org/10.1007/s40653-018-0231-y

Oculus, V. R. (2020, November 11). Introducing the accessibility VRCs. *Oculus for Developers.* https://developer.oculus.com/blog/introducing-the-accessibility-vrcs/

Pyrooz, D. C., & Sweeten, G. (2015). Gang membership between ages 5 and 17 years in the United States. *Journal of Adolescent Health, 56*(4), 1–6. https://dx.doi.org/10.1016/j.jadohealth.2014.11.018

Schkade, J., & McClung, M. (2001). *Occupational adaptation in practice.* Slack.

Spradley, J. P. (1970). *You owe yourself a drunk: An ethnography of urban nomads* (Rev. ed.). Waveland Press.

Taylor, R. R. (2017). *Kielhofner's model of human occupation* (5th ed.). Wolters Kluwer.

Tonks, S., & Stephenson, Z. (2019). Disengagement from street gangs: A systematic review of the literature. *Psychiatry, Psychology, and Law, 26*(1), 21–49. https://dx.doi.org/10.1080/13218719.2018.1482574

5 Compartmentalizing Evaluation Information to Understand How Activities and Occupations Relate to a Person's Story

Laurie Knis-Matthews and Margaret Swarbrick

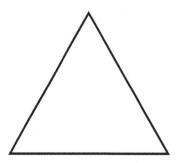

Figure 5.1

Occupations
Activities

Voices of the Practitioners: Understanding and Using Occupations During the Evaluation and Intervention Approach

I know there are protocols for different injuries, and in some professions this makes sense because you are working on a muscle or endurance deficit. However, it doesn't make sense in occupational therapy until you tie it to the person's occupation because otherwise why are you doing it? (Julie)

True OT is using occupations. If you're not going to use an occupation as an end goal, you're not an OT. (Morgan)

How Activities and Occupations Are Conceptualized Within MMCR

Throughout the literature, the constructs of activity and occupation often appear in different combinations with slightly different meanings based on the authors and time it was published (AOTA, 2020; Bauerschmidt & Nelson, 2011; Golledge, 1998; Pierce, 2001; Polatajko et al., 2004). The MMCR describes activities and occupations in two distinct manners: first as a construct to help

DOI: 10.4324/9781003392408-6

further understand a person's life story during the evaluation process and then as a way to help guide effective interventions. *There is more detailed information about occupation-based intervention in the next section of the book.*

As previously mentioned, during the evaluation process, practitioners begin formulating a general understanding of the person's life story by gathering information about relevant activities. When the practitioner collaborates with the person served, they gather information using the occupational profile by exploring, clarifying and restating information to gain a full understanding of relevant activities and occupations.

Take a step back and first explore how these constructs shape an understanding of a person's story during the evaluation process. Following Pierce's perspective (2001), this begins with a review of the basic understanding of activity and occupation (Figure 5.2). According to Pierce (2001), there are clear distinctions in subjectivity, context and value between the two constructs.

Activities

Activities are viewed as a general idea held in the minds of a culture or society (Pierce, 2001). These general and broad descriptions make it easier for people to visualize and talk about activities within a shared society. A person does not need to engage in the activity to discuss it with others. For example, hiking, painting a mural or riding a horse are activities that most people can visualize and discuss without having experienced it. As a starting point to understand a person's story, activities provide a common idea in terms of physical context, timing, value, and feelings (Pierce, 2001).

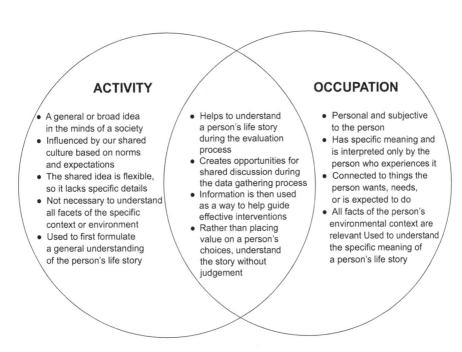

Figure 5.2 Similarities and differences between activities and occupations.

In terms of activity, such characteristics immediately come to mind:

It is a general idea.
It is a collective idea in the minds of a society based on norms and expectations.
There is flexibility in the shared idea so it lacks specific details.
This general meaning is influenced by our shared culture.
Culture and society influence our perception of the right or wrong way to do something.
It is not necessary to understand all facets of the specific context or environment.

Following the MMCR, the practitioner gathers initial information about general activities that are *meaningful* to the person. They will not spend time discussing the activity of scuba diving if the person has no interest or desire to pursue this activity. However, if scuba diving is relevant to the person, then the practitioner would begin a conversation or learn more about the sport of scuba diving. These preliminary discussions will provide the practitioner with a general awareness before asking specific questions of how it relates to the individual person's experiences.

Occupations

According to Pierce (2001), learning about the specific person is central to understanding their occupations. Understanding the meaning, distinct value, and emotional connection of an occupation can only be told from their perspective. Explore all facets of the environment (location, physical, temporal, cultural, social and virtual) to gather further context about the person's occupations.

To further expand on Pierce's view, let's return to additional explanations of occupation. In a position paper on human displacement, the World Federation of Occupational Therapy (WFOT) (2012) describes how, in part, occupational therapists' responsibility is to work with people to participate in occupations that they want, need or are expected to do. As a profession, we tend to focus our emphasis on occupations that people want to do. It is a very positive perspective as we use the terms chosen, valued and meaningful occupations. However, in reality, many people engage in occupations because it is necessary for survival or expected by others rather than chosen.

Hammell (2017) further develops this idea as she states that occupations are not always positive and based on personal choice, but instead can be illegal, demeaning or even jeopardize a person's health status. Hammell (2017) proposes the future of occupational therapy lies in viewing occupational engagement as central to human's well-being, which is a human right. These human rights can be basic such as having clean water, adequate food, and proper shelter. Well-being also refers to a person's connectedness with others, belonging and value. She states that doing occupations with other people provides the foundation for relationship building, decreases stressful life experiences and provides value to the person's sense of self.

In terms of these worldviews, such characteristics of occupations come to mind:

It is personal and has specific meaning to a person.
It is connected to things the person wants, needs or is expected to do
It is subjective and interpreted only by the person who experiences it.
There is an attached emotional connection for the person.
It is embedded in all facets of the environmental context.
There is a beginning and an ending.
It can be completed alone or with others.

TRY IT: Looking at Occupation With a Different Lens

Imagine you are working with Tammy who is a fifty-year-old woman living with her seventy-year-old mother in a two-bedroom apartment. Tammy identifies her mother as her best friend and confidant. Despite Tammy's identified interests such as walking for exercise, watching old movies and painting, she is hesitant to leave the apartment and pursue these interests in order to remain at home with her mother.

What specific questions can you ask Tammy to learn more about her *occupations* related to this story of what she wants, needs or is expected to do?

How might this situation be viewed by others in our society?

How does the practitioner understand Tammy's occupations more fully, emphasizing her well-being over societal stigma?

Voices of the Practitioners: Learning About a Person's Occupations During the Evaluation

During the evaluation I am talking to them about occupations that they love or what they want or need to do. Based on this information, this challenges me as a practitioner to be more creative with the intervention plan. It's not easy, but it also shouldn't be. (Rose)

When I'm first getting to know a person, I write down those big idea concepts on my card that I keep with me. I have a section for what their biggest deficit areas are and what their occupations are. My treatment plans are to merge those two categories. (Rose).

How Activities and Occupations Are Used Together to Understand a Person's Story

Each classification provides different but useful information to learn more about the person's story. During the evaluation process, the practitioner gathers information about both a person's activities and occupations. Casting a wide net, the practitioner strategically begins with a general understanding of the activities relevant to a person's story. This provides a common language, general understanding and creates a collective perception of these activities between the practitioner and person served. Activities are necessary, because they provide a general guide for the practitioner to discuss and understand an individual's story.

Once this wide net of information is collected, the practitioner, using the art of practice, begins exploring those most important general activities using open-ended questions, probing, clarifying and restating pertinent information. Understanding the most relevant, meaningful and specific details about the person's story transitions into learning more about a person's occupations.

To explain activity and occupation further, imagine a family eating breakfast together in the Western world. What do you visualize? Children seated in chairs around a kitchen table eating eggs, toast, cereal, juice or coffee during the early morning hours. An adult is standing at the stove, cooking bacon and eggs, using a large frying pan. The smell of the fresh brewed coffee that is about to be poured in a coffee mug. The family members may be dressed in their pajamas while eating at the table and are talking about their plans for the day.

While your image may be slightly different, the general idea of these activities is somewhat flexible to understand this point. Activities help to paint a collective image in our minds so we can follow the story based on the typical culture and norms in our society. While this information is extremely helpful to begin learning about a person's story, it falls short of understanding their occupations.

To gather occupation-based information about a specific person eating breakfast, the occupational therapy practitioner might ask some follow-up questions:

Tell me what you usually eat and drink for breakfast? Who prepares this meal?
Whom specifically do you eat breakfast with?
What time do you usually eat breakfast and for how long?
What are some of the specific topics of conservation discussed at the kitchen table?

These questions only scratch the surface of this personal experience, but it helps to illustrate how a simple activity such as eating breakfast is understood from an activity or occupation perspective.

Activities and Occupations Are Both Necessary to the Evaluation Process: A-HA Moment

Occupational profiles or top-oriented evaluations are intended to learn more about the specific details of the person's life story. In turn, this information guides the practitioner to learn more about the person's occupations and move past a general idea of activities. As a result, intervention focusing on the person's well-being will become more meaningful and occupational based. Without gathering knowledge about a person's occupation in his or her unique facets of environment, interventions will become more disconnected, less relevant and less functional.

This basic understanding of a person's relevant activities is important to uncover during the initial gathering process and serves as a starting point of conversation during the occupational profile. It is necessary for practitioners to ask specific probing questions to more deeply understand the context, value and subjectivity of how/which of these activities would be considered occupations.

Value Judgements May Cloud an Understanding of a Person's Activity and Occupational Choices

As previously mentioned, activities are deeply connected to our cultural expectations. Our society holds some activities in higher regard, thus influencing others to favor these views over a person's personal choices. For example, from a societal perspective, paid work is highly valued, but the specific paid job of prostitution is viewed as negative.

While the general and flexible characteristics of activities create opportunities for shared discussions during the data gathering process, the practitioners must be cautious of placing value on a person's activity and occupational choices. Labeling a person's choices as desirable or undesirable can ultimately influence how practitioners perceive a person's activities and occupations. Rather than listening to the person's story, this may lead to a practitioner immediately beginning to formulate judgements while gathering information about the person's general activities.

Reflect on the general activities associated with a person who is homeless. Perhaps this image is connected to a person who spends the day looking for food in dumpsters or garbage cans, constantly asks bystanders for extra money, carries all of their belongings with them and sleeps in an alley or under a bridge. This might not be a desirable image. Would you be surprised to learn, upon deeper discussion, that each person who is homeless does not describe a similar picture as stated here? Instead, a person may be part of a family unit and living in a long-term shelter. They are part of a larger community at the shelter and spend their days searching for a paid job while their children attend public school. Yet another person who is identified as homeless might be sleeping on their best friend's couch at night and spend their days completing the necessary paperwork to secure government benefits. There are no black and white explanations to people's life experiences, but it is all a gray area. It is necessary for the practitioner to move beyond common labels and stereotypes to uncover a person's occupations related to what they want, need or are expected to do.

Take the Time and Learn the Specifics About Each Person's Occupations

There are numerous obstacles contributing to why practitioners do not fully explore a person's occupations such as reimbursement issues, limited time, scarce resources, productivity expectations, length of stay, intervention environments that encourage a reductionist approach and negative perceptions of colleagues to exploring a person's occupations (Colaianni & Provident, 2010; Di Tommaso et al., 2016; Eschenfelder, 2005; Estes & Pierce, 2012; Grice, 2015; Nayar et al., 2013; Wong & Fisher, 2015). Without additional inquiry into a person's occupations, practitioners can easily fall into the trap of determining intervention priorities without the valuable and essential input from the person served. How can the person benefit if the practitioner sets the priorities? If the person does not see the value, the intervention may not be successful and no one benefits.

For example, dressing is often a common activity emphasized in an adult rehabilitation practice area. It is common for a practitioner to conclude that each person needs to get dressed in order to "go somewhere", so it is emphasized during intervention. The practitioner must then take this information to probe, clarify and question how these general ideas of dressing activities are understood and performed, in context, to advance a person's well-being. Does the person have a specific uniform to wear? A specific type and style of shoe? Need to quickly and efficiently change clothes moving from one event to another? Have a favorite outfit? Is it personal and has a specific meaning to a person?

Summary

Learning more about a person's activities and occupations is a necessary part of the evaluation process and subsequently sets the stage for an occupational-based intervention plan. During the occupational profile, practitioners first begin formulating a general understanding of the person's story by asking about activities that are purposeful, necessary and meaningful. Activities are broad descriptions that allow for common understanding between people in a general culture or society. Within the occupational therapy evaluation process, these activities provide a starting point for discussion and further collaboration during the therapeutic process. Once a general understanding of the person's activities is identified, the practitioner then begins asking more probing and clarifying questions to determine which of those activities reach the level of occupation. Occupations are best described directly from the persons served to understand the unique meaning, distinct value and emotional connection central to their human rights.

References

American Occupational Therapy Association. (2020). Occupational therapy practice framework: Domain and process (4th ed.). *American Journal of Occupational Therapy*, *74*(Suppl. 2), 7412410010. https://doi.org/10.5014/ajot.2020.74S2001

Bauerschmidt, B., & Nelson, D. L. (2011). The terms occupation and activity over the history of official occupational therapy publications. *American Journal of Occupational Therapy*, *65*(3), 338–345. https://doi.org/10.5014/ajot.2011.000869

Colaianni, D., & Provident, I. (2010). The benefits and challenges to the use of occupation in hand therapy. *Occupational Therapy in Health Care*, *24*(2), 130–146. https://doi.org/10.3109/07380570903349378

Di Tommaso, A., Isbel, S., Scarvell, J., & Wicks, A. (2016). Occupational therapists' perceptions of occupation in practice: An exploratory study. *Australian Occupational Therapy Journal*, *63*(3), 206–213. https://doi.org/10.1111/1440-1630.12289

Eschenfelder, V. (2005). Shaping the goal setting process in OT: The role of meaningful occupation. *Physical & Occupational Therapy in Geriatrics*, *23*(4), 67–81. https://doi.org/10.1080/J148v23n04_05

Estes, J., & Pierce, D. E. (2012). Pediatric therapists' perspectives on occupation-based practice. *Scandinavian Journal of Occupational Therapy*, *19*(1), 17–25. https://doi.org/10.3109/11038128.2010.547598

Golledge, J. (1998). Distinguishing between occupation, purposeful activity and activity, part 1: Review and explanation. *British Journal of Occupational Therapy*, *61*(3), 100–105. https://doi.org/10.1177/030802269806100301

Grice, K. O. (2015). The use of occupation-based assessments and intervention in the hand therapy setting—a survey. *Journal of Hand Therapy*, *28*(3), 300–306. https://doi.org/10.1016/j.jht.2015.01.005

Hammell, K. W. (2017). Opportunities for well-being: The right to occupational engagement. *Canadian Journal of Occupational Therapy*, *84*(4–5), 209–222. https://doi.org/10.117/0008417417734831

Nayar, S., Gray, M., & Blijlevens, H. (2013). The competency of New Zealand new graduate occupational therapists: Perceived strengths and weaknesses. *Australian Occupational Therapy Journal*, *60*(3), 189–196. https://doi.org/10.1111/1440-1630.12027

Pierce, D. (2001). Untangling occupation and activity. *American Journal of Occupational Therapy*, *55*, 138–146. https://doi.org/10.5014/ajot.55.2.138

Polatajko, H. J., Davis, J. A., Hobson, S. J. G., Landry, J. E., Mandich, A., Street, S. L., Whippey, E., & Yee, S. (2004). Meeting the responsibility that comes with the privilege: Introducing a taxonomic code for understanding occupation. *Canadian Journal of Occupational Therapy*, *71*(5), 261–268. https://doi.org/10.1177/000841740407100503

Wong, S. R., & Fisher, G. (2015). Comparing and using occupation-focused models. *Occupational Therapy in Health Care*, *29*(3), 297–315. http://doi.org/10.3109/07380577.2015.1010130

World Federation of Occupational Therapists. (2012). *Position paper: Human displacement*. http:/www.wfot.org/ResourceCentre.aspx

6 Putting It All Together to Identify Occupational Performance Issue(s)

Laurie Knis-Matthews and Margaret Swarbrick

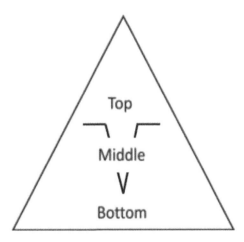

Figure 6.1 Visual representation of generic top-middle-bottom occupational performance issues.

Voices of the Practitioners: How to Determine the Occupational Performance Priority Issues

Sometimes my evaluation shows an immediate problem like a safety risk. I found out the person fell three times this month getting out of the shower. Am I going to spend my first day asking him to take a shirt and put it on? No. I am going to get him into the bathroom to figure out what is the situation and why is he falling. (Pam)

When I worked in acute care, I had to check in with nursing because you wanted to make sure that everything was copasetic. Something could have happened the night before that I should be aware of first. So I always checked in with the staff and then I did my occupational profile. (Abigail)

During the evaluation findings we gather top and bottom information to make the goals. I still think of those steps and I can picture that part of the OTPF. That part of the OT process where I decide on those client factors and connect it to the top part. (Julie)

We are looking at so many things related to the person, environment and occupation to get to occupational performance. Taking all this information determines a person's occupational success and occupational validation. (Morgan)

DOI: 10.4324/9781003392408-7

I like to emphasize function. Play is functional with kids, but we want to know what's getting in the way with play. Vision? Fine motor? I'm figuring it out most of the time from something the parent has repeated enough to me that this is what's clearly getting in the way. (Jackie)

I synthesize the individual information immediately and think about how it applies to the person's occupational performance. At the end of the day, I take the time to pull those components together, make more connections between different things that might be happening and how all those facts intertwine to impact the occupational performance. (Rose)

Understanding the Person's Story, Occupational Performance Issues and Eventual Intervention Priorities

Occupational performance issues are derived from the dynamic connection between the person, environmental context and occupations with relevant activities (AOTA, 2020; Baum et al., 2015; Knis-Matthews et al., 2017; Law et. al., 1996). In the MMCR, occupational performance issues are visualized as the center of the triangle using the labels top-middle-bottom to identify the most pressing part of the person's story relative to the occupational performance issues.

The MMCR Guide to Understanding a Person's Story (Triangle) in Appendix 1 provides a systematic way for practitioners to organize the specific information collected during the evaluation process. This is a messy process, as the information often crosses over all three constructs of person, environment and occupation and may not neatly fit into one section of the story. There is no definitive cookbook to this process, as the practitioner must decide how the information is organized and interpreted.

In the center of the triangle, there is a square root or letter V–looking symbol ($\sqrt{}$). In the MMCR, this ($\sqrt{}$), or occupational performance issue, symbolizes the first and then subsequent set of life changes that will eventually lead to an intervention plan. These configurations vary each time the practitioner begins the evaluation process with each new person served. The completed clinical reasoning guidesheet provides visual feedback about the person's story in order to consider/clarify what are the first most pressing top-middle-bottom occupational performance issues. The initial occupational performance issues are not set in stone, but it is a place to begin the process. If certain sections of this clinical reasoning guidesheet have minimal information or appear vague, then the practitioner should consider engaging with the person served using open-ended questions or using probes to deepen their understanding of the person's story.

The initial top-middle-bottom occupational performance issues eventually help shape intervention priorities. Fight the urge to immediately begin planning intervention to facilitate the change process. Before a practitioner can begin planning intervention, they must first understand the person's story, determine goals for change in collaboration with the person served, and determine what might be getting in the way. The intervention process is discussed in the following chapter.

What Does $\sqrt{}$ Symbolize and How Does It Relate to Occupational Performance? A-HA Moment

$\sqrt{}$ symbol reflects a person's specific occupational performance issues. It is determined from the person-environment-occupation information gathered during the evaluation process. A person's story might uncover multiple $\sqrt{}$ $\sqrt{}$ $\sqrt{}$ occupational performance issues that are necessary to the change process. However, this *first* $\sqrt{}$ occupational performance emphasizes the most pressing issue to be addressed in the person's life. This begins the transition into designing an intervention that matches the needs and desires of the person served.

Taking a Closer Look at Each Top-Middle-Bottom Occupational Performance Issue

Up into this point, three important constructs of person-environment-occupation that contribute to understanding a person's life story have been discussed. The practitioner has mentally shifted through the incoming evaluation data to compartmentalize the specific information around the constructs of person-environment-occupation. The next step is to analyze all the evaluation data, prioritizing which occupational performance issues contribute to formulating eventual intervention priorities. Occupational performance issues are derived from the dynamic connection between the person, environmental context and occupations with relevant activities (AOTA, 2020; Baum et al., 2015; Knis-Matthews et al., 2017; Law et al., 1996).

In the MMCR, occupational performance issues are visualized as the center of the triangle using the labels top-middle-bottom to identify the most pressing part of the person's story relative to the occupational performance issues. For example, reflect on an adolescent graduating from high school. For those entering high school, this goal might be a few years away, as there are hundreds of smaller accomplishments to be obtained along this journey. Other students are nearing the end of this multiyear journey, and their top goal is closer to achievement.

Occupational Performance Issue: Top

The top may be a goal accomplished in the long term or is an overarching goal within the bigger picture. How long does it take to accomplish a top or longer-term goal? Well, that depends. Putting parameters on the time it takes to achieve a top goal is tricky and needs further clarification to understand how this fits into the person's story. For example, some students' top goal of graduating high school is still many years away if they are entering the school as a freshman. Other students perceive graduating from high school as a top goal (see Figure 6.2 as an example) but are closer to achievement if they just successfully finished their final exams in senior year.

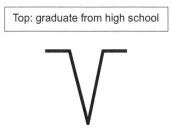

Figure 6.2 Visual representation of a student's top goal of graduating from high school as part of the occupational performance issue.

Occupational Performance Issue: Middle

The middle also represents a part of a person's occupational performance issues. Similar to the top, this information may come from an occupational profile or top evaluations that facilitate opportunities for practitioners to learn about the person's unique life story, occupations and environmental facets. While the top focuses on the longer term or big picture, the middle highlights those goals or accomplishments that can be achieved during a shorter period.

Let's return to the scenario of a student graduating from high school. Now if the top goal was just to graduate, then it might become frustrating, stressful or discouraging to continue working on this long-term goal without acknowledging those important but smaller accomplishments along the way. To illustrate this point, perhaps the student considers the ending of each marking period as an accomplishment? Or a sports season? An annual band concert? An art show? Spring break? A senior prom? While these smaller accomplishments will be different for each student, each goal (middle) provides smaller opportunities for accomplishment and reflection.

Following the MMCR, the middle is identified as these smaller goals or periodic accomplishments. The middle represents part of a person's occupational performance issues that are shorter-term plans, steppingstones or accomplishments that are achieved while working toward the ultimate top. These accomplishments or middles can serve as motivators and help the person work on smaller goals while working toward the top. In the MMCR, the middle is not a method to be used during the intervention approach to reach the top. Before moving toward an intervention approach, the practitioner must understand the person's story and how it relates together.

Back to the previous example, while all high school students are working toward an ultimate goal of graduating, each student is working on different middles, as some are trying to successfully finish a marking period, make a varsity sports team or prepare for potential colleges. In these diagrams that follow, review some potential middle examples representing different students who are graduating from high school (see Figure 6.3).

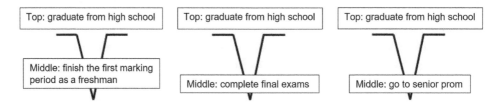

Figure 6.3 Visual representation of various middles of a person's occupational performance issue with a similar top being to graduate from high school.

The selection of tops and middle is complicated. There is no cookbook to follow, and it is different for each person served. For example, Mark wants to get a good paying job at a local box store (top) but first wants to develop a plan to consistently get a good night's sleep, so he is not late for work (middle). He is worried that if he cannot implement healthier sleep habits then he will be consistently late for work or tired while on the job. In this situation, Mark is able to identify his top and middle and provide a connection from one to the other.

In contrast to Mark's situation, it is unlikely that all people served will directly identify their top and middles during the occupational profile. At times, the person may discuss parts of their story during the evaluation process, but the area for change or importance is inferred by the practitioner. A person might have a longer-term plan but does not see those immediate goals to be addressed along the way. For example, Sonia dreams of opening up her own hair salon (top) but she is currently in danger of becoming evicted from her apartment for constantly disturbing her landlord at night. While Sonia has identified a long-term goal, she did not view the connection to how an eviction from her apartment will disrupt her lifestyle and longer-term goals. In this scenario, the practitioner made the connection and addressed the current issue or middle (see Figure 6.4).

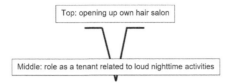

Figure 6.4 Visual representation of the person served identifying the top occupational performance issue while the practitioners identifies the middle.

Other times it is the opposite, as the person served can only identify immediate goals for the next day or week and is unable to examine the bigger picture. For example, Pedro is experiencing shortness of breath and a constant cough after a recent hospitalization due to COVID-19. His immediate goal is to continue picking up his daughter from school. While the practitioner may understand the larger picture of Pedro fulfilling his parental responsibilities, he is only concerned that his daughter returns home safe when she attends school (see Figure 6.5).

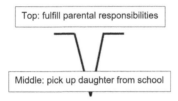

Figure 6.5 Visual representation of the person's immediate middle occupational performance issue when the practitioner views the bigger picture by identifying the top.

Identifying the top and middle can be confusing because it is in such a gray area; at times, the middle is determined by the practitioner and other times by the person served. In order to stay person-centered in this process, *either the top or middle (ideally both) must be based on the person's desire for performing the specific tasks or relearning the new skill to be successful in their occupational performance issues.* Without input from the person, then the motivation will not be a guiding factor during the intervention process, potentially leading toward intervention based on activities rather than occupation.

The practitioner collaborates with the person served to select the top or middle. For example, a person who identifies as homeless and lives in a car reports her most important issue is to find a safe place to park at night. The practitioner, respecting the person's goals, must help the person to problem-solve safe places to park during the nighttime hours with the location of her car and not use this as an opportunity to independently assume she wants to now stay in a temporary shelter (see Figure 6.6).

Occupational Performance Issue: Bottom

The bottom also represents part of a person's occupational performance issues. Bottom information typically comes from analysis of performance or bottom-oriented evaluations that facilitate opportunities for the practitioner to measure specific client factors and/or performance skills that

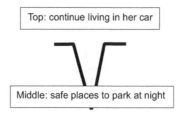

Figure 6.6 Visual representation of the practitioner identifying a middle occupational performance issue while respecting the person's wishes to continue living in her car.

may strengthen or hinder the person's top/middle. The practitioner typically selects the relevant bottom(s) and connects how it will align with the middle and top occupational performance issues.

Laypeople are often less familiar with the reasons why bottoms may impact their goals so there is more input from the practitioner. For example, it is not common for parents to identify how proprioception issues are impacting their child's ability to do jumping jacks during gym class. While administering numerous bottom-oriented evaluations during the evaluation process, the practitioner must prioritize which bottom(s) are most important to address at the start of the intervention process. Being transparent about this with the person served will be very important—especially discussing in lay terms the person understands.

Returning to our previous example of the high school student, perhaps after the pandemic, the student is returning to school but is struggling. Based on bottom evaluations, it is determined the student has high levels of stress, panic attacks during examinations, a shortened attention span for the length of typical classes and lacks the confidence to ask the instructor questions. All of these are potential bottoms that may impact the person's goal of being successful in school and eventually achieve their goal of graduating. However, from this extensive list of challenges, the practitioner might work with the student to select one or two challenges they think would be most important initially.

Note: A bottom is not a diagnosis such as hip replacement, cerebrovascular accident (CVA), traumatic brain injury, or schizophrenia. In the MMCR, diagnosis is viewed as part of a person's story (and should be placed under the Person construct) but not the sole emphasis of a person's story. This clinical reasoning can be followed, even in the medical model setting, where diagnosis is given much attention. Our domain of concern, the practice framework, does not highlight diagnosis first, nor do occupation-based practice models.

Additional examples of hypothetical tops, middles and bottoms:

A person who wants *to eventually get a part-time weekend job as a cashier at a grocery store* (top) but first needs to make decisions (bottom) to determine the best bus route to get there in the most efficient way (middle) (see Figure 6.7). In past attempts, she has been impulsive in her decision making and unsuccessfully tried to walk to work.

Note how specific the top information is. A cashier working in a grocery store is not the same position as working in the grocery store warehouse and requires a different skill set. The weekend hours might be busier than during the weekend daytime.

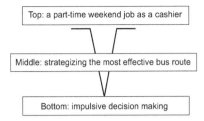

Figure 6.7 Visual representation of a person who needs to learn how to strategize the most effective bus route in order to get a part time job as a cashier.

A **caregiver** wants her daughter to eventually live in a group home as a young adult (top). The caregiver has collaborated with their daughter to initiate (bottom) brushing her teeth (middle) without asking for parental assistance (see Figure 6.8). The caregiver reports this will help her daughter be more independent when she moves into the group home.

Following her daughter's goals, the caregiver's first middle is for her daughter to brush her teeth without parental assistance. Over time, there will be many more middles to facilitate the eventual independence expected while living in a group home (top), but this middle was specifically identified as important to address first.

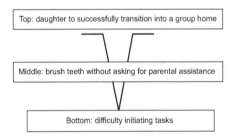

Figure 6.8 Visual representation of identifying the first middle occupational performance issue for the daughter to begin initiating tasks in order to transition into the group home.

A **father** whose daughter just had a baby and is excited to be a new grandfather (top) but due to left-sided upper body weakness (bottom), he is very nervous about holding this granddaughter (middle) (see Figure 6.9).

While the grandfather is excited about this new role, he was particularly nervous about holding his new granddaughter because of his upper body weakness. Holding an infant requires different positioning and movement of the body vs. other potential grandparent duties such as changing a diaper or feeding.

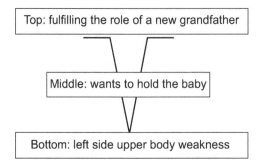

Figure 6.9 Visual representation of a grandfather new to this role who first wants to hold the new baby but has ongoing left-sided upper body weakness.

Understanding and Selecting the Top-Middle-Bottom Parts of Occupational Performance: A-HA Moment

The top-middle-bottom all contribute information necessary to prioritize the person's occupational performance issues.

The top or the middle uncover the person's specific interests and goals to identify where the change process may begin in both the long and short term.

Top: This information comes from a top or occupational profile type of evaluation. It is specific to the person's story, identifying the person's longer-term goals and specific interests. At times, the person served identifies the top, while other times it is determined by the practitioner.

Middle: This information also comes from a top-oriented evaluation tool or occupational profile. It is specific to the person's story, identifying the person's shorter-term goals or accomplishments that may be achieved before reaching the top.

Sometimes the top and/or middle information is not explicitly stated by the person served, but instead implicitly stated. The practitioner discusses this information with the person for more clarity and direction.

Bottom: This information comes from a bottom-oriented or analysis of performance type of evaluation. It is usually selected by the practitioner, in collaboration with the person, to identify what might be getting in the way of a person's goal achievement.

Top-middle-bottom does not need to align directly together in a neat package. This is where the practitioner uses clinical reasoning to understand the person's story and interpret how all the occupational performance parts relate together to the story.

Summary

After the practitioner mentally conceptualizes the information about the person, environment and occupation, now it is time to determine the initial top-middle-bottom intervention priorities. This first set of occupational performance issues will ultimately set the stage for the intervention plan. Derived from the occupational profile, the top and middle occupational performance issues highlight a part of a person's story, occupations and environment. While the top focuses on the longer term, overarching goals or big picture plan, the middle highlights those smaller and more immediate accomplishments or plans that can be achieved during a shorter period. The bottom also represents part of a person's occupational performance issues and typically comes from analysis of performance evaluation that measures specific client factors and/or performance skills.

References

American Occupational Therapy Association. (2020). Occupational therapy practice framework: Domain and process (4th ed.). *American Journal of Occupational Therapy*, *74*(Suppl. 2), 7412410010. https://doi.org/10.5014/ajot.2020.74S2001

Baum, C. M., Christiansen, C. H., & Bass, J. D. (2015). The person-environment-occupation performance (PEOP) model. In C. M. Baum, C. H. Christiansen, & J. Bass-Haugen (Eds.), *Occupational therapy: Performance, participation and well-being* (4th ed., pp. 49–55). Slack Incorporated.

Knis-Matthews, L., Mulry, C. M., & Richard, L. (2017). Matthews model of clinical reasoning: A systematic approach to conceptualize evaluation and intervention. *Occupational Therapy in Mental Health*, *33*(4), 360–373. http://doi.org/10.1080/0164212X.2017.1303658

Law, M., Cooper, B., Strong, S., Stewart, D., Rigby, P., & Letts, L. (1996). The person-environment-occupation model: A transactive approach to occupational performance. *Canadian Journal of Occupational Therapy*, *63*, 9–23. http://doi.org/10.1177/000841749606300103

Section 2

Intervention

7 MMCR Five-Step Guide to Infusing the Frame of Reference/Practice Model Into a Person's Story

Laurie Knis-Matthews and Lynne Richard

Voices of the Practitioners: Guidelines for Actions Influence the Evaluation and Intervention Plan

I have a good understanding of the different frames of references and practice models and am able to pick the ones that are a good fit. I lean towards certain ones because it just made sense for me. (Kristen)

It's an important question to ask students about this because the ability to identify a FOR and work through why you feel like that's the one that should be applied is the beginning of clinical reasoning. (Rose)

All I've learned about the frame of references helps guide my treatment . . . I'm applying what I've learned in the knowledge base to apply to my interventions. (Pam)

Many professionals use guidelines to assist in the decision-making process. For example, a person who is not feeling well might make an appointment to see a medical professional. After asking a series of questions and performing some tests, the professional will begin formulating a diagnosis and determine a plan of action such as prescribing a medication or recommending further testing. The medical professional identifies this course of treatment based on guidelines for action.

Occupational therapy is also a profession that follows guidelines for action. Practitioners utilize their clinical reasoning skills to strategically select evaluation tools, conduct interviews, and implement intervention plans unique to the person's life story and goals. In the occupational therapy profession, a frame of reference and/or practice model both serve under the umbrella term: guidelines for action. However, a frame of reference and practice model have differences in terms of scope, applicability to the person served, evaluation tool selection and intervention focus.

Occupational therapy students learn about frames of references and practice models early in their academic programs. This knowledge is often the focal point to their occupational therapy education, yet it appears to be an abstract and misunderstood process when applying these guidelines to a specific person's evaluation and intervention process. The concept of a guideline for action will be used to indicate when a frame of reference or practice model is selected and used to guide subsequent decision making in the therapeutic process.

DOI: 10.4324/9781003392408-9

It is not within the scope of this textbook to review common frames of reference or practice models for content mastery. There are numerous textbooks written about various frames of reference and practice models rich in depth and breadth. It is recommended that the reader first gain a thorough understanding of each frame of reference and/or practice model. Rather, the purpose of this chapter is to follow the MMCR to illustrate a five-step reasoning process suitable for use with any frame of reference/practice model, serving as a guideline for evaluation and intervention for any person served.

This five-step process will facilitate a practitioner's speed and efficiency in selecting and incorporating the frame of reference and/or practice model in real time. Steps 1, 2, and 3 break down the cognitive process that is occurring simultaneously while the practitioner is gathering and analyzing evaluation information. Steps 4 and 5 are completed after the evaluation information is analyzed and emphasize how this information is specifically applied to the person served.

A Five-Step Guide to Infusing a Frame of Reference/Practice Model Into a Person's Evaluation Selection and Intervention Plan

There is a common saying, "there are no cookbooks in occupational therapy!" A cookbook is a kitchen reference term that provides specific information on how to make a meal. Cookbook recipes suggest specific ingredients and explain how to combine those ingredients together in a sequential manner. Guidelines for actions are necessary because there are no cookbooks in occupational therapy. A practitioner cannot open a book to follow techniques for improving a child's handwriting or ways to incorporate memory aids for an older adult. These techniques are modified and implemented based on the context of a person's life story, goals, and intervention priorities. This is why a frame of reference and/or practice model serves as a guideline for action and is not a specific guaranteed recipe for success.

However, a sequential clinical reasoning process occurs when a practitioner formulates how a frame of reference and/or practice model will guide the process from abstract constructs into an action plan with evaluations and an intervention plan. As practitioners begin the evaluation process with a person, they use guidelines for actions to begin compartmentalizing the evaluation data and emerging intervention plan around the three core constructs of person, environment, and occupation within the guideline for action. Seasoned practitioners make this look effortless, but it is a complicated process. Some common questions to consider when initiating a potential plan:

When do practitioners begin selecting relevant frames of reference and/or practice models specifically for a person served?
Why is this frame of reference and/or practice model selection important?
How many frames of reference and/or practice models can be used for a person served?
Which top- or bottom-oriented evaluations align with specific frames of reference and/or practice models?
How does the general idea of the frame of reference and/or practice model influence the intervention plan?

Outlined is a five-step process to guide practitioners to apply a frame of reference and/or practice model during evaluation and intervention. Refer to Figure 7.1 to view the MMCR clinical reasoning guidesheet (also found in Appendix 2) entitled "MMCR Five Step Guide to Infusing a Frame of Reference/Practice Model Into a Person's Evaluation Selection and Intervention Plan" to complete the steps.

MMCR Five Step Guide to Infusing a Frame of Reference/Practice Model into a Person's Evaluation Selection and Intervention Plan

Step 1: Frame of Reference (FOR)/Practice Model (PM):

Step 2: Words in a Box:

Step 3: Frame of reference and/or practice model party paragraph:

Step 4: Succinct summary of person's story emphasizing relevant occupational performance
      ∇   issues

Step 5: Explanation of how the frame of reference and/or practice model will directly influence the specific intervention plan:

Figure 7.1 Clinical Reasoning Guidesheet: MMCR Five-Step Guide to Infusing a Frame of Reference/ Practice Model Into a Person's Evaluation Selection and Intervention Plan.

Steps 1, 2, and 3 will mentally assist the practitioner to choose the most relevant frame of reference and/or practice model specific for the person served. This choice also assists in selecting relevant evaluation tools. For example, a practitioner following the Cognitive Disabilities Model would typically select the Allen Cognitive Level Screen (ACLS) as one of the bottom-oriented evaluations (Allen, 1985).

Step 1: Identify the Specific Frame of Reference and/or Practice Model to Guide the Evaluation and Intervention Process

Frame of reference and/or practice model selection is one of the initial decisions a practitioner considers guiding the overall evaluation and intervention process. This decision involves cognitively sifting through potential guidelines for action while identifying the pros and cons of each for the specific person served. At times, the practitioner may follow one guideline for action or combine a few internally consistent ones. While there are distinct characteristics of a frame of reference and a practice model, both can be used together if there is congruence between them. These initial decisions are always set "in wet sand", as this process is fluid and ever changing depending on numerous factors such as the person served, practice area location, intended goals for achievement, etc.

Frames of Reference and Practice Models Are Both Considered Guidelines for Action, But Each Have Unique Distinctions

There are similarities and differences in each occupational therapy frame of reference and practice model. Both are considered a guideline for action because they delineate part of our domain of concern and have some connection to the constructs of person, environment or occupation. However, upon closer inspection, each frame of reference and practice model offers a unique perspective in scope, theoretical base, evaluation selection and the occupational therapy practitioner's role in the change process (Mosey, 1981). Following the work of Cole and Tufano (2020), several specific distinctions are highlighted here.

Frames of reference:

- emphasize a specific age group or disability, making the areas narrow in scope.
- include methods to conduct evaluations and specific evaluations influenced by the frame of reference.
- include a function and dysfunction continuum presented as opposite ends of a continuum, starting with a deficit-driven perspective.
- outline an intervention moving the continuum from dysfunction toward function.
- relate to applied scientific inquiry, where research investigates the efficiency of specific techniques and strategies for change.

Practice models:

- are applicable to all age groups, people (with or without disability) and practice areas so they are broader in scope and content.
- include methods to conduct evaluations that emphasize occupations and consider the person's unique life story.
- outline intervention plans that emphasize the interconnectedness of the person, environment and occupation constructs.

Step 2: Words in a Box

During step 2, the practitioner creates a mental picture of a box, as seen in Figure 7.2, by then adding words in the box, to highlight the most important words, phrases, definitions, evaluations or change processes that are the essence of the frame of reference and/or practice model. Mentally grouping those words, phrases, definitions, evaluations and intervention ideas will help the practitioner to remember and connect these relationships to the bigger picture. *If you are selecting more than one frame of reference and/or practice model, then create a box for each one.

Figure 7.2

Step 3: Frame of Reference and/or Practice Model Party Paragraph

Think about the last time you attended a party. Many people may be moving around the room and engaging in short conversations that are meaningful and specific. Imagine that someone at the party asks you about a favorite frame of reference and/or practice model. Yes, I suppose this is an OT party or no one would ask this question! How would you describe the frame of reference or practice model in a few minutes describing abstract constructs in layman's terms? What key points would be necessary to highlight?

Reflecting on these words in a box, the practitioner begins crafting full paragraphs to link these ideas together into a unifying message. The purpose of the party paragraph is for the practitioner to write and eventually spontaneously visualize a general understanding of this frame of reference and/or practice model that highlights the core constructs, phrases, definitions, evaluations or intervention ideas (previously written in your words in a box) to determine how it all relates together. It is not necessary to write down every single detail, but focus on the parts that represent a core understanding of the frame of reference and/or practice model.

This party paragraph assists the practitioner to recall and then articulate the frame of reference or practice model to others with speed and accuracy. This is a common reasoning practice and is sometimes referred to as a heuristic. A heuristic is a decision-making strategy or "rule of thumb" approach. It is the method that experienced practitioners use as a kind of mental shortcut. The more familiar and comfortable you are with the concepts (the party paragraph helps that happen), the more you will be able to produce solutions in a more efficient manner.

The challenging part of this step is to create a detailed but concise explanation of the frame of reference and/or practice model. At times, practitioners add in too much information and get lost in the details. While all parts of the frame of reference and/or practice model are important, these steps represent a snapshot of what the practitioner is thinking about when making these initial choices in real time.

TRY IT: Using Alonzo's Story to Practice Using This Five-Step Process

Information from Alonzo's intake report: Alonzo is a twenty-year-old man who lives with his mom, dad and younger sister in a one-family house with a fenced yard. Alonzo is diagnosed with cerebral palsy. He displays an unsteady gait and uses a cane due to left-sided weakness. Alonzo enjoys being with his dog, Spike, spending time outside in nature, and listening to music.

This brief information might be all the information a practitioner has to begin identifying a potential frame of reference or practice model, creating your words in a box, and then putting it together into a party paragraph. Steps 1, 2 and 3 will assist the practitioner to select a frame of reference and/or practice model.

Step 1: Identify one or two potential frames of reference and/or practice models to guide Alonzo's plan. For example, the Model of Human Occupation, Kawa Model, Dimensions of Wellness Model, cognitive disabilities, biomechanical frame of reference, sensory-motor frame of reference, rehabilitation frame of reference, etc.

*Reflect on the characteristics of a frame of reference vs. practice model. If selecting more than one, make sure both flow well together.

Step 2: Visualize the constructs, phrases, definitions, evaluations or change process highlighted in the selected frame of reference/practice model(s). In your box, write down all the information (as words or phrases) that come to mind.

Step 3: Use these words in a box to construct a concise but coherent party paragraph highlighting the frame of reference and/or practice model in relationship to this person and context.

Note: Eventually you will not need to use the clinical reasoning guidesheet, as it will become an automatic way of thinking.

Step 4 and step 5 assist the practitioner to align how the selected frame of reference and/or practice model guides the interpretation of the evaluation results and plans for intervention. These steps move into the application phase and are often the most challenging to combine an understanding of the frame of reference and/or practice model with the person's specific story.

Step 4: Succinct Summary of the Person's Story Emphasizing Relevant Occupational Performance Issues ∇

Complete step 4 *after* the top- and bottom-oriented evaluations are completed for the person served. You have selected and administered the evaluations based on your choice of frame of reference and/or practice model. At this time, the practitioner uses all of the information gathered during the evaluations to determine the initial top-middle-bottom occupational performance issues and can summarize the person's story from this perspective. This step reminds the practitioner that a person's unique story and goals are the center point of the intervention plan.

An example of *step 4* after an analysis of Alonzo's evaluations:

Alonzo is satisfied living with his mom, dad and younger sister, but is looking for opportunities to do more things by himself. He states that his mom is always worried about him and tends to discourage him from being more independent. Alonzo loves all animals and has a fish, bird, rabbit and dog in the house. He is very fond of his German Shepherd named Spike. Alonzo constantly asks his mother for permission to walk Spike around the neighborhood, but his mother wants Alonzo to stay in the fenced backyard with Spike. She is worried that using his cane to support his left-sided lower body weakness (bottom) makes it unsafe (bottom) for Alonzo to control Spike when he is excited during the neighborhood walk. Alonzo hopes that if he proves to his mother that he is capable of walking the dog around the neighborhood (middle), then she might feel more comfortable letting him do other things such as go on a nature hike with his two best friends (top).

Step 5: Explanation of How the Frame of Reference and/or Practice Model Directly Influences the Specific Intervention Plan

Now that you have an increased understanding of the frame of reference/practice model from your words in a box and party paragraph, plus a concise summary of the person's initial top-middle-bottom performance issues, it is time to combine this information and apply it to guide the person's specific intervention plan. Reflect on the information gathered during the evaluation process from the occupational profile and analysis of performance(s). Based on this information, the practitioner learned about the person's unique life story, goals and challenges. A person's unique life story and goals DO NOT change based on the frame of reference and/or practice model selected, but rather the practitioner uses these guidelines to strategize how to facilitate change to reach those goals.

TRY IT: Using Alonzo's Story to Practice Using This Five-Step Process

Reflect on the information provided in *step 4*. Alonzo's unique story does not change depending on which frame of reference and/or practice model guides the intervention plan. In other words, he still wants to show his worried mother that he can safely walk Spike around the neighborhood, even with an unstable gait and use of his cane.

Step 5: Align all the previous steps to reflect on your action plan to help Alonzo create change. Use the specific language of the frame of reference and/or practice model in your explanation.

For example, as guided by the biomechanical frame of reference, Alonzo's decreased strength and endurance create challenges in his ability to walk Spike beyond the fenced yard. Considering he wants to walk Spike around the neighborhood (middle) and go on a nature hike with his best friends (top), Alonzo would benefit from exercises that will increase his strength. To keep the exercise occupation-based, he can walk around the fenced yard for multiple repetitions throughout the day, which will also increase his endurance. Balance activities should also be incorporated to increase his safety and prevent a fall due to his unsteady gait. Passive and active range of motion will reduce any potential pain he may experience due to left-sided weakness. Alonzo will need to work toward being able to support himself walking while also having the strength and balance to walk Spike. Increasing his strength and endurance will allow for proper body mechanics during his neighborhood walks with Spike.

Summary

While guidelines for actions are common in most health professions, the occupational therapy profession categorizes these guidelines into frames of reference or practice models. A five-step reasoning process has been introduced to assist practitioners in selecting and incorporating the most suitable guideline for action for each person served. Steps 1, 2 and 3 help the practitioner to reflect on suitable guidelines for action that can be utilized while the practitioner is gathering and analyzing evaluation information. Steps 4 and 5 are completed *after* the evaluation information is analyzed and emphasize how this information is specifically applied to the person served.

Step 1: Identify the specific frame of reference(s) and/or practice model to guide the evaluation and intervention process.

Step 2: Add your words in a box.

Step 3: Use the words in a box to formulate a frame of reference and/or practice model party paragraph.

Step 4: Describe a succinct summary of person's story emphasizing relevant occupational performance issues.

Step 5: Explain how the frame of reference and/or practice model directly influences the specific intervention plan by combining steps 3 and 4.

References

Allen, C. K. (1985). Cognitive levels. In C. K. Allen (Ed.), *Occupational therapy for psychiatric diseases: Measurement and management of cognitive disabilities* (pp. 31–78). Little, Brown & Company.

Cole, M. B., & Tufano, R. C. (2020). *Applied theories in occupational therapy: A practical approach* (2nd ed.). Slack Incorporated.

Mosey, A. C. (1981). *Occupational therapy: Configuration of a profession*. Raven Press.

8 Overview to Intervention Planning: Spiraling *Within* the Top-Middle-Bottom Occupational Performance Issues

Laurie Knis-Matthews and Lynne Richard

Voices of the Practitioners: The Importance of Mentally Strategizing the Entire Intervention Plan Process

After the evaluation I have a chance to step back. I am normally not writing the short-term goals yet. I need to stay aware and think about those goals. What is appropriate for them to do in 3 days, in 5 days, in a week from now to make benchmarks? (Morgan)

I think about where this child is now and where they need to be by the end of this session or where I need them to be in 10 sessions from now. (Rebecca)

You cannot effectively provide treatment without making a plan. If you don't have a reason for the things that you are doing or if you're not able to process why someone needs to do it, that means you don't really know or potentially don't care. If you're not going through that process at all, you are doing a disservice to the profession. (Rose)

MMCR Overview Guide to Intervention Planning

At times, there is a misconception that upon completion of the evaluation process, the next step for the practitioner is to document an evaluation summary, including goals, prior to strategizing the intervention plan. Rather, seasoned practitioners, using their clinical reasoning skills, begin mentally formulating the overall intervention plan when the evaluation data collection has paused. They begin mentally planning an overall intervention approach BEFORE solidifying the initial goals on the evaluation summary.

Once the intervention plan is set (in wet sand) then the practitioner creates goals directly from this proposed intervention plan. Strategizing the intervention plan before developing the goals will facilitate a more thoughtful, occupation-based approach that is connected to a person's specific life story. It will also allow the practitioner to take into consideration the context of the setting (i.e., length of stay) and what is possible within that context. While it appears natural for seasoned practitioners to conceptualize intervention first, this clinical reasoning process must be taught to novice practitioners and students.

Before delving deeper into intervention planning, it is helpful to be familiar with a few of the symbols and sections of the next clinical reasoning guidesheet: MMCR Overview Guide to Intervention Planning. This clinical reasoning guidesheet was created based on the types of questions novice practitioners ask when learning how to strategize intervention. Expect a certain level of confusion, as these new symbols and terms are introductory in this stage of the book. Trust the

DOI: 10.4324/9781003392408-10

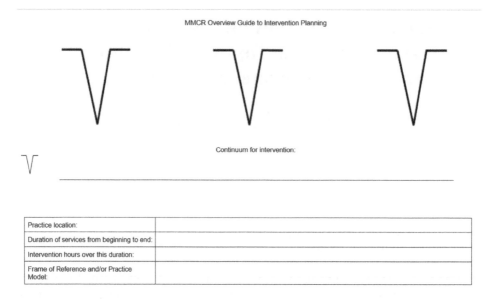

Figure 8.1 Clinical Reasoning Guidesheet: MMCR Overview Guide to Intervention Planning.

process and it will eventually make sense with more knowledge and practice. Please refer to Figure 8.1 (also found in Appendix 3) to review the MMCR Overview Guide to Intervention Planning. This clinical reasoning guidesheet will be discussed in the next few chapters.

A Return to the Top-Middle-Bottom Occupational Performance Issues

It is important to keep the top-middle-bottom(s) occupational performance issues at the center of intervention planning. Based on the person's story, goals and potential challenges, the practitioner should address the initial top-middle-bottom(s) during intervention to promote a plan that is client-centered and occupation-based.

Now this is a complicated process, so this is where clinical reasoning comes in. At times, the person served is able to identify an immediate goal or middle while not being able to visualize a longer-term plan or top. Other times, the person served has a definite long-term plan but is not able to identify all the short-term accomplishments or middles while working toward the top goal. To stay client centered throughout the intervention process, the person identifies either the top, middle or both during the occupational profile.

Voices of the Practitioners: During Intervention Planning, Priorities Are Strategic and Client Centered

I might ask the client what else [do] we need to do to get you home? They might say that "I need to be the one to make the coffee in the morning. My wife can't do it and I need to turn on the pot of coffee, pour it into a coffee mug and bring it into the living room". And so that is what we will work on. (Morgan)

Sometimes parents identify 10 goals they want us to work on, but I try to have them focus on the ones that are most important right now. Most times the parents' goals are based on things that are very functional. For example, I have a child whose goal is to put on a jacket so we do this in every single session. (Casey)

Why Are There Three Symbols (∇) Representing Occupational Performance Issues on This MMCR Overview Guide to Intervention Planning Guidesheet?

There are three blank (∇) symbols representing occupational performance issues on the MMCR intervention planning clinical reasoning guidesheet. Once the practitioner has collected data using a top-oriented evaluation and multiple bottom evaluations, then it is time to prioritize the level of importance. The initial occupational performance issue has already been determined (from the triangle clinical reasoning guidesheet introduced in Section 1) and will be addressed first in the intervention plan.

Rarely does a person have just one top-middle-bottom to address during intervention, as real life is more complicated and messier. However, the practitioner does need to sort out what comes first or what is addressed over a longer time period. A person's goals are not equal in time, as some take years to accomplish and others may take a few days. The second, third and fourth (∇) symbols provide a space for the practitioner to plan subsequent occupational performance issues addressed during the intervention process. How many occupational performance issues the practitioner will address during intervention is multifaceted and depends on many factors described throughout this section of the book.

Spiraling *Within* Each Set of Top-Middle-Bottom Occupational Performance Issues

Visualize a spiral. Do you imagine a shape that is curvy, continuous and has winding lines? Perhaps you are thinking of common objects such as a spiral staircase, a spiral notebook or a tornado. In the MMCR, the image of a spiral visualizes intervention in two ways: up and down *within* each set of occupational performance issues and *across* the entire process from the beginning to the end. Please refer to Figure 8.2 to visualize the intervention spiral within each occupational performance issue.

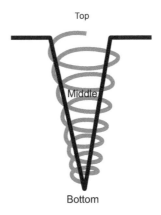

Figure 8.2 Intervention spiral.

First examine how the initial top-middle-bottom(s) occupational performance issues spiral up and down during intervention. To create a plan that is client centered and occupation based, the elements of the top-middle-bottom are incorporated (or spiraled) throughout the intervention approach. This is tricky. Some practitioners are comfortable focusing on bottoms and may describe using a bottom-up approach, but in reality, do not reach "the up" (the middle or top) during intervention. Why is this a problem? Rarely are people motivated to improve some aspect of their client factors or performance skills identified solely from bottom-oriented evaluations. When was the last time a person was excited to perform range-of-motion exercises?

Rather, people are motivated to enhance what is meaningful to their lives, and this is typically identified through the middle or top occupational performance issues. If the practitioner facilitates intervention emphasizing the bottom only, then it will simply not be meaningful or understood by the person. Consider this potential reason the next time a person refuses or is hesitant to participate in occupational therapy services.

To expand on this somewhat abstract explanation, two case examples, Moana and Dakota, are presented with intervention explanations.

Case Example: Moana's Story

Moana, an eleven-year-old girl diagnosed with cerebral palsy, has left-sided weakness. She is about to enter middle school and describes being very nervous about making new friends. Upon probing during the occupational profile, Moana describes feeling embarrassed that she cannot carry her own lunch tray back to the table in the middle school cafeteria, as an aide carries the tray for her. While Moana's top or long-term goal is to make new friends at the middle school, she specifically stated an immediate uncomfortable situation occurring in the cafeteria, especially with the aide carrying her lunch tray (middle). Based on the manual muscle testing (Lovett & Martin, 1916; Wright, 1912), Assessment of Communication and Interaction Scale version 4.0 (ACIS) (Forsyth et al., 1998) and the Pediatric Balance Scale (Franjoine et al., 2003), the bottoms are related to balance issues, difficulty with supination, left-sided weakness and sustaining a conversation with others.

TRY IT: Ideas for Moana's Intervention Plan

Before you continue reading this example, based on the information provided, describe three or four ways to implement Moana's intervention plan.

Following this example, a practitioner may begin intervention with a focus on the bottom such as strengthening left-sided weakness by providing arm supination exercises or playing a conversation starter game to increase her chances of making friends at the lunch table. The practitioners might assume these bottom-oriented intervention plans will eventually improve Moana's skill set to be successful carrying her lunch tray in the cafeteria and making new friends at middle school.

However, this bottom-oriented plan would not keep Moana's interest, as she would not perceive exercises or game playing as connected to her desire to be more independent in the cafeteria. In the MMCR, these types of intervention approaches are "peripheral" to the actual top-middle-bottom spiral. Peripheral means the plan for change is somewhat related to the person's story but does not directly address the top-middle-bottom.

Instead of a bottom-up approach, begin the intervention plan with the middle and then spiral both up and down. This spiral includes some elements of all three occupational performance issues. For example, carrying her own lunch tray in the cafeteria (middle) is most important to Moana. With an individualized intervention plan, Moana's confidence in carrying her lunch tray may eventually or simultaneously lead to the practitioner being able to spiral upward to the top of creating opportunities to make new friends. As Moana is becoming more independent in carrying her tray, she might feel increasingly comfortable starting conversations with peers at the lunch table (spiral up from the middle). Addressing the left-sided weakness, forearm supination, balance and conversing with peers are absorbed or spiraled through the middle of carrying her lunch tray (spiral down from the middle). The emphasis is placed on the middle that is more meaningful to the person, rather than the bottom.

The example here describes WHY the practitioner is planning intervention with a focus on the middle first, but HOW does the practitioner actually make this happen? Conceptualizing the intervention process by consciously separating the why from the how will assist the practitioner to begin with occupations and activities that are meaningful to Moana from the *first day* of occupational therapy services. Interventions need to reflect the context of Moana's environment and task—creating an authentic experience. When addressing how to help Moana carry the lunch tray in the cafeteria, the practitioner should consider the following during the intervention plan:

- using the same lunch tray Moana would carry in school so it is similar in weight and size,
- placing similar types of food on the tray that she would have to carry in the cafeteria,
- practicing how far she will need to walk to her table with the tray and food during lunch,
- anticipating and creating contingency plans if she spills food on her clothes or in general,
- emphasizing speed, efficiency and effectiveness in carrying her lunch tray and eating, as there is limited time to eat during lunch,
- practicing in similar clothes and shoes that she would wear to school while carrying this tray,
- identifying and practicing safe conversation starters that could be maintained with peers for the duration of the lunch period,
- anticipating and practicing ways she can respond to questions about the way she walks or uses her left hand,
- practicing multitasking so she can sustain a conversation with peers while carrying a tray of food,
- practicing and creating plans in which she needs to place the tray down to pay for lunch.

TRY IT: Using the MMCR as a Guide, Explain the WHY for Each Bulleted Intervention Suggestion Listed Above

There are 10 bulleted intervention ideas for Moana's intervention plan. Add more ideas to spiral the top-middle bottom. Consider how different practice locations influence these intervention ideas.

Reflect on these 10 ideas and explain why each intervention idea will represent a part of the top-middle-bottom spiral.

While it is ideal to implement this plan in the actual school cafeteria, this is not always realistic. Perhaps this plan occurs while Moana is participating in occupational therapy services in a specialized summer camp or in a rehabilitation setting for children. The practitioner can utilize many of these ideas listed even if not in the actual cafeteria. While it is not occupation-based intervention in the purest description, it is certainly more meaningful than doing exercises or playing a conversation starters game with the practitioner.

Being able to provide these types of intervention ideas requires a detailed understanding of Moana's middle school cafeteria. The practitioners can gather this information from multiple people such as Moana, lunch aides at the school, a school representative on the child-study team, a caregiver, etc. Creating intervention plans following the MMCR model is more challenging and time consuming for the practitioner because it demands the practitioner take the time to listen to the person's story and tailor the intervention to include those specific meaningful facets of the story. Practice these actions during each session and not as a one and done event. This is much harder to do than pulling cones out of the closet or playing a board game without any context, but is more meaningful for the person served and the practitioner.

Once Moana is satisfied with carrying her food tray without assistance from the aide, then the emphasis on this middle is minimized, but not completely resolved yet. For example, perhaps there is a special lunch in the cafeteria that will require Moana to carry a bowl of soup or make her own ice cream sundae with speed and efficiency. Once this middle (carrying the lunch tray) requires less emphasis, then perhaps the top (making new school friends) moves to the middle, as this is the next area of importance to address, with the top remaining to become more comfortable in a new middle school. See the top-middle-bottom visual representation of Moana's first two occupational performance issues in Figure 8.3.

Case Example: Dakota's Story

As mentioned earlier, sometimes a person is able to identify a longer-term goal but has difficulty recognizing the initial issues to be addressed along the way. For example, Dakota is a forty-eight-year-old woman overwhelmed with sadness after the recent loss of her wife, Linda, from a long illness with cancer. Using the Barth Time Construction (BTC) (Barth, 1998) as an

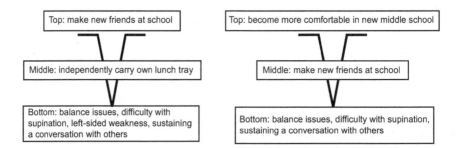

Figure 8.3 Visual illustration of Moana's top-middle bottom occupational performance issues. The first middle emphasizes Moana's primary concern of "fitting in" the school cafeteria while carrying her lunch tray. Once she gains confidence and skill, the next emphasis of intervention (middle) is helping Moana to make more friends at school. The bottoms shift in levels of emphasis and importance during the overall intervention plan.

occupational profile, Dakota reported that while she has been anticipating life without her partner for a long time, she was unprepared for the daily activities of living alone. Dakota described household activities that Linda was responsible for, specifically paying the weekly bills, mowing the lawn and doing the laundry. Although Dakota did not directly state these occupations and activities as immediate needs, these three potential middles emerged often through Dakota's story telling. Dakota described a flowerbed in her backyard that was very special to Linda and occupied much of their time together. She described specific gardening tasks to maintain a small section of the garden.

This is an example of the person identifying the overall top while the practitioner selects the first middle goal to be addressed during intervention. In this situation, the practitioner can still create the intervention plan by emphasizing the middle as the center point and then spiraling up and down as needed. The spiral from the middle to the top is extremely important here. Dakota's top, adjusting to her life without Linda and eventually transitioning into the role of a widow, is an overarching event to all aspects of her story and most meaningful to her. One of Dakota and Linda's occupations was keeping up with the flower garden (noted on the occupation section of the triangle). This occupation, connecting their lives together, is a motivating presence throughout the entire intervention plan and will provide added meaning to the other middles.

Selected by the practitioner and in collaboration with Dakota, the first middle is to create a system to pay the weekly bills, as there are long-term financial and societal consequences for late payments. See Figure 8.4 for a visual representation of Dakota's first top-middle-bottom occupational performance issues. The next middle might be learning how to wash, dry and fold laundry at the laundromat. Dakota has enough clean clothes for the next few weeks, so it does not need to be a priority. Finally, taking on the responsibility of mowing the lawn is next, as the spring season is still a few months away. See Figure 8.5 for Dakota's next top-middle-bottom occupational performance issues.

Based on the Kohlman Evaluation of Living Skills (KELS) (Kohlman & Robnett, 2016), Dakota had difficulty with the money management section connected to paying bills and writing out checks. Dakota again described gardening in Linda's flower bed during the leisure participation section of the KELS. At this time, she emphasized the flowerbed as a past interest when her wife was alive. Dakota was tearful throughout the evaluation process and often asked for frequent breaks to collect her thoughts.

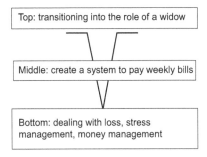

Figure 8.4 Visual illustration of Dakota's first top-middle-bottom occupational performance issue.

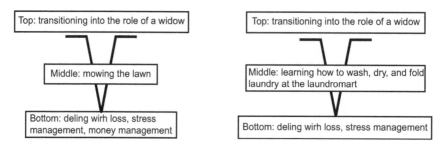

Figure 8.5 Visual illustration of Dakota's subsequent top-middle-bottom occupational performance issues. The top remains the same throughout the intervention plan. as adjusting to this role transition may take a long time. The emphasis on the middles is constantly changing in emphasis during the intervention plan.

Similar to tops, some bottoms might take years to accomplish, while others are quicker and shorter term. Dealing with the stress and loss of a loved one may be part of Dakota's story for a long time. These stress levels might intensify when experiencing new learning without her partner or during certain times of the year such as anniversaries or birthdays. Based on the KELS evaluation results, Dakota's bottom may be emphasized for some time throughout the intervention plan, as the practitioner teaches Dakota about check writing, maintaining a savings account and/or coping with the stress of losing a loved one.

As mentioned earlier in this chapter, it is important for the practitioners to reflect on why they are creating a specific intervention plan, but it is equally important to strategize how this plan is implemented. For example, listed next are some possible intervention approaches (the bulleted sections describe how this intervention approach is conducted and is followed with an explanation of why):

- Introduce, select and practice various stress management techniques such as deep breathing, journaling, progressive muscle relaxation, visualization of a calming place, meditation, etc. The practitioner will model one technique at a time and create a practice schedule. The practitioner will create a rating scale for Dakota to monitor the efficiency of each technique. Once Dakota decides on one or two techniques, then she will practice it (under the direction of the practitioner) until it becomes habitual.

This is an important skill to address during the intervention plan (bottom), as it will take some time to identify which technique is most comfortable for Dakota and then practice it until it becomes more habitual. Based on her situation, certain techniques might be more relevant such as meditating in Linda's garden or deep breathing when at the bank or laundromat. Dakota will utilize this skill while she is experiencing the stress of new learning such as bill paying, doing laundry, mowing the lawn (middles) or working in the garden where she feels closest to Linda's memory (top).

- Focus on bill paying by learning about Linda's system first. Dakota will decide what part of Linda's system she will continue to follow and what needs to be adjusted into her own system. In collaboration with Dakota, the practitioner will create a system (new learning and old learning) that includes written directions for clarity and reminders. The practitioner is active in the bill paying process until Dakota slowly practices taking over these steps with confidence. Selected stress management techniques are practiced in real time throughout the intervention plan.

Starting with a sharing of Linda's bill paying system may create a sense of familiarity and comfort (top and middle). These activities will keep a connection to Linda, as she and the practitioner will discuss her method of paying the bills (top) but are also beginning the process of Dakota creating her own system (middle).

Dakota and the practitioner will work on parts of this system during each session. Over time, Dakota will continue to increase her responsibility for bill paying and the practitioner will have less. As part of the healing process, stories about Linda will be encouraged throughout these sessions (bottom) and specific stress management techniques are incorporated in real time (bottom).

*These sessions require paying Dakota's actual bills while using her new system.

• In collaboration with the practitioner, Dakota may create a small savings plan to purchase a few of Linda's favorite flowers for the upcoming planting season. This will require Dakota to monitor planting websites and/or catalogs. It will require her to review and begin strategizing how much money is currently in their savings.

Gardening was very important to both Linda and Dakota throughout their relationship and may be a good way to stay connected to Linda's memory (top). In addition to the money management system being created, setting aside money into a savings account to prepare for the purchases of flowers, special gardening tools or gardening clothes will reinforce money management or savings for a meaningful occupation (middle), and this may help her decrease the stress experienced after losing a loved one (bottom).

How to Begin Conceptualizing the Intervention Plan: A-HA Moments

Data gathering for the person's initial evaluation pauses, as it is never definitively completed. The practitioner is always evaluating for changes and adjustments to the top-middle-bottom throughout the intervention process.

The practitioner should be mentally planning an overall intervention approach BEFORE solidifying the initial goals on the evaluation summary.

To create a plan that is client centered and occupation based, the elements of the top-middle-bottom are spiraled throughout the intervention approach in two ways: spiraling *within* each set of top-middle-bottom occupational performance issues (discussed in this chapter) and spiraling *across* the entire process from the beginning to the end (discussed in the next chapter).

Be mindful of implementing interventions that are peripheral to the actual top-middle-bottom spiral. At times, the peripheral plan for change only somewhat relates to the person's story but does not directly address the top-middle-bottom. This may lead to intervention plans that are less meaningful to the person served and that focus on the bottom only.

Instead of a bottom-up approach, begin the intervention plan with the middle and then spiral from the middle up and from the middle down. Rather than emphasize the bottom of the intervention plan, instead absorb it through the middle. This will help facilitate a more occupational-based and meaningful intervention plan for the person served.

Be mindful of the person's triangle information. The intervention plan must align with the person, facets of environment and occupations to promote well-being.

Summary

Once the data gathering nears a pause, the practitioner begins strategizing how the top-middle-bottom occupational performance issues will be addressed throughout the intervention plan. To remain client centered and occupation based during the intervention approach, the top-middle-bottom is first spiraled within the occupational performance issues. As the middle occupational performance issues represent an immediate need to be addressed by the person served or the practitioner, it is important to emphasize this middle while incorporating parts of the top or bottom. At times, practitioners appear more comfortable emphasizing the bottom occupational performance issues with the intention to eventually move up toward the top, but this may lead to interventions that are more preparatory without context and less occupational based.

References

Barth, T. (1998). Barth time construction. In B. Hemphill (Ed.), *Mental health assessment in occupational therapy: An integrative approach to the evaluation process* (pp. 115–129). Slack Incorporated.

Forsyth, K., Salamy, M., Simon, S., & Kielhofner, G. (1998). *A user's manual for the assessment of communication and interaction skills (ACIS)* (version 4.0). MOHO Clearinghouse.

Franjoine, M. R., Gunther, J. S., & Taylor, M. J. (2003). Pediatric balance scale: A modified version of the berg balance scale for the school-age child with mild to moderate motor impairment. *Pediatric Physical Therapy, 15*(2), 114–128. https://doi.org/01.PEP.0000068117.48023.18

Kohlman Thomson, L., & Robnett, R. (2016). *KELS Kohlman evaluation of living skills* (4th ed.). AOTA Press.

Lovett, R. W., & Martin, E. G. (1916). Certain aspects of infantile paralysis with a description of a method of muscle testing. *JAMA, LXVI*(10), 729–733. https://doi.org/10.1001/jama.1916.02580360031009

Wright, W. G. (1912). Muscle training in the treatment of infantile paralysis. *Boston Medical and Surgical Journal, 167*, 567–574. https://doi.org/10.1056/NEJM191210241671701

9 Overview to Intervention Planning

Spiraling the Top-Middle-Bottom Occupational
Performance Issues *Across* the Intervention Plan

Laurie Knis-Matthews

Introducing the Parts of the Continuum for Intervention

Now it is time to discuss the second spiral. While the explanation of the first spiral focused on the connection of the top-middle-bottom *within* occupational performance issues, this explanation provides more detail of the symbolic spiral *across* the intervention plan. Continue reviewing Appendix 3, "MMCR Overview Guide to Intervention Planning" clinical reasoning guidesheet introduced in the last chapter. The explanation continues by introducing the solid straight line printed under the Continuum for Intervention heading on the MMCR Overview Guide to Intervention Planning clinical reasoning guidesheet.

While strategizing the intervention process, visualize a horizontal straight line that starts with a top-middle-bottom symbol reminder and periodic vertical lines dividing the horizontal line into smaller segments. This generic visual example will help you to strategize the process and see the bigger picture.

Generic example: Continuum for intervention

$$\bigvee \underline{\qquad\qquad}/\underline{\qquad\qquad}/\underline{\qquad\qquad}/$$

Note: This illustration represents a *tentative* intervention guide. As the practitioner is working in a real practice setting with real people, there are many reasons for these tentative intervention plans to change. All aspects of the continuum for intervention are fluid and dynamic throughout the process, as initial top-middle-bottoms are resolved or changed, services terminate earlier than expected, or people progress faster or slower than originally anticipated. For example, people can change their mind on a goal. This change in goal direction could alter the top-middle-bottom, causing a restructuring of the entire plan.

The horizontal line. $\bigvee \underline{\qquad\qquad}$

This horizontal line represents the overall continuum of intervention created specifically for each person served. This line represents a person's total intervention plan from the beginning until the end of services. This line may represent a person who is participating in services within any time frame on any practice location such as seven days in the hospital, a shelter, or hospice; three months of outpatient services in a community-based program or at a summer camp; or a year of occupational therapy services in a nursing home, long-term rehabilitation unit, or school year.

DOI: 10.4324/9781003392408-11

For example, the horizontal line represents a person participating in OT services:

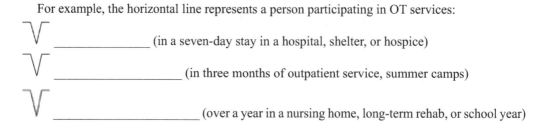

$\underline{\qquad\qquad\qquad}$ (in a seven-day stay in a hospital, shelter, or hospice)

$\underline{\qquad\qquad\qquad\quad}$ (in three months of outpatient service, summer camps)

$\underline{\qquad\qquad\qquad\qquad}$ (over a year in a nursing home, long-term rehab, or school year)

The Occupational Performance Issue (Top-Middle-Bottom) Is at the Beginning of the Continuum for Intervention

Reflect on traditional visualizations of the intervention continuum representing a sideways hierarchy or staircase. Both of these visual illustrations presented in Figure 9.1 highlight the intervention process beginning with a focus on bottom-oriented information and working up through the middle and eventually to the top. Challenges occur when the practitioner begins at the bottom and for many reasons (philosophy of the program, time constraints, or productivity rates) never reaches the middle or the top during the intervention plan. This strategy leads to an abundance of interventions that support occupations but are not occupation based.

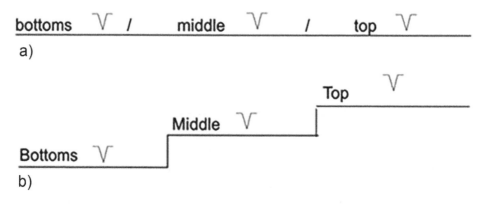

Figure 9.1 a) Traditional sideways hierarchy imagery and b) traditional stairway hierarchy imagery. Conceptualizing the top-middle-bottom occupational performance issues illustrated during the intervention process as a staircase.

Using these traditional approaches, the practitioner may reason these interventions will eventually generalize this new learning toward the middle or top. Sometimes there is an unsubstantiated expectation that a generalization of skills naturally occurs after discharge from services, when the person is in their original environment or no longer has access to occupational therapy services.

MMCR spiral imagery

Now reflect on the visual illustration presented in Figure 9.2. Placing this familiar symbol at the beginning of the continuum is a reminder for the practitioner to emphasize some combination of this initial top-middle-bottom occurring throughout the entire duration of the intervention plan. As previously mentioned, visualize the top-middle-bottom as a spiral with the practitioner entering through the middle. This spiral, incorporating some elements of the top-middle-bottom, continues throughout the entire duration of the intervention plan. By spiraling across, considerable intervention attention is placed on the middle and/or top occupational performance issues in addition to the bottom.

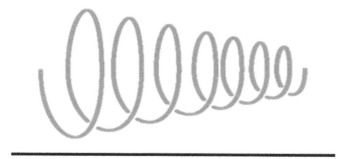

Figure 9.2

Other Factors to Consider When Conceptualizing the Continuum of Intervention or the Horizontal Line

Refocus your attention back to the horizontal line. To be clear, a person's story and personal goals *do not* change based on where they are participating during intervention or for how long. However, a number of factors influence HOW they prepare and implement this intervention approach. This intervention preparation begins with the practitioner reflecting on some basic questions relating to practice location, the duration of services from beginning to end, number of intervention hours over this duration, and the guiding frame of reference and/or practice model(s).

Voices of the Practitioners: Perspectives on the Uniqueness of a Person's Intervention Plan

Intervention is not a one-way process. After the evaluation, I pinpoint barriers and discuss that with the person to make sure that we [are] on the same page and create a plan together. Then I spend time reflecting about the activities or occupations that they have told me are important to them to figure out how those can be incorporated. (Rose)

One client's goal might not be the other client's goal. Let's say they have the same diagnosis, but the interventions are definitely going to be unique to the client. (Kristen)

I want to see what their values and beliefs are to incorporate that into the intervention plan. Once I felt like I understood their story, then I was able to develop interventions that were motivating. This is what the core of what OT is; being client-centered, creative, and out of the box. (Kristen)

Practice Location

Location, location, location. Where intervention happens really does matter. Occupational therapy practitioners face unique opportunities and challenges to be more or less occupation based related to each practice location. Some locations are medically model based, with more pressure to be diagnosis driven, fostering a sense of dependency on staff, reimbursement focused and discharge conscious (Gentry & Snyder, 2018). Meanwhile, other practice locations may follow a wellness model that emphasizes the individual, promotes an equal collaboration between the therapist and person served, and facilitates a plan that emphasizes wellness and prevention (Swarbrick, 1997). The characteristics of each model are equally important depending on the practice location of where the person is served. The practitioner's awareness of these characteristics is vital to strategizing a reflective intervention plan within the pros and cons of each practice location.

Repeating this message again: a practice location *does not* change a person's story (that is why a practitioner needs to learn about the person's story before planning intervention). During the occupational profile, a person's interests and goals are explored with tops or middles identified. However, the practitioner must adjust the intervention plan to address the person's top and/or middle even within the challenges of the practice location. It appears such a simple idea, yet it is difficult to follow while implementing an intervention plan.

Unfortunately, some practitioners actually build the intervention plan based on the practice location or administrative obstacles rather than the person served. For example, it is common for people receiving OT services in a rehabilitation program to work on dressing skills or participate in a feeding program. This intervention emphasis might be influenced by third-party reimbursement guidelines and suggested protocols. Pursuing these areas as part of this intervention plan might be completely necessary to certain people, but it is doubtful that it is relevant for every single person in a rehabilitation setting.

To explore another example, consider an inpatient setting where the practitioner, out of habit, offers a weekly group focused on helping participants shop for nutritious meals. This same group (method of intervention), with rotating sequential topics, has been offered in this same group format with the same worksheets (interventions that support occupations) for the last fifteen years. It does not matter what the person's goals are or if there is even an interest in the topic of nutrition. It does not matter if some of the group members did not do the food shopping, need to adjust their buying choice due to supplemental nutrition assistance from the government, or are now buying their groceries online instead of at the store, as the rotation of topics does not change. This example illustrates a practice location that is emphasized more than the person served.

This is further complicated as there appears to be a misapprehension that certain practice locations (such as home care) are automatically occupation based no matter what the intervention plan entails. For example, Kayla, who is an editor of a magazine, is recovering from a cerebrovascular accident (CVA) and participating in occupational therapy services at home. During the occupational profile, Kayla describes typing her monthly column on her computer as a priority task (middle) to help her return to work at the magazine (top). Rather than embrace Kayla's goal of returning to work as a magazine editor, the practitioner selects art projects to enhance fine motor skills for speed and efficiency. The practitioner describes this intervention as occupation based because the art project was completed at Kayla's kitchen table. There was an assumption these fine motor skills would eventually generalize into Kyla's work goals without actually typing on her computer. While this home care location affords the opportunity to conduct occupation-based intervention, this intervention selection is not relevant to Kayla's story, even if completed in her home and at her kitchen table.

TRY IT: Incorporating Characteristics of Occupation-Based Intervention

Reflect on the core characteristics of occupation- and client-centered principles to begin strategizing how this information aligns into the intervention plan.

What occupation characteristics and client-centered principles are apparent, if any, in Kayla's intervention plan listed earlier?

Based on these characteristics, describe ways the practitioner can alter this suggested intervention plan to become more meaningful and occupation based.

Duration of Service From Beginning to End

There is a misconception that practitioners always determine when intervention begins and ends. It is actually not that black and white. Yes, a practitioner has the expertise, based on ongoing evaluation, to determine if a person has achieved the goals or reached a status where services will no longer promote change. However, the length of time a person can participate in occupational therapy services is complex and multifaceted. Does the practice location have a typical length of stay? How long can the person pay for the services? Does the person served have a personal timeline for goal achievement? Does an outside agency, such as an insurance company or federal mandate, dictate the intervention plan priorities?

The length of time the practitioner has to work with a person influences how fast or slow intervention moves toward competency, how much can realistically be accomplished during the intervention plan, not overwhelming the person with an abundance of new learning, and determining if the intervention focus should be based on compensatory strategies or if there is enough time for a deeper learning. Although the length of time cannot cause the person to move any faster toward competency, it does influence how much change is attempted and the order of priority. For example, practitioners who work on a medical floor may only have a few days to implement the intervention plan. However, another practitioner may then work with the same person in a nursing home facility and have the opportunity of working with a person multiple times a week over the time span of a year.

Amount of Intervention Hours Over This Duration

The purpose of occupational therapy intervention is to assist people in making meaningful life changes, maintain abilities, and/or slow down a decline. It is the responsibility of the practitioner to use relevant teaching-learning principles embedded in occupation-based practice using a variety of methods and to assist the person or caregiver through the change process of developing awareness, identifying the reasons to change and creating a plan to formulate habits (Nemec et al., 2015). Lally et al. (2010) conducted a research study investigating the habit formation patterns of a daily life activity with ninety-six participants. The researchers estimated it took approximately two months of regular performance to become habitual. Nemec et al. (2015) described that a range of factors (motivation, willpower, and reward) influences a person's ability to create and sustain new habits.

Once the practitioner has a general timeline of the intervention process from beginning to end, reimagine the duration in terms of hours and not days or months. A person might participate in occupational therapy services for two months. Based on the study described earlier, this initially sounds like adequate time to develop habits and create lasting change, especially if it taps into the person's motivation and internal reward system. However, the structure of our healthcare system typically suggests services once per week in blocks of time anywhere from one hour, to forty-five minutes, or even thirty minutes. Although the ability to practice over time while still engaged in eight hours of services is helpful (one time a week for sixty minutes over two months), it does not sound as appealing as sixty days, nor does it reach the range to sustain habit formation.

Nemec et al. (2015) also distinguishes a difference if the person is developing a new habit or eliminating a well-established habit within the person's daily routine. Consider how many habits a person who has been institutionalized needs to eliminate while moving into the community setting. All of these habits cannot be changed at one time, as this may create anxiety. Perhaps starting the change process by eliminating one habit (the next middle) will be the emphasis of the next occupational performance issue.

Reflect on the bigger picture during an intervention plan and how the cultural environment of a location may be enabling those "undesirable" habits. Consider this information the next time an intervention plan encourages a person to fist bump rather than shake hands upon introduction. What about a person who has been simulating mopping a floor as part of a vocational training program for five years and then is blamed for not performing well on the actual task once he secured a job outside of the program, or a young adult diagnosed with autism spectrum disorder who is not grasping the skills of working in a flower shop because she secretly wants to go to college, but the individualized education plan (IEP) team members discouraged this path. Yes, this is complicated.

Frame of Reference and/or Practice Model(s)

Our guidelines for action are an extremely important part of the evaluation and intervention planning process. It is necessary to keep the frames of references and/or practice models in mind when beginning to strategize an overall plan. The selection of a frame of reference or practice model is based on many factors such as the practice location, the person served, the practitioner's level of expertise, and life views (Mosey, 1981). Please refer back to the earlier chapter emphasizing how frames of references and/or practice models align with evaluation selection and intervention planning.

Considerations When Spiraling Across the intervention continuum: A-HA Moments

When creating the intervention plan, imagine a continuum, symbolized with a horizontal line, representing a person's total intervention plan from the beginning until the end of services. All interventions must focus on some aspect of the top-middle and/or bottom(s).

The top-middle-bottom occupational performance issue is situated at the beginning of the horizontal line as a reminder that intervention is spiraled throughout the plan, with the practitioner entering through the middle. This spiral, incorporating some elements of the top-middle-bottom, continues throughout the entire duration of the intervention plan.

A person's story and personal goals *do not* change based on who the practitioner is or what the service is. However, a number of factors influence HOW the practitioner prepares and implements this intervention approach such as the practice location, the duration of services from beginning to end, the number of intervention hours over this duration, and the guiding frame of reference and/or practice model(s).

Summary

Once the evaluation information has been conceptualized, compartmentalized, and prioritized, then it is time to think about executing the overall intervention plan. As previously stated, to create a plan that is client centered and occupation based, the elements of the top-middle-bottom are spiraled throughout the intervention approach in two ways: spiraling *within* each set of top-middle-bottom occupational performance issues and spiraling *across* the entire process from the beginning to the end. Using the MMCR Overview Guide to Intervention Planning clinical reasoning worksheet, practitioners are able to visualize the overall intervention planning and strategize spiraling the top-middle-bottom within and across the process. During the occupational profile, a person's interests and goals are explored with tops or middles identified. Peoples' stories and personal goals often *do not* change based on where they are participating in intervention or for how long. However, a number of factors (practice location, duration of services from beginning to end, amount of intervention in terms of hours, and frame of reference/practice model) do influence how the intervention will be carried out by the practitioner.

References

Gentry, K., & Snyder, K. (2018). The biopsychosocial model: Application to occupational therapy practice. *The Open Journal of Occupational Therapy*, *6*(4). https://doi.org/10.15453/2168-6408.1412

Lally, P., van Jaarsveld, C. H. M., Potts, H. W. W., Wardle, J. (2010). How are habits formed: Modelling habit formation in the real world. *European Journal of Social Psychology*, *40*, 998–1009. https://doi.org/10.1002/ejsp.674

Mosey, A. C. (1981). *Occupational therapy: Configuration of a profession*. Raven Press Books.

Nemec, P., Swarbrick, M., & Merlo, D. (2015). The force of habit: Creating and sustaining a wellness lifestyle. *Journal of Psychosocial Nursing*, *53*(9), 24–30. https://doi.org/10.3928/02793695-20150821-01

Swarbrick, M. (1997). A wellness model for clients. *Mental Health Special Interest Section Quarterly*, *20*(1), 1–4.

10 Overview to Intervention Planning

Spiraling the Top-Middle-Bottom Occupational Performance Issues *Across* the Intervention Plan Continued

Laurie Knis-Matthews and Margaret Swarbrick

Explanation of This Process With an Example of High School Preparation

To begin this discussion, let's return to the familiar example of academic preparation of a high school student. Imagine this experience by including all four years of high school from entering as a freshman until senior graduation. Viewed this way, this conceptualization may seem lengthy, overwhelming, and distant.

_____

Freshman   Senior

Consider the four years of high school on a horizontal continuum divided into four sections representing each academic year.

_____/_____/_____/_____

Freshman   Sophomore   Junior   Senior

Focusing on smaller achievements or increments of the experiences appears more manageable and approachable. To focus on smaller achievements in this example, students often emphasize one year at a time. Within each academic year, students delineate smaller successes by emphasizing one marking period at a time or even one month within that marking period at a time.

Now consider a more focused conceptualization of each academic year such as a student's senior year:

marking pd 1/   marking pd 2/   marking pd 3/   marking pd 4/

Consider an even more focused conceptualization of a student's activities during marking period 1:

month 1/   month 2/   month 3/

The Practitioner Can Apply a Similar Reasoning Process to Planning a Person's Intervention Plan

Vertical lines $\vee$ _____ / _____ / _____

DOI: 10.4324/9781003392408-12

Following the MMCR, all intervention plans focus on making changes toward some aspect of the top, middle and/or bottom (spiraling from within and across) to remain aligned with the person's story. The vertical lines added throughout the horizontal line delineate and emphasize various sections of the overall intervention plan to make it more manageable, similar to the high school example provided earlier.

Conceptualizing the overall intervention plan into smaller sections will create a sequential awareness of the process from the beginning to the end. These vertical lines further assist the practitioner to chunk or group relevant methods into smaller sections of the intervention plan while reinforcing top-middle-bottom(s) performance issues during occupational-based practice.

For example, possible sections of intervention during:

V _____/_____/_____ (a seven-day hospital stay)

    1–2 days   3–4–5 days   6–7 days

V _____/_____/_____ (three months of OT outpatient services)

    1 month   2 months   3 months

V _____/_____/_____/_____ (a year of OT services in a nursing home)

    1–3 mo   3–6 mo   6–9 mo   9–12 mo

These examples are generic suggestions to guide problem solving and planning based on the individual's experiences, needs, goals, and expected length of stay. Determined by the practitioner, the amount of time needed to promote skills development to help the person accomplish their goal varies within each section in terms of days, months, or years.

Reasons Why the Vertical Lines Are Not Predetermined on the Clinical Reasoning Guidesheet

There are no predrawn vertical lines on any of the "MMCR Guide to Intervention Planning" clinical reasoning guidesheets, as this configuration is dynamic, unique to the person served, and evolves based on many factors. The vertical lines are placed on the continuum for intervention by the practitioner to determine when, where, why, and how smaller changes are made across the overall plan. Once practitioners identify the smaller sections of the intervention plan, they then select relevant methods utilized within each section to reinforce occupation-based practice. This is a complicated process, and it is definitely another gray area.

There are two clinical reasoning guidesheets to address this part of the process: the previously discussed "MMCR Overview Guide to Intervention Planning" (Appendix 3) and a new "MMCR Guide to Address Specific Sections of the Overall Intervention Plan" (see Figure 10.1, also found in Appendix 4). Review both of these clinical reasoning guidesheets side by side. The purpose of the "MMCR Overview Guide to Intervention Planning" is to help practitioners reflect on the big picture to identify where to place the vertical lines and label the central ideas for each specific section. This helps the practitioner to strategize the overall intervention.

The purpose of the "MMCR Guide to Address Specific Intervention Sections of the Overall Intervention Plan" is for practitioners to determine when, where, why, and how to create conditions for skills development. This clinical reasoning guidesheet assists practitioners to drill down

∇ _____

Circle the section of this plan: Beginning Part of Plan   Middle Part of Plan   Ending Part of Plan

Identify the specific section in terms of time:

┌───┐
│   │
└───┘

Label and briefly describe the central idea of this specific section of the plan:

┌───┐
│   │
└───┘

How does this specific section connect to the overall intervention plan? Describe the ways these intervention ideas are related to ∇

┌───┐
│   │
└───┘

Describe the plan for creating awareness and/or skill building?

┌───┐
│   │
│   │
└───┘

Select specific methods used to promote change:(therapeutic use of occupations and activities, interventions to support occupations, education, training, advocacy, self-advocacy, group intervention and virtual interventions)

┌───┐
│   │
└───┘

Identify and describe the specific teaching-learning principles to promote change:

┌───┐
│   │
└───┘

Figure 10.1 Clinical Reasoning Guidesheet: MMCR Planning Guide to Address Specific Sections of the Overall Intervention Plan

into each section of the continuum for intervention. This encourages practitioners to think about how they will design the conditions and specific methods and how each section will highlight the top-middle-bottom(s).

Note: Use a separate clinical reasoning guidesheet to reflect on each specific intervention section of the overall intervention plan. For example, in addition to the "MMCR Overview Guide of Intervention Planning", the practitioner will use three MMCR guides to address *specific* intervention sections for the hospital stay and outpatient services. There will be four guidesheets used to plan the four sections of the group home example that follows.

Case Example: Manny's Story

To provide more clarity to these abstract points with my students, I often begin by introducing and discussing Manny's story. Manny is a man in his late twenties, diagnosed with autism spectrum disorder, who has lived in the same group home for over ten years. Manny was unsuccessful in the previous vocational training program completed immediately after high school. Based on the occupational profile information, he wants a job at the community grocery store in the deli department (middle). He wants to save enough money from this job to meet a potential boyfriend and take him on dates (top). Based on the social skills observation and scoring portion of the Comprehension Occupational Therapy Evaluation (COTE) scale (Brayman et al., 1976), he has difficulty initiating and sustaining conversation with others (bottoms). He tends to be more comfortable conversing with perceived authority figures, such as the staff, rather than peers (even though they have lived together for ten years).

After reviewing the evaluation findings, completing the "MMCR Guide to Understanding a Person's Story (Triangle)", and determining the first set of top-middle-bottom occupation performance

---

Incorporating Specific Details Makes a Difference: A-HA Moment

Mentioned in Manny's story were specific details to provide the practitioner with information to be client-centered and occupation-based during the intervention plan. For example, he specifically identified wanting to work in a specific community grocery store. This is significant, as grocery stores are not the same and each location has different physical layouts, routines, and processes. Manny identified pursuing a job in the deli department. Departments run differently even within the same store. For example, the routine, social groupings, and physical environment at the deli is different from the seafood or bakery departments.

The practitioner needs to probe and clarify Manny's story to uncover those specific details to make this intervention plan more meaningful than simply working in a generic department at any grocery store. At times, people served may not have all the information predetermined. Manny is still unclear as to what specific job he wants to pursue in the deli department. However, if you are having difficulty creating specific intervention plans, consider that you need more information about the person's story and goals before you can move forward to create change. It never hurts to ask more questions.

---

issues, my OT students begin developing a potential intervention plan. It was recommended that Manny participate in occupational therapy services for one year (three times a week for sixty- to ninety-minute sessions) within his community. Initially, the students' ideas are scattered all over the intervention continuum without a sequential awareness of the change process. Students tend to address an issue once or twice during the intervention plan rather than clustering similar types of interventions together for deeper learning.

Three Examples of Typical Initial Intervention Responses From Students

Typical response 1: Manny will participate in a cooking group at the group home. He will be responsible for selecting a deli dish for the weekly menu. He will continue to gain more leadership skills by taking over more of the responsibilities of the cooking group and eventually fulfill the role as a potential co-leader. He will be encouraged to socialize with his peers during this group.

In what section of the overall intervention plan would this be addressed?

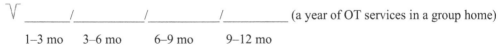

1–3 mo   3–6 mo   6–9 mo   9–12 mo

Actually, there is no X placed on the continuum because this intervention idea is not relevant to any section, as it is "peripheral" or does not directly relate to his top-middle-bottom. Participating in a cooking group is not going to help Manny get a job in the deli department or a boyfriend. He has been living with the same peers for ten years, so it will not be motivating for him to be more comfortable speaking to them more often. This plan does not utilize the location he wants to be in (grocery store), but keeps him in the location of the group home. To further relate this point, imagine the frustration if an occupational therapy student was ready to begin level two fieldwork but had to continue performing simulated OT tasks with their peers in the classroom.

Typical response 2: Take Manny to the nearest grocery store with the other members of the group home in the group home van. Manny will be responsible for purchasing the deli order for the meal while another member buys a dessert and another person buys coffee, etc.

V _____/__**X**__/_____/_____ (a year of OT services in a group home)

     1–3 mo   3–6 mo   6–9 mo   9–12 mo

While it is positive in that this example gets Manny into the community (at the grocery store), he is not ready to order the deli food. While it is relevant to his top-middle-bottom occupational performance issue, it is not starting from the beginning. This is an example of entering through the middle without addressing the bottom. The practitioner needs to address Manny's difficulty initiating and sustaining conversation with others to increase his confidence and successful experiences at the grocery store. The practitioner needs to strengthen Manny's awareness of the amount, type, and frequency of social conversations occurring at the deli counter. Perhaps the practitioner can model specific social skills while ordering the deli food a few times, create an observation list as a visual cue to direct Manny's attention toward specific social interactions, or teach Manny how to begin taking over smaller parts of the direct ordering and interactions at the deli counter.

Be Mindful of Unintentionally Creating Situations Where the Actions of the Persons Served Stand Out to Others

Practitioners need to be mindful of the stigma that still exists in the community. For example, a vehicle that displays the name of the agency transporting Manny to the store can be a trigger for stigma (negative attitudes and stereotypes) among other persons in the area if parked in front of the store. In this case, the practitioner could consider parking away from the entrance.

TRY IT: How Often Does This Happen During Intervention Sessions?

As a practitioner and advocate, question actions taken during intervention sessions that create uncomfortable situations for the person served. For example, it might be commonplace for staff and persons served to use informal gestures (e.g., fist bump rather than handshake). These actions can become habitual while the person is in the program, but this needs to be replaced with a formal gesture for a meeting such as a job interview or meeting with a probation officer, etc.

What potential factors or situations have you observed in healthcare programs? What actions or messages can you take to create a more typical situation? Identify a few subtle changes to make it less noticeable (such as not pulling up to the front door with the program van or wearing your badge while on a community outing).

Typical response 3: The majority of students immediately propose helping Manny to get a job and begin completing a job application or going on an interview within the first three months of intervention.

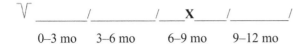

0–3 mo   3–6 mo   6–9 mo   9–12 mo

This intervention section, emphasizing working at the deli counter by filling out job applications and preparing for the job interview, is addressed later in the year-long plan, near month seven or eight. There are earlier issues to first be accomplished relating to getting a job, while also considering that Manny does not consistently initiate and sustain conversations with peers. There is also much to achieve in the first months in terms of understanding a deli job at the grocery store and typical social conversations sustained at the deli counter. Clustering these intervention methods is practiced by first observing the types of conversations occurring at the deli department, implementing a system where Manny can coordinate the weekly deli order by asking peers, going to the deli department, learning how to sustain short conversations with "safe" topics, etc. These examples focus on Manny's bottom while spiraling through the middle of the deli counter.

TRY IT: Understanding the MMCR Guidesheets to Conceptualize Manny's Overview of Intervention Planning and Specific Intervention Sections

The practitioner should become familiar with both of these clinical reasoning guidesheets to strategize why and how the change process will occur. Each section of the intervention plan has a different focus, methods, and duration of time.

A sample of Manny's guidesheet can be found at the end of this chapter in Figure 10.2. Before reviewing the sample, try it yourself first.

Note: The practitioner should use these clinical reasoning guidesheets until they are able to mentally formulate intervention plans.

Using the MMCR overview guide to intervention planning:

Identify all potential practice locations relevant to Manny's intervention plan.

Identify the duration of services from beginning to end: how long will you have to collaborate with Manny?

How many hours do you anticipate collaborating with Manny?

What potential practice models and/or frames of reference are you considering guiding Manny's intervention plan?

Over the year-long intervention plan, label how you will move through Manny's top-middle-bottom occupational performance issues (using the three occupational performance symbols on the page).

Reflect on all of this information to draw vertical lines (always with a pencil) to begin planning how Manny's year-long intervention plan will be divided into sections that represent a beginning, middle, and end part of the plan. How long will each vertical section be?

Summary

Conceptualizing an intervention plan can be a complicated process for the practitioner to determine where to start and how to facilitate steady progress toward goal attainment consistent with the person's top-middle-bottom occupational performance issues. To remain aligned with the person's story, it is important to spiral the top-middle-bottom intervention plan from both within and across the continuum. To make this process more manageable, practitioners mentally group or chunk smaller sections of the overall intervention plan. These specific sections help the practitioner to determine when, where, why, and how smaller changes are strategically made across the overall plan.

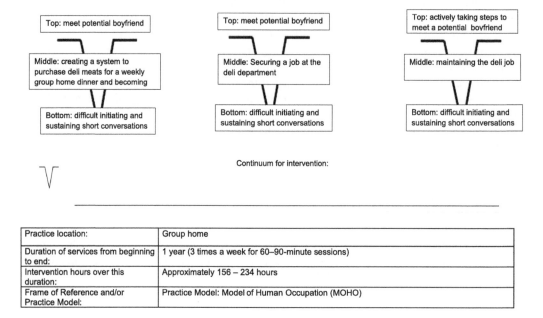

Practice location:	Group home
Duration of services from beginning to end:	1 year (3 times a week for 60–90-minute sessions)
Intervention hours over this duration:	Approximately 156 – 234 hours
Frame of Reference and/or Practice Model:	Practice Model: Model of Human Occupation (MOHO)

Figure 10.2 MMCR Overview Guide to Intervention Planning: Manny.

Reference

Brayman, S. J., Kirby, T. F., Misenheimer, A. M., & Short, M. J. (1976). Comprehensive occupational therapy evaluation scale. *American Journal of Occupational Therapy*, *30*(2), 94–100.

11 Strategizing the Beginning-Middle-Ending of the Specific Intervention Plan

Laurie Knis-Matthews and Margaret Swarbrick

Voices of the Practitioners: Reasons Why Practitioners Reflect on Specific Interventions Plans

The first day in the hospital environment is most important because it is always going to influence the things you do and how you are able to do it. But soon after that, where the person is going to be discharged and then that becomes the most important factor. (Rose)

It is important to combine experience, knowledge, and research to provide a logical argument and a full rationale as to why you are doing a specific intervention. (Pam)

It's great if they function really well in the clinic, but that doesn't matter if they can't do it at home. (Rebecca)

Every person is different and every person is going to need a different approach. This idea is threaded through every decision we make. What would happen if we took clinical reasoning out of OT? It would just be a cookie cutter. (Casey)

While reflecting on the plan, most experienced practitioners are simultaneously conceptualizing the reasons why they are selecting certain types of interventions. It is a complex clinical reasoning skill, and seasoned practitioners make it look effortless, but it is not. Understanding the reasoning why (cognitive process) a practitioner intends to do something during intervention is a very different skill than how (psychomotor process) the practitioner implements interventions. The following sections will attempt to explain the *why* and *how* factors of intervention more fully. These considerations occur simultaneously during the clinical reasoning process. The *why* and *how* factors are presented separately in this book for learning purposes only.

Continue to review the two clinical reasoning guidesheets side by side to address this part of the process: the "MMCR Overview Guide to Intervention Planning" (Appendix 3) and the "MMCR Planning Guide to Address Specific Sections of the Overall Intervention Plan" (Appendix 4). While the purpose of the "MMCR Overview Guide to Intervention Planning" helps the practitioner strategize the overall intervention process, the purpose of the "MMCR Guide to Address Specific Intervention Sections of the Overall Intervention Plan" is for the practitioner to determine why and how to create change.

The "MMCR Planning Guide to Address Specific Sections of the Overall Intervention" aids practitioners to think about *how* they will facilitate change, what specific methods are used, and how each section highlights the top-middle-bottom(s). This chapter will focus on this specific clinical reasoning guidesheet.

DOI: 10.4324/9781003392408-13

Considerations When Identifying Sections and Grouping Methods Within the Vertical Lines: The *Why* Factor

In each section, divided by the vertical lines, the practitioner has a central idea to describe the intervention emphasis related to the identified top-middle-bottom occupational performance issues. Labeling each central idea assists the practitioner to first explain the *why* factor. This cognitive process taps into mental skills and knowledge that guide the rationale for selecting interventions and methods. The practitioners ask themselves questions such as:

- What specific section of the overall intervention plan am I executing?
- What is the central idea of this specific section of the overall plan? How can I label this section to incorporate the goals to be accomplished and what needs to be learned?
- How does this section connect to the overall intervention plan? How does it relate to the top-middle-bottom occupational performance issue spiral?

Answering these questions is important so the practitioner connects the intervention to the person's unique life story in order to strategize ways to foster skill development to impact change and reinforces a combination of the top-middle-bottom occupational performance issues. To keep this process somewhat manageable, conceptualize three comprehensive or main parts (beginning, middle, and ending) to the intervention process, which includes specific sections to each part of the plan. Review these examples from a variety of intervention durations and practice locations. Depending on the practice location, the range and duration will differ.

Beginning   Middle   Ending
X_____/_____/_____ (a seven-day hospital stay)

1–2 days   3–4–5 days   6–7 days

Beginning   Middle   Ending
X_____/_____/_____ (three months of OT outpatient services)

1 month   2 month   3 month

Beginning   Middle   Ending
X_____/_____/_____/_____ (a year of OT services in a nursing home)

1–2 month 3–6 month 6–9 month 10–12 month

Start Intervention at the Beginning

Determining how to begin the intervention plan can be complicated. During the beginning part of the intervention plan, the practitioner creates a process or system that will be incorporated or spiraled throughout the entire plan. The process might be to set up a person's new room upon relocation to a group home, nursing home, or shelter. Another process might develop specific relaxation techniques a person can implement when any new learning is introduced. In collaboration with the person served, the practitioner explores the most effective ways to set up these processes for eventual change by using trial and error, preferred learning styles, and relevant teaching-learning principles. One size does not fit all. Each person served has a different life story and goals, and despite the practice location or amount of time available to engage in the intervention process, this implementation starts at the beginning.

Starting intervention at the beginning of the continuum is much easier to do when the practitioner is leading with the middle or top occupational performance issue (rather than the bottom) to create change. In isolation, bottom-focused intervention plans are more disconnected from real life and non-functional, so it is more challenging to create processes for any length of time, leading to the "one and done" types of intervention plans. This means that the practitioner is constantly changing topics, activities, or methods throughout the intervention plan to keep a person's interest. For example, referring to the example of Manny in the previous chapter, it is difficult to create a process that emphasizes Manny's increased ability to initiate and sustain conversations with others. Perhaps Manny could play a conversation starter game, participate in a weekly cooking group, create a generic resume, or role-play a mock interview. Over time, these types of interventions are repetitive and boring. In isolation, these common intervention ideas are bottom-focused interventions, steeped in non-functional outcomes, and at times peripheral to the top-middle-bottom.

Instead, the practitioner who taps into a person's motivation may be able to engage initial and sustained determination and interest. The practitioner will not need to change the topics, activities, or methods throughout the intervention plan to keep a person's interest. Middle and/ or top occupational performance issues connect to context and are relevant to the person's story.

To provide more clarity on the beginning part of the intervention process, return to Manny's story in Chapter 10. Using the "MMCR Planning Guide to Address Specific Sections of the Overall Intervention" process guidesheet, reflect on the section, title of the section, and provide a brief overview of what will be included in the intervention. Review Figure 11.1, Manny's MMCR Planning Guide to Address Specific Sections of the Overall Intervention Plan.

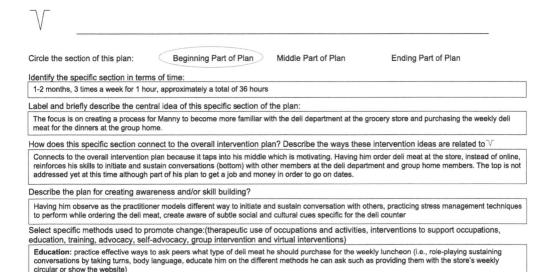

Circle the section of this plan: (Beginning Part of Plan) Middle Part of Plan Ending Part of Plan

Identify the specific section in terms of time:

1-2 months, 3 times a week for 1 hour, approximately a total of 36 hours

Label and briefly describe the central idea of this specific section of the plan:

The focus is on creating a process for Manny to become more familiar with the deli department at the grocery store and purchasing the weekly deli meat for the dinners at the group home.

How does this specific section connect to the overall intervention plan? Describe the ways these intervention ideas are related to ∨

Connects to the overall intervention plan because it taps into his middle which is motivating. Having him order deli meat at the store, instead of online, reinforces his skills to initiate and sustain conversations (bottom) with other members at the deli department and group home members. The top is not addressed yet at this time although part of his plan to get a job and money in order to go on dates.

Describe the plan for creating awareness and/or skill building?

Having him observe as the practitioner models different way to initiate and sustain conversation with others, practicing stress management techniques to perform while ordering the deli meat, create aware of subtle social and cultural cues specific for the deli counter

Select specific methods used to promote change:(therapeutic use of occupations and activities, interventions to support occupations, education, training, advocacy, self-advocacy, group intervention and virtual interventions)

Education: practice effective ways to ask peers what type of deli meat he should purchase for the weekly luncheon (i.e., role-playing sustaining conversations by taking turns, body language, educate him on the different methods he can ask such as providing them with the store's weekly circular or show the website)
Interventions to support occupation: create and use an observation sheet to assist him in determining the quality and quantity of social conversation occurring at the deli department (this will allow Manny to reflect on interactions), create and use of a cheat sheet with socially acceptable

Identify and describe the specific teaching-learning principles to promote change:

Modeling: The practitioner will first demonstrate asking staff and group members if they have any deli requests for the weekly luncheon
Trial and error: Manny will try asking the practitioner to prepare himself. This will provide him with the safe space to try different methods and adding his own style.
Repetition and practice: Manny will begin by asking staff members their requests for the weekly luncheon since he is most comfortable with them. He will have repeat similar interactions with the staff members first and then with his peers. Repeated practice with the staff members will increase his

Figure 11.1 Sample of the beginning part of Manny's intervention plan using the MMCR Planning Guide to Address Specific Sections of the Overall Intervention Plan.

Explanation of Figure 11.1: The Beginning Part of Manny's Intervention Plan Using the MMCR Planning Guide to Address Specific Sections of the Overall Intervention Plan

Beginning   Middle   Ending

XXXXXXX/_____/_____/_____

1–3 month   3–6 month   6–9 month   10–12 month

Identify the specific section in terms of time: One to two months, meeting three times per week for approximately one hour, consisting of approximately 36 hours to address the beginning part of this intervention plan.

Label and describe the central idea of this beginning part: The first three months will focus on creating a process for Manny to become more familiar in his preferred location at the deli department in the grocery store. This process will include:

- polling group home members about the type of deli meat to purchase at the grocery store for the weekly luncheon,
- determining the grocery store location to purchase the deli meat,
- finding and using cost-effective transportation means to get to the grocery store,
- observing how the practitioner will model different ways to initiate and sustain conversation with others,
- becoming aware of subtle social and cultural cues specific for the deli counter,
- practicing taking over small parts of ordering the deli meat,
- initiating greetings and very short conversations with customers and employees,
- practicing stress management techniques to perform while ordering the deli meat.

How does this specific section connect to Manny's overall intervention plan? Describe the ways these intervention ideas are related to his $\bigvee$ *for eventual intervention choices and method selection*:

Manny wants to get some type of deli job at the grocery store, so the intervention plan starts with the practitioner setting up a situation where Manny is responsible for selecting the deli meat for the weekly luncheon at the group home. He selects the deli portion of the meal, with input from the other group home members and staff, while participating in the actual in-store purchase. Going to the actual deli department taps into Manny's motivation (middle) but remember that he has difficulty initiating and sustaining conversation with peers (as you will need to spiral down to the bottom). Having Manny go into the store (rather than ordering the deli meat online) directly reinforces his skills to initiate and sustain conversations with others. He is interested in learning more about the deli department, so he is motivated to be in the grocery store. The practitioner creates a system, or process, for Manny to order deli meat at the grocery store and reinforces his social skills in a creative and individualized intervention way. This also helps him to become familiar with his future environment at the grocery store (including all the facets of this location such as physical, cultural, social, temporal, and virtual).

During this intervention plan, the practitioner will:

- teach Manny effective ways to ask his peers what type of deli meat to purchase for the weekly luncheon,
- identify potential grocery stores in the neighborhood and explore different ways to get to the store such as walking, taking the bus, or taking the group home van (instead of just taking the group home van to any store),

- create and use an observation sheet to assist Manny in determining the quality and quantity of social conversation occurring at the deli department,
- encourage Manny to begin practicing greetings with others at the group home until he is confident to also greet unfamiliar people at the deli counter,
- role-model behaviors such as how to place a deli order, sustain short side conversations while waiting for an order, and ask potential questions about the deli meat.

It may take about 3 months of the 12-month intervention plan incorporating the right amount of teaching-learning principles, reinforcing his preferred learning style, and constant trial and error. This attention to detail and setting up processes in the beginning stages of the intervention process might appear time consuming, but once these processes are created, the remainder of the intervention plan becomes more meaningful, habitual, and less stressful.

Moving Into the Middle Part of the Intervention Plan

During the beginning part of the intervention plan, the practitioner identifies and creates processes to initiate the change process related to the top-middle-bottom occupational performance issues. For Manny, the beginning of the intervention plan focused on him becoming familiar with the deli department at the grocery store and participating in ordering the weekly deli meat. He was able to increase his awareness of the types and frequency of social skills in this location, leading to initiating and sustaining conversations with others. The practitioner has not addressed the top (finding a boyfriend) yet, so as to not overwhelm Manny with too much new learning.

Once the processes have formed, now it is time to move into the middle parts or "heavy lifting" of the intervention plan. Over the duration of the intervention plan, the practitioner uses the middle part for practice and reinforcement with an increase in task demands. This is an example of spiraling across the continuum. At times, the middle part of the intervention plan is a longer section than the beginning or the end because a majority of new learning is occurring in this part. The middle is the heart of occupation-based practice emphasizing the top-middle-bottom performance issues. The practitioner may begin spiraling through the middle, down to the bottom, but also up to the top illustrating the spiral within.

Occupational therapy practitioners are agents of change. Our professionals implement these changes with clever intervention plans that are innovative, outside the box, adaptable, and ever changing. Our clever approaches to intervention planning are one of our profession's greatest strengths. However, although a person served is interested in pursuing some aspect of change in their lives, this can be scary, uncertain, unfamiliar, and stressful.

Based on the MMCR, reimagine what an effective intervention plan means to the person served. This comes from strategizing how to spiral the person's top-middle-bottom across the intervention plan directly. A practitioner taps into a person's motivation (middle or top), so the person pursues this new learning without realizing or caring what challenges or stressors lie ahead. In other words, the motivation for change becomes greater than the fear of change.

Using Another Example to Describe a Clever Approach to an Intervention Plan: A-HA Moment

Ronnie recently underwent surgery for a total hip replacement. During the occupational profile she described wanting to continue cooking her famous meatballs for the weekly family Sunday dinner (middle). Getting back to this occupation symbolizes her sense of self and well-being as a productive member of the family unit (top). Due to the total hip replacement, she has temporary movement restrictions such as not bending at her hips greater than 90 degrees, crossing her legs, or turning her toes inward (all bottoms).

The practitioner focuses on setting up processes to assist Ronnie to make these meatballs with her preferred ingredients, using her family recipe, and preferably in her kitchen. The practitioner will introduce, practice, and reinforce topics related to conserving energy, best places to store the ingredients and equipment in the kitchen, and following hip precautions while preparing the meatballs. Some practitioners might be "creative" by making similar meals such as lasagna one week, spaghetti another week, or a cup of tea to get her back into the kitchen. If Ronnie is motivated and wants to make her famous meatballs, then make the meatballs rather than trying these different food dishes.

These other food items, not mentioned during Ronnie's occupational profile, are peripheral to the plan and not viewed as creative, but a distraction. Ronnie will be motivated to address facets of this intervention plan for her special meatballs during every single occupational therapy session. The practitioner uses the middle of making the meatballs as the cornerstone of the plan while infusing other bottoms into the sessions. This intervention plan will facilitate Ronnie's increased sense of purpose in her family unit (top). This is a clever and realistic intervention plan that will capture her motivation every time she participates in a session.

Yes, this type of intervention plan requires more thought and preparation in the beginning, but once the processes are set and a routine is established, the rest of the intervention planning process becomes more efficient.

The Middle Part of Manny's Intervention Plan

To provide more clarity on the middle part of the intervention process, we return to Manny's story. Using the "MMCR Specific Planning Guide to Sections of the Overall Intervention" process guidesheet, reflect on the section, title of the section, and provide a brief overview of what will be included in the intervention.

Beginning   **Middle**   Ending

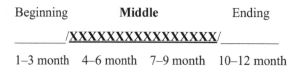

1–3 month   4–6 month   7–9 month   10–12 month

Identify the specific section in terms of time: months 4–9, meeting three times per week for approximately 1 hour, consisting of approximately 72 hours to address the middle part of this intervention plan.

Label and describe the central idea of this specific section of the plan: The next six months will focus on reinforcing the processes in the beginning of the intervention plan, so it is more comfortable initiating and sustaining conversations in Manny's preferred location at the deli department in the grocery store. While this ongoing process is becoming more familiar and habitual, the practitioner begins addressing Manny's desire to obtain employment at the deli department in the grocery store.

• Exploring types of jobs and responsibilities available in a deli department,
• Learning how to create a resume and complete other necessary paperwork,
• Practicing interview skills specifically for the deli job,

- Identifying topics to sustain longer conversations with others,
- Practicing sustaining longer conversations with the interviewer,
- Implementing specific stress management techniques while at the interview,
- Beginning to apply for jobs!

How does this specific section connect to Manny's overall intervention plan? Describe the ways these intervention ideas are related to his √ *for eventual intervention choices and method selection*:

Processes initiated during the beginning of Manny's intervention plan will continue as the practitioner moves into the middle part of the plan. Manny will continue to initiate asking the other group members to poll their deli choice and take on more responsibility ordering the deli meat at the grocery store. He will continue to practice making side conversations with other customers or deli staff about safe topics such as the daily weather or a sports game. While reinforcing the specific social skills and deli ordering for the luncheon is becoming more habitual, it is time to begin addressing the social skills of initiating and sustaining conversations with others in preparation for an actual deli job. The practitioner lessens the amount of modeling at the grocery store and becomes more of a support and resource. Eventually, the practitioner will transfer this beginning intervention to another staff member at the group home to concentrate on the next section (middle) of intervention.

The practitioner again leads with the middle by methodically introducing typical job search activities such as:

- identifying and searching for specific jobs available in the deli department such as counter help, cleaning up, transporting the deli meat, etc. Consider job responsibilities that do not require as much social interaction such as counter help vs. cleaning up in the back during less busy hours.
- deciding on the specifications of the intended job such as paid or unpaid, part time vs. full time, and day or evening hours. Consider working hours that tend to be less busy at the deli counter such as nighttime or during the week may assist with decreased stress surrounding initiating or sustaining conversations with others.
- creating a resume and/or completing the necessary application process. Gathering all forms of identification and past work experiences, references, and contact information. Discuss legal and illegal questions that might appear on a job application.
- practicing interview skills with particular attention to initiating and sustaining a conversation (this will be different from quick greetings at the deli department).
- identifying and practicing stress management techniques that will be suitable to implement during a job interview.

At times, this new learning related to a job search will be stressful and challenging, but Manny will be motivated to continue because it is his personal goal. All of these intervention ideas require a lot of practice to become habitual, so be careful of the "one and done" intervention plan.

Preparing the Plan to End Intervention

At this point, processes initially set up at the beginning of the intervention continuum and continued throughout the middle part of the intervention plan have been introduced, practiced, and reinforced, working toward some level of competency. The ending part of the intervention plan, nearing discharge or termination of services, includes specific sections that emphasize preparation to sustain skills gained. Where occupational therapy intervention ends is more complicated, as it is influenced by numerous factors such as progress made by the person, relevancy of intervention approach to the suggested top-middle-bottom, location of services, person's perception of goal achievement, and overall duration of the intervention. At times, the intervention may end abruptly due to external forces connected to reimbursement issues, typical length of stay, changes in medical condition, etc. Other times, services terminate when the person achieves designated goals or achieves desired lifestyle changes.

The practitioner prepares for the next transition process during the ending sections of intervention, as the person will be transferring from services with an increased knowledge and/or skill set. The practitioner will reflect on some of these following questions:

- What is driving this termination of services? Did the person accomplish the goal or did another factor positively or negatively impact?
- What location (environment) is the person going to next? Consider the physical, temporal, social, cultural, and virtual facets of this next location. How prepared is the person for this next location and environmental facets?
- Did the practitioner sufficiently address all aspects of the top-middle-bottom occupational performance issues?
- What still needs to be addressed during the intervention plan (including compensatory techniques) prior to ending services?

The Ending Part of Manny's Intervention Plan

To provide more clarity on the ending part of the intervention process, return to Manny's story. Using the "MMCR Specific Planning Guide to Sections of the Overall Intervention" process guidesheet, reflect on the section, title of the section, and provide a brief overview of what will be included in the intervention.

Beginning   **Middle**   **Ending**

_____/_____/_____/**XXXXXXXXX**

1–3 month   4–6 month   6–9 month   9–12 month

Identify the specific section in terms of time: months 9–12, meeting three times per week for approximately one hour, consisting of approximately 36 hours to address the middle part of this intervention plan.

Label and describe the central idea of this ending part: During the final three months of the intervention plan, Manny continues to order the deli meat for the weekly luncheon without any assistance from others. He has secured a part-time evening maintenance job in the deli department at a grocery store 30 minutes away from the group home.

Intervention does not end with Manny beginning employment, but the practitioner continues to assist Manny with the actual transition into work and while preparing to pursue a potential boyfriend. During this ending part of the intervention plan, Manny will:

- practice time management strategies to get to work on time using his preferred method of transportation,
- initiate asking for assistance when unsure of work tasks,
- identify and practice sustaining conversations with co-workers during breaks,
- implement specific stress management techniques during break time,
- create an awareness of how to meet others and/or a potential boyfriend with similar interests.

How does this specific section connect to Manny's overall intervention plan? Describe the ways these intervention ideas are related to his √ *for intervention choices and method selection*:

During the middle part of the intervention plan, the practitioner helped Manny look for and secure a job at the deli department (in a perfect world). The practitioner incorporates the top-middle and bottom occupational performance issues during Manny's ending part of the intervention plan. In collaboration with the practitioner, the final three months provides Manny with more time to handle the transition into the deli department at the grocery store. While exciting, this shift in location and all the environmental associated facets may create additional stress and self-doubt. Realistically, the practitioner is not on the job site with Manny but facilitating the intervention plan when he returns to the group home.

While Manny has been practicing initiating and sustaining conversations with others for the last year, the frequency and depth of these conversations will change. He is no longer able to simply poll other group home members for their deli choice, keep conversations short around a few typical safe topics, or stay task-focused such as ordering deli meat. Now Manny socializes with the same co-workers each week, and he identifies dinner break time with co-workers as the most stressful part of the job. Typically, co-workers get to know each other during break time and ask personal questions about family, interests, or outside activities. Peers will observe Manny's non-verbal communication in terms of eye contact, shifting in a seat, or rocking when nervous.

Manny will:

• converse with co-workers during dinner break,
• identify cues when someone is no longer interested in talking,
• identify one or two places to go for a quiet dinner break with fewer opportunities for socialization,
• practice stress management techniques to implement while talking with co-workers.

The practitioner will use a variety of modeling, role-play, and script writing to help Manny engage in conversations during the dinner break. While these methods are interventions to support occupations, it appears to be the most effective choice, as the practitioner cannot go onsite to the deli department. However, all of these interventions to support occupations must directly relate to Manny's situation at the grocery store.

In time, Manny may make a few friends at the deli department requiring more sustained conversation, possibly outside of work. He is ready to save money and begin learning how to meet potential partners. The practitioner will assist Manny in:

• determining how much money to save so he is able to take out a person on a date,
• how to approach a person that he is interested in talking to at work,
• discussing the pros and cons of dating others at work,
• where to meet others with similar interests.

TRY IT: Using the Guidesheet to Complete the Middle and Ending of the Intervention Plan

It is helpful to become more familiar with these clinical reasoning guidesheets, as you will eventually begin thinking about intervention while conducting the evaluations.

Make a copy of the MMCR Planning Guide to Address Specific Sections of the Overall Intervention Plan clinical guidesheet found in Appendix 4 to complete Manny's middle and ending part of the intervention plan based on the information provided in this chapter.

When to Spiral Up to the Top

Knowing when to incorporate the top is tricky and depends on the person's life story and identified goals. As mentioned in earlier chapters, during the intervention process, the person determines the top and/or middle. To embrace a person-focused approach, some connection of the top is addressed: from the beginning of the intervention plan if the practitioner solely identifies the middle; if the person served identifies both the middle and top (as in Manny's story), then the practitioner might have more time to begin incorporating the top into the middle or even at the end of the plan.

Yes, There Is a Beginning-Middle-Ending to All Intervention Plans, Even in Short-Term Placements: A-HA Moment

Manny's example illustrated the MMCR intervention approach over a year. This time frame shows the many intricate facets to help a person make change using trial and error, preferred learning styles, and relevant teaching-learning principles.

The MMCR also guides a practitioner in a much shorter-term stay. To illustrate this consider a seven-day, inpatient rehabilitation unit with a medical model philosophy. A short inpatient stay consists of two quick transitions: the beginning, where the person served learns about occupational therapy, functional implications of a diagnosis, routine of the rehab facility, results of the top- and bottom-oriented evaluations, etc. It is a shortened time, as the person only has a few hours of direct intervention time to become familiar with occupational therapy services. The second transition out of services occurs at the end of the week. The practitioner has about one hour left of direct intervention time to tie up loose ends, make referrals to interprofessional partners, and make recommendations to continue the change process depending on where the person is going next. The middle or bulk of the intervention practices and reinforces the top-middle-bottom occupational performance issues introduced during the first two days and concluded on day seven.

_____/_____/_____

1–2 days	3-4-5-6 days	7 day
Beginning	Middle	End

While this is not nearly as ideal to create change as the year-long intervention plan, it is the reality of our healthcare system. The turnaround time is very fast, creating the appearance that the beginning-middle-ending occur simultaneously. While the practitioner may continue evaluating for a baseline measure well into the third or fourth day, those initial processes need to begin on day one to promote some sense of normalcy, routine, and familiarity with the intervention process.

Summary

Before executing the intervention plan, practitioners often reflect on why they are proposing a specific direction to address a person's occupational performance issues. To make these plans more manageable and assist the practitioner to spiral the occupational performance issues across the continuum, mentally separate the overall interventions plan into specific sections consisting of a beginning, middle, and ending. Within each of these sections, practitioners then highlight central ideas that guide the rationale for selecting interventions and methods. During the beginning part of the intervention plan, the practitioners identify and create processes to initiate the change process related to the top-middle-bottom occupational performance issues. Once the processes have formed, it is time to move into the middle parts or "heavy lifting" of the intervention plan. Over the duration of the intervention plan, the practitioner uses the middle part for practice and reinforcement with an increase in task demands. The practitioner prepares for the next transition process during the ending sections of intervention, as the person will be transferring from services with an increased knowledge and/or skill set.

12 Strategizing How to Create Change During the Intervention Plan

Laurie Knis-Matthews and Margaret Swarbrick

Distinguishing Where the Person Is in the Change Process: Intervention Emphasizing Skill Building or First Creating an Awareness

Evaluation information guides the practitioner to establish a baseline measure for change related to the first top-middle-bottom(s). In other words, it helps the practitioner and person served or caregiver to determine intervention priorities to create change. The evaluation results also assist the practitioner to determine where the person is in this change process. Following the steps of the change process leading to development or elimination of habits, the person develops an awareness of the change, identifies reasons for this change and creates an action plan (Nemec et al., 2015). A person or caregiver needs to be aware of what change is taking place before carrying out the actions of this change.

The practitioner begins the intervention plan by identifying where the person is in the change process and uses this information to create increased awareness or skill building. However, addressing a person's self-awareness issues may not always occur at the start of the intervention plan, as it depends on multiple factors. Some people seek occupational therapy services with the awareness of an area to improve, strengthen or develop but are not sure how to pursue it. For example, a caregiver may know a child's handwriting is difficult to decipher but does not know how to make it more legible. A person diagnosed with a traumatic brain injury identifies difficulty in concentrating on tasks at work when more people enter a room but does not know how to change the office environment to minimize outside distractions.

Other times, people seek services without an awareness of what needs to be developed, improved or changed prior to making a plan of action. To clarify this point, consider the following examples: a tenant who is about to be evicted for loud nighttime activities but does not connect the late-night activities with an angry landlord who lives in the apartment downstairs; a parent whose child was just diagnosed with cancer and is just entering the healthcare arena but does not know anything about services or the diagnosis; a person who does not understand why the courts have mandated her to attend an anger management course.

Where the person is in this change process will influence the intervention plan in terms of where to begin, what processes to create, how long it takes for the change to occur, how much progress can be made over the duration of the intervention plan, what type of methods are selected and what type of teaching-learning principles are utilized.

The Role of Intervention When Individuals Are Facing Life-Threatening or Life-Ending Conditions: A-HA Moment

Traditionally, interventions, including those described in the intervention chapters, focus on improvement and skill building. However, there are times when an individual will not

---

DOI: 10.4324/9781003392408-14

be able to build skills and is actually in the process of losing abilities in movement, cognition and speech. These conditions can include Alzheimer's disease, amyotrophic lateral sclerosis, end-stage disease processes such as cancer or other chronic conditions. In these circumstances the intervention goals are focused on identifying meaningful life roles and occupations and addressing barriers to participation. The focus is often on pain management, symptom relief and supportive care that can optimize their quality of life for as long as possible through meaningful participation.

TRY IT: Intervention Plans Influence Where a Person Is in the Change Process

Based on the evaluation results, the practitioner determines if the intervention plan begins with assisting the person to create an awareness for change or if the person has already identified what needs to be changed but needs to develop the skills to implement this change.

Let us return to Manny's story to clarify this point. Manny is now working at the deli department and experiencing problems at work, especially sustaining conversation with others during dinner breaks.

Scenario 1: Manny articulates the reason for these problems at work but does not know how to change his behavior.

Scenario 2: Manny is having repeated problems at work but is unable to articulate why this keeps happening.

The first scenario suggests that Manny has awareness but not yet the skills to make change, while the second scenario implies Manny does not have the awareness or skills to make a change.

How will the intervention plan (specific sections, methods, teaching-learning principles) differ in scenario 1 and scenario 2? Explain the reasons for these differences in your suggested approach.

Addressing a Person's Awareness Can Happen During the Beginning, Middle and/or End of the Intervention Plan

This process is complicated and definitely a gray area. Intervention plans focusing on awareness and/or skill building do not fit into compartmentalized check-off columns; rather, parts of this plan constantly move between an emphasis on awareness and skill building. Almost every time a person experiences new learning, the practitioner first creates an awareness of this new technique, skill or method. For example, a person learning to use a sock aid first needs to understand why this adaptive device is important and how to use it during dressing. Once there is an increase in self-awareness, the skill building through practice, repetition and reinforcement eventually becomes habitual.

To make this more of a gray area, there are times where skill building takes priority over awareness. A practitioner collaborating with a person who has a safety concern will first implement a plan for action and then address the awareness later. For example, a person who constantly forgets to take his or her medication may pose a safety risk. The practitioner first implements specific memory aids to help the person remember to take these daily medications. Once a medication routine is created, then the practitioner may address the reasons (awareness) for this plan.

An Intervention Plan, Starting With Creating an Awareness for Change, Does Not Imply the Practitioner Determines What Needs to Be Changed: A-HA Moment

While it is helpful for the practitioner to conceptualize the process in terms of awareness and skill building across the intervention continuum, this does not imply that the practitioner solely determines what or how this process occurs. The person is the most central figure in the intervention plan. This person must be motivated to endure this often complicated and emotional process to sustain the desired behavior, habit or routine after services are discontinued.

Selecting and Incorporating Suitable Methods During the Intervention

The practitioner carefully selects relevant methods for each person served, and these methods differ depending on the section of the overall intervention plan. A seasoned practitioner uses multiple methods to reinforce change while spiraling the top-middle bottom across the duration of the intervention plan. This combination of methods continuously changes depending on the person's top-middle-bottom occupational performance issues, the segment of the intervention plan and how much awareness and/or skill building needs to be addressed.

For example, a practitioner begins Manny's intervention plan by *educating* him about social norms at the deli counter such as waiting for your number to be called to place a deli order or standing at a socially acceptable distance from the other customers while in line. Once Manny begins practicing for his interview at the grocery store during the middle of the intervention section, the practitioner may focus on *incorporating interventions to support occupations* such as role-playing interview scenarios. Finally, the method might emphasize *self-advocacy* as Manny begins to speak up for himself at work during dinner breaks or starts a conversation with a potential boyfriend.

Voices of the Practitioners: Incorporating Client-Centered and Occupation-Based Interventions

I have a patient who has terminal cancer. We are not necessarily working on every single one of those things that I originally outlined. We are also having conversations about how she can engage in the most meaningful occupation, but all in the context of what she is in at this moment in terms of safety, function and desire. (Morgan)

The majority of my caseload is in the day center, and I try to be as occupation based as I can, but I am stuck in the gym. I catch my clients if they need to go to the bathroom while switching groups. I walk into the bathroom to do toileting or hand washing. It required being more creative to make it functional. (Pam)

If I have all these amazing activities planned for my client and they are not interested, then I'm doing something wrong. I need to refocus, reprioritize and redistribute the time we're spending on certain things. (Rose)

Why does my father need to have a lift? Why does he need this customized shower chair or wheelchair? I often explain to the family members why they need a particular piece of equipment. To do this, I'm pulling my knowledge from treating people, with my knowledge of insurances and discharge planning. I need to explain the reason why, whether I'm talking to a family member or the vendor. (Louise)

> In an acute care hospital, the productivity, standards and overall pace of everything [are] so fast. There is an emphasis on talking less and doing more to get in and out quickly. But you miss so much if you don't stop to take the time to build that rapport, use your therapeutic use of self and obtain that occupational profile to guide the intervention plan. (Jackie)

Before moving deeper into a discussion about intervention planning along the continuum, it is necessary to revisit information about occupations. In MMCR, the practitioner must consider the construct of occupations in two related but distinct ways. First, as part of the person-environment-occupation data gathering process, the practitioner must understand the meaningful activities and occupations related to the person's story and context. Once this is determined (as identified on the MMCR triangle under the occupation and activities section), the practitioner uses this information to begin formulating a plan incorporating a combination of methods to support purposeful occupations central to their well-being.

According to the *Occupational Therapy Practice Framework* (OTPF), there are a variety of methods to select from when implementing occupation-based practice, including therapeutic use of occupations and activities, interventions to support occupations, education, training, advocacy, self-advocacy, groups and virtual formats (AOTA, 2020). The type of method(s) selected for intervention depends on multiple factors such as the person's story, environmental context, goals and/or practice location, etc. As each situation is unique, the methods are carefully selected and unique for each person.

TRY IT: Incorporating Different Types of Methods Into the Intervention Plan

In your own words, describe the eight suggested types of methods and provide examples of ways these methods, used alone or in combination, can guide a person's intervention plan.

Next, reflect on Manny's story to identify how each method can be used in some combination throughout the intervention plan for the suggested year-long intervention or identify ways these methods would change if the duration of intervention was shorter.

Therapeutic use of occupations and activities
Interventions to support occupations
Education
Training
Advocacy
Self-advocacy
Group intervention
Virtual interventions

Let's Examine Another Case Example Emphasizing the "How" to Intervention Planning: Sojourn's Story

A practitioner working on a detox unit may be allotted forty-eight to seventy-two hours of intervention time prior to the person being discharged to the next location. This shortened amount of time is a crucial factor when deciding which method a practitioner can offer to benefit the person served. To illustrate this point, Sojourn is a twenty-year-old female who is experiencing her first hospitalization for drug detox. In this situation, it would be essential for the practitioner to gather data about Sojourn's story and occupations so the next practitioner is ready to begin intervention in a place that will be client centered, meaningful and occupation-based from day one. However, when interviewed in her room, Sojourn appeared fatigued, agitated and tearful while experiencing intense withdrawal symptoms from a heroin addiction. During this short interview, she described limited interest in recovery, but she has agreed to transfer to a longer-term drug rehabilitation inpatient unit after detoxification.

Top: some willingness to pursue recovery by cutting down or quitting use of substance
Middle: transition from the role and responsibility of a patient in a detox unit into a drug rehabilitation inpatient unit
Bottom: coping with intense withdrawal

Groups are a common method of intervention in this practice location. In combination with an educational format, groups are an effective arrangement for many people to share their story, create a sense of belonging and discuss resources for recovery. However, due to the intense withdrawal symptoms, the group format may not be the most effective approach for Sojourn. Instead, within this short time, her intervention plan emphasizes an education method done at bedside or alone. The practitioner will provide Sojourn with general knowledge (to create an awareness) about the benefits of recovery, the expectations of the drug rehabilitation inpatient unit and examine immediate strategies to help her manage withdrawal.

Undeniably, occupation-based practice is viewed as the preferred method of intervention, representing our core value of care (Gillen et al., 2019). According to Golledge (1998), the practitioner should use activities minimally or not at all, as it may lead to selection of interventions that are preparatory activities and not occupation based. While there is a place for these types of interventions (hot packs, role-play scenarios, completing topic worksheets, splint construction), practitioners do not always use these techniques as intended steppingstones to reach occupation-based interventions. For example, following Sojourn's story, a practitioner could offer interventions that support occupations such as learning how to pause and breathe when feeling anxious or overwhelmed by withdrawal symptoms and fear of the restrictions on the inpatient setting.

In the Choosing Wisely Campaign, Glen Gillen uses the label non-purposeful to describe a classification of activities that are less effective and unnecessary when used by a practitioner to help a person facilitate change (Gillen, 2013; Richardson, 2018). The examples of non-purposeful activities such as moving cones around, putting pegs on boards or running your fingers up and down a wall ladder does not promote personal choice—it creates disconnects to the person's actual life story and lacks eventual support toward a person's occupations (Gillen, 2013; Golledge, 1998). Most people are not professional cone stackers or call their families after a long day in therapy to talk about how many pegs they put on a board. Following Sojourn's story, a practitioner could implement non-purposeful activities such as making a collage depicting people engaging in different types of coping skills. (Note: The collage is not a recommended activity for Sojourn but is listed to provide an example.)

While occupation-based practice is the gold standard of care, many obstacles can influence the degree to which how occupational based an intervention can be such as practice locations steeped in the medical model tradition, shortened intervention times and external factors including reimbursement and productivity pressures. Instead of viewing occupation-based as an all-or-nothing type of intervention, perhaps it is important for the practitioner to consider how many occupation-based characteristics are incorporated throughout the intervention plan.

For example, in the earlier example of collaborating with Sojourn on a detox unit, it is undeniable that the practitioner will not achieve the ideal implementation of occupation-based intervention in two to three days while on a medically focused unit. Do not be discouraged and default to non-purposeful activities, steppingstones that support occupations without any intention of reaching the middle or top or following norms of using the same old intervention methods placing the responsibility on Sojourn to assimilate. Consider how a practitioner can collaborate to create an intervention plan that incorporates some characteristics of occupation-based intervention.

TRY IT: Incorporating Characteristics of Occupation-Based Intervention

Review the core characteristics of occupation- and client-centered principles to begin strategizing how this information can be infused into the intervention plan.
What client-centered characteristics are apparent in Sojourn's intervention plan listed earlier?
   Based on these characteristics, describe one or two other intervention ideas that the practitioner can implement on a two- to three-day detox unit or on a slightly longer five- to seven-day inpatient unit.

Since Sojourn is experiencing intense withdrawal, consider dividing the expected sixty minutes of occupational therapy services per day (she probably cannot manage that much at one time) into fifteen-minute segments. The practitioner will be able to reinforce these intervention plans four times a day over eight sessions if she is discharged in two days. The practitioner decided to approach this plan with an emphasis on educating Sojourn at bedside or in her room. This will also allow more time to understand her story and communicate it to the next practitioner working with Sojourn in the inpatient unit. The practitioner will

- introduce and practice one or two relevant coping skills for the withdrawal symptoms at bedside such as deep breathing or visualization,
- gather information about the implicit and explicit rules of the future inpatient unit to share with Sojourn before discharge. This written list incorporates understandable language with lots of white space and large font, so she can take it with her upon discharge,
- begin short conversations about what life in recovery would look and feel like and what occupations she would want to focus on to support her recovery such as sleep and rest, activities of daily living (ADLs), work, school, etc.

Reflecting back on some of the characteristics of occupation relevant to this suggested intervention approach, imparting information on Sojourn's next specific inpatient unit, practicing coping skills to be done in bed and beginning a short conversation about the twelve-step program for addiction recovery are relevant, meaningful and unique to Sojourn's life story. The emphasized educational method is a good match to implement this client-centered intervention plan (and it did not include a group format).

Reflecting on Occupation-Based Intervention: A-HA Moment

All aspects of the intervention continuum are fluid and dynamic throughout the process, as initial top-middle-bottoms are resolved or changed, services are terminated earlier than expected or a person progresses faster or slower than originally anticipated.

The construct of occupation is a central part of the person-environment-occupation data gathering process. The practitioner must understand the meaningful activities and occupations related to the person's story and context. The practitioner uses this information to begin formulating a plan incorporating a combination of methods to support occupations that are purposeful to the person and central to his or her well-being.

There are a variety of methods to implement occupation-based practice, including therapeutic use of occupations and activities, interventions to support occupations, education, training, advocacy, self-advocacy, groups and virtual formats. As each situation is unique, the methods for creating change are carefully selected and vary with each person seeking services.

While occupation-based practice is the gold standard of care, there are many obstacles that can influence the degree to which how occupational based an intervention can be. Instead of viewing occupation based as an all-or-nothing type of intervention, consider how many occupation-based characteristics are incorporated throughout the intervention plan.

Additional Considerations for Method Selection

Do not always begin the continuum with interventions that support occupations, as sometimes this method will be more effective toward the middle or even at the end of the intervention plan. There is a misconception that intervention supporting occupations should primarily be introduced at the beginning of the intervention plan and then follow a progression to activities and then finally to occupations. Incorporate interventions that support occupations when new learning is introduced, the person is transitioning to a new location or a task is becoming increasingly complex, as it may ease a person's stress levels.

Select methods based on the person's learning style, top-middle-bottom occupational performance issues and life story rather than the practice location. While practitioners have clinical reasoning skills to determine the methods that are best for each person served, outside influences related to practice settings, medical concerns or reimbursement guidelines often dictate preferred methods. For example, reflect on why a group format is a common method for use in certain practice locations. Will every person served benefit from this method of intervention, or is it influenced by administrative policy?

Incorporate different methods for each section of the beginning-middle-ending part of the intervention plan. Each section of the intervention plan has a different focus and goals (determined by the why), so adjust the methods accordingly. Carefully combining different types of methods will solidify a person's learning process and keep them motivated at the same time.

Suitable methods selected relate to where the person is within the change process (awareness and/or skill building) and relevant teaching-learning principles to match the person's learning style and life experiences. Each of these areas are equally important to consider when implementing a relevant intervention plan.

Selecting and Incorporating Suitable Teaching-Learning Principles During Intervention

Once the practitioner has an overall sense of what the person wants to change (ꝏ) and where in the change process the person is (awareness or skill building), the next step is to incorporate relevant teaching-learning principles throughout the methods chosen for each section of the intervention plan. The intention of occupational therapy intervention is to assist people in making meaningful life changes that will be sustained upon termination of services. It is the responsibility of the practitioner to use relevant teaching-learning principles embedded in practice to assist the person to move through the change process to develop competency and sustainable habits.

Teaching and learning are at the core of all intervention. Practitioners spend considerable amounts of time teaching people new and creative ways to perform meaningful tasks, such as teaching someone how to insert a tampon with the use of one arm, maneuvering an electric wheelchair around the park for participation in a family outing, cleaning and maintaining a splint to use during work, washing and keeping clean while using a public restroom or completing an application for a Social Security card. Most people served will not be motivated to "learn" how to stack cones, play games or do passive range-of-motion exercises.

Review the teaching-learning process guidelines listed next. These guidelines were compiled by multiple sources (American Psychological Association, 2015; Carnegie Mellon University, n.d.; DiPietro, n.d.; Dumont et al., 2010; Mosey, 1986; Principles of Learning, n.d.). Practitioners should carefully select those principles that align with the peoples' learning preferences, prior experiences and where they are in the change process in order to guide the development of the intervention plan and intervention methods.

Guidelines to the Teaching-Learning Process

Characteristics of the **person** that influence learning:

1. It is more motivating for the person to identify what needs to be learned rather than being told by other people.
2. Age, gender, race, culture and life experiences.
3. Active involvement.
4. A person's attention and perception influence learning.
5. The person should understand what needs to be learned, why this is necessary and how specifically it will relate to their life situation.
6. Learning should begin at the person's current level and proceed at a steady but comfortable progression. The learning process cannot be rushed. The person will be bored if the learning is too basic and overwhelmed if the learning is too complicated.
7. Each person experiences some degree of stress during a new learning situation.

Characteristics of the **environment** that influence learning:

1. Each time people change locations, their stress level increases.
2. Reflect on all facets of a person's environment (location, physical, temporal, social, cultural and virtual) and consider the pros and cons of each location where learning will take place.
3. Organize the physical environment to support the person's ability to learn.
4. Create a supportive collaborative learning environment.
5. Generalizing learning to new environmental contexts is not a spontaneous process, but needs to be facilitated, practiced and nurtured.

Considerations to promote learning during an intervention plan:

1. Setting goals that are short term, specific, clear and moderately challenging enhances motivation more than goals that are long term, general and overly challenging.
2. Start with small accomplishments of simplified information and then build it up to complex information.
3. Focus on skills the person wants to learn and use in their everyday lives.

4. Show interest in the person's thoughts and opinions, even if they differ from others.
5. Utilize such techniques as trial and error, shaping and modeling others.
6. Provide reinforcement and positive feedback throughout the learning processes that lays the foundation for subsequent experiences.
7. Frequent repetition and practice solidify learning.
8. Provide clear, explanatory and timely feedback.
9. Body language sends powerful messages during the teaching-learning process.
10. Carefully select relevant teaching methods to support each specific person's preferred learning style.

TRY IT: Infusing Teaching-Learning Principles Into the Intervention Plan

While this is not an exhaustive list, many of the teaching-learning principles discussed throughout the book might be familiar. Reflect on and discuss each of the identified teaching-learning principles. Research and identify more teaching-learning principles you can try and apply in your work.

Teach Information Directly Related to the Person's Top-Middle-Bottom for the Intended Location(s)

Very often practitioners select the same activity or methods to use with a majority of people they serve without careful attention to the individual's experiences, perceptions and goals. Using activities, methods or teaching information that is peripheral or unrelated to a person's top-middle-bottom won't engage and benefit the person served. It requires less time and energy for the practitioner to teach information more aligned to their experiences and comfort level, rather than focus on what the person served needs to learn. While practitioners are not experts on all worldviews and occupations, they will need to become familiar with any new learning before teaching it to others. There are many ways to become more familiar with new learning before teaching it to others such as reading research about the topic, interviewing others with similar experiences, watching videos or practicing the skill directly.

Be Mindful of Locations and Fluctuating Stress Levels When Incorporating New Learning Into the Intervention Plan

Even if the practitioner provides the person with opportunities for direct learning, generalizing new information from one situation or environmental context does not automatically occur, but requires time, attention and practice. When teaching a new skill, place careful attention on a person's environmental context and consider motivational factors. The practitioner considers all relevant locations from the person's story and where intervention occurs. The practice location may not align with the person's locations associated with their life story. The practitioner must keep in mind the intended location(s) when selecting relevant teaching-learning principles.

While being mindful of the varied locations, each time a person changes location, stress levels increase, even if considered good stress. For example, while an occupational therapy student excitedly anticipates the beginning of fieldwork, there is a certain comfort level being in the classroom in terms of instructor expectations, peer groups and classroom familiarity. In the classroom, students may be able to sustain new and complicated learning for a longer time, because all other facets of the environment are familiar and predictable. A new location (environment) consisting of different social groups, norms and expectations creates elevated stress at the beginning of the fieldwork experience, influencing a student's skill performance. It may take a while to reach competency of skills (this is why occupational therapy students complete months, not days or weeks, of fieldwork).

This increase in stress level is similar for people served. Each time a person changes locations, expect new learning to be slower and challenging until other environmental facets become more familiar. If the practitioner has the opportunity to work with a person in multiple locations throughout the duration of the intervention, consider introducing the new learning and increasing expectations first in a familiar location. For example, Manny's group home is a safe and familiar location where new learning is first introduced and then incrementally practiced within the food store location. While this location was very motivating for Manny it also created elevated levels of stress. Over time, the food store location became more familiar, and the expectations gradually increased.

TRY IT: Incorporating Teaching-Learning Principles and Methods Into Lola's Intervention

Lola identifies as a woman who is thirty years old, homeless and living under a bridge with two other people. After eating rotten food, she experienced a severe bacterial infection leading to hospitalization and subsequent occupational therapy services. Lola spends her day collecting food from dumpsters and garbage cans near the bridge but has difficulty deciding which food is good or spoiled to eat (bottom related to decision making and problem solving). Because she had negative experiences with food banks and does not want governmental assistance upon discharge, Lola plans to return to living under the bridge (top) and will continue similar practices of securing and eating available food near the bridge (middle). She has not made a direct connection to eating rotten food with her current bacterial infection (focus on increasing awareness of the change process) but is open to suggestions on how to stop getting so sick after eating (motivation for change).

Upon reading this information, the intervention plan will focus on making decisions and solving problems while securing non-spoiled foods in the surrounding neighborhood near the bridge.

Following Lola's story, the practitioner may teach her:

1. how to purchase healthier and safer foods to eat on a very limited budget,
2. how to cook healthier foods in a safer manner,
3. about available resources such as shelters, potential disability assistance and food banks
4. how to recognize the differences between spoiled and unspoiled foods.

The first three teaching areas are peripheral to her plan. It appears that Lola is interested in returning to her home under the bridge and continuing to secure food by frequenting dumpsters and garbage cans. Healthy food is expensive, and she might not have the money to purchase healthy food or proper equipment to cook foods.

She already mentioned a disinterest in pursuing homeless shelters, applying for government assistance or buying food, so spending time teaching her about these resources may not be relevant to her immediate future location.

The last teaching area directly relates to her plan. Spending time teaching Lola about specific types of spoiled and unspoiled food commonly found in the nearby dumpsters and garbage cans will be more meaningful. This new learning has more chances to carry over from one location into the next. The practitioner could review and discuss YouTube video clips demonstrating these practices or bring in spoiled food to demonstrate comparisons.

Reflect on Lola's story. Identify what information you need to learn before teaching it to Lola. Identify various teaching-learning principles and methods you will use throughout the intervention plan.

Summary

Practitioners simultaneously consider the reasoning why they are developing an intervention plan in a certain way while also strategizing how to create this change for the person served. Strategizing how this change will occur throughout the intervention plan involves planning for such factors as determining how to increase a person's self-awareness or skill building, incorporating suitable intervention methods, utilizing relevant teaching-learning principles and upgrading and downgrading activities based on the person's status. As each person and situation are unique, these factors are carefully selected for each person. This continuously changes depending on the person's top-middle-bottom occupational performance issues, the segment of the intervention plan and how much awareness and/or skill building needs to be addressed.

References

American Occupational Therapy Association. (2020). Occupational therapy practice framework: Domain and process (4th ed.). *American Journal of Occupational Therapy, 74*(Suppl. 2), 7412410010. https://doi.org/10.5014/ajot.2020.74S2001

American Psychological Association. (2015). *Top 20 principles.* www.apa.org/ed/schools/teaching-learning/top-twenty-principles.pdf

Carnegie Mellon University. (n.d.). *Learning principles: Theory and research-based principles of learning.* Eberly Center. www.cmu.edu/teaching/principles/learning.html

DiPietro, M. (n.d.). *How learning works: The seven learning principles.* https://cetl.kennesaw.edu/how-learning-works-seven-learning-principles

Dumont, H., Istance, D., & Benavides, F. (Eds.). (2010). *The nature of learning: Using research to inspire practice.* www.oecd.org/education/ceri/50300814.pdf

Gillen, G. (2013). A fork in the road: An occupational hazard? *American Journal of Occupational Therapy, 67*, 641–652. https://doi.org/10.5014/ajot.2013.676002

Gillen, G., Hunter, E. G., Lieberman, D., & Stutzbach, M. (2019). AOTA's top 5 choosing Wisely® recommendations. *American Journal of Occupational Therapy, 73*, 302420010. https://doi.org/10.5014/ajot.2019.732001

Golledge, J. (1998). Distinguishing between occupation, purposeful activity and activity, part 1: Review and explanation. *British Journal of Occupational Therapy, 61*(3), 100–105. https://doi.org/10.1177/030802269806100301

Mosey, A. C. (1986). *Psychosocial components of occupational therapy.* Raven Press.

Nemec, P., Swarbrick, M., & Merlo, D. (2015). The force of habit: Creating and sustaining a wellness lifestyle. *Journal of Psychosocial Nursing, 53*(9), 24–30. https://doi.org/10.3928/02793695-20150821-01

Principles of Learning. (n.d.). www.ednet.ns.ca/files/curriculum/Prin-of-Lrn.pdf

Richardson, H. (2018). *Choosing Wisely® Q&A: Glen Gillen on non-purposeful intervention activities.* www.aota.org/publications-news/otp/archive/2018/choosing-wisely-nonpurposeful-activities.aspx

Section 3

Documentation

13 Documentation Overview and the Evaluation Summary

Laurie Knis-Matthews and Ashley N. Fuentes

The Four Basic Ingredients to Effective Documentation

This chapter will begin with a review of the four basic ingredients to effective documentation. Each ingredient is essential to form the foundation for an overall documentation plan.

1. Strengths
2. Challenges
3. Raw data
4. Interpretation

Strengths and Challenges

It is vital for occupational therapy practitioners to capture and embrace a person's strengths. All human beings have strengths, but they may present in different ways such as traits, behaviors, attributes, skills, accomplishments and/or satisfying life experiences. A person's strengths, first documented during the evaluation summary, are included in all subsequent progress notes and discharge summaries. Too often, documentation tends to highlight the challenges or what a person needs to "fix", rather than creating a balance. Unfortunately, rather than integrating a person's strengths fully throughout a person's story, it is often reduced to a few sentences at the end of an evaluation summary or progress note.

A practitioner's ability to learn about the person's story and highlight strengths and goals distinguishes occupational therapy from other professions. Accentuating a person's strengths in all forms of documentation will provide other professional partners with a balanced perspective and help formulate intervention strategies more efficiently. In other words, an occupational therapy practitioner might be the best person on the interprofessional team who can articulate strengths with specificity to a person's story. Using the MMCR, a practitioner reflects and documents those strengths related to the top-middle-bottom occupational performance issues.

However, there needs to be a balance of both strengths and challenges in documentation. Most times, a person seeks therapy to overcome some type of challenge(s). In documentation, these identified challenges form the basis of the intervention plan, with progress periodically monitored. Rather than documenting every challenge a person is currently experiencing, the practitioner strategically identifies and prioritizes relevant challenges to the person's story based on top and bottom evaluations selected, the person, environmental facets and occupations.

Raw Data and Interpretation

Raw data are factual or objective statements that paint a picture about a person's behaviors, skills and/or verbal statements. These objective statements, or the raw data, are necessary to provide the

DOI: 10.4324/9781003392408-16

reader with synthesized information of what occurred during the evaluation and intervention process without subjective interpretation. A practitioner carefully documents these factual statements in a neutral stance (without personal bias) and without interpretation. Just state the facts. Raw data can come from a variety of sources such as informal observations, the occupational profile documenting the person's own words or actions taken during a bottom-oriented evaluation that eventually determines a standardized assessment score.

It is important for the practitioner to be as factual as possible. Words and actions matter. For example, does the person consistently cry when discussing the reasons for hospitalization? Does a person consistently discuss the loss of his wife during conversations with others? Documenting observable skills and/or behaviors when presenting evaluation data is also equally important. For example, when administering the money management section of the Kohlman Evaluation of Living Skills Evaluation (KELS) (Kohlman & Robnett, 2016), in addition to the score, it is equally relevant to describe how that score (based on interpretation) was determined. In other words, what did the practitioner observe? It may be equally important to describe other observations such as how the person manipulates the coins or calculates change from a purchase.

However, documenting the raw data, or just the facts, alone is not enough. Interpretations represent the practitioner's subjective understanding about the person's behaviors, skills and/or verbal statements documented within the raw data. As experts in our profession, practitioners should make interpretations about the data collected during the evaluation process within our domain of concern. Interpretations form the basis for types of probing questions asked during an occupational profile or how an evaluation score connects to a specific person's story. Interpretations are based on sound clinical reasoning and evidence, rather than personal experience or bias.

Along with a balance of strengths and challenges, both raw data and interpretation statements form the foundation for effective documentation. A practitioner providing only raw data does not connect the dots about the person's story based on our area of expertise. In contrast, a practitioner providing only interpretations does not provide the necessary raw data to support potential hunches.

TRY IT: Distinguishing the Four Essential Ingredients of Effective Documentation

In your own words, describe how strengths, challenges, raw data and interpretation each uniquely contribute toward communicating the evaluation findings to others.

Distinguishing the difference between raw data and interpretations is more challenging than it may appear. Review these "hypothetical" situations to determine if it is raw data or interpretations. Underline the word(s) that are interpretations, and rewrite the statement using only raw data information.

The client refuses to shower, so she was unkempt and malodorous.

The patient was very unsafe during the wheelchair transfer to the chair.

Max's difficulty with concentration is affecting his handwriting skills.

The consumer was hesitant to start the activity.

Christine appeared stressed during the interview session.

Patient has a delusion that he is married with three children.

Visual Overview of the Documentation Process From the MMCR Perspective

At this point in the process, using specific frames of reference and/or practice models as a guideline for action, the practitioner has completed the evaluations, identified the initial top-middle-bottom occupational performance issues, has mentally formulated an intervention plan and is now preparing the evaluation summary. The evaluation summary also includes long-term and short-term goals aligned with the top-middle-bottom occupational performance issues. The practitioner monitors the progress of these goals over the duration of the continuum for intervention.

Evaluation summary _____x_____/PN_____/PN_____/PN & discharge summary

*PN stands for progress note.

This horizontal continuum and vertical lines should be familiar from the previous chapters about intervention planning. Conceptualize the same visual overview, but now emphasize the documentation process. The evaluation summary is information taken from the occupational profile and analysis of performance selections. Placed at the beginning of the horizontal line, the evaluation summary emphasizes the most pressing top-middle-bottom occupational performance issue(s) for the specific person served.

How the Evaluation, Intervention and Documentation Processes Work Together: A-HA Moment

The practitioner selects occupational profiles (tops) and analysis of performance (bottoms) as part of the evaluation process for each person served. Once the evaluation information is formulated around the constructs of person-environment-occupation, the most pressing top-middle-bottom occupational performance issue(s) are determined. While practitioners begin constructing the evaluation summary, they simultaneously mentally plan the intervention process in terms of the beginning, middle and ending sections. Relevant documentation such as long-term/short-term goals, progress notes and discharge summaries mirror this intervention process.

Evaluation Summaries

At this point, the practitioner is aware that strengths, challenges, raw data and interpretations centered around the occupational performance issues form the foundation to effective documentation (evaluation summaries, progress notes, discharge summaries, etc.). Typically, evaluation summaries are the first comprehensive piece of occupational therapy documentation written about the person seeking services and can be the most complicated.

An evaluation summary provides a snapshot of a person's baseline centered on the initial top-middle-bottom(s) occupational performance issues. A practitioner does not need to include every small detail about the person served nor include areas peripheral to the top-middle-bottom occupational performance issues. For example, from this perspective, reexamine a typical medical chart for entries that are peripheral to the top-middle-bottom occupational performance issues. Typical medical chart entries focus on how well a person slept or if they ate all of their meal, but this is peripheral to a person's story unless they are struggling with insomnia or eating a meal due to body image issues or gastroenterology issues.

Relevant areas to the person's evaluation findings	Strengths	Challenges	Raw Data	Interpretation

Figure 13.1 Clinical Reasoning Guidesheet: MMCR Guide to Evaluation Summaries.

How does the practitioner mentally shift through all the information obtained during the evaluation process to determine what is included in the evaluation summary? Actually, following the MMCR, this part of clinical reasoning is completed (in wet sand). Refer back to Appendix 1, "The MMCR Guide to Understanding a Person's Story (Triangle)." Using this clinical reasoning guidesheet, the practitioner has compartmentalized all the incoming evaluation findings around the three constructs of person, environment and occupation leading to the first top-middle-bottom occupational performance issue(s).

Now it is time to determine what specific information from the person-environment-occupation triangle will be used to create the evaluation summary. Expand on parts of the specific information taken from the triangle to include all four ingredients to effective documentation (strengths, challenges, raw data and interpretations). To help conceptualize this process, refer to Figure 13.1 (also found in Appendix 5: "MMCR Guide to Evaluation Summaries" clinical reasoning guidesheet).

Divided into five columns (relevant areas to the person's evaluation findings, strengths, challenges, raw data and interpretations), the guidesheet highlights the most important parts of the person's story that will be transferred into the evaluation summary.

To begin this process, the practitioner brainstorms some important detailed areas that might be included in the evaluation summary around the previously selected top-middle-bottom(s) occupational performance issues. Moving across each row, the practitioner identifies if each area is considered a strength, challenge or both. This check-off visual will help keep the practitioner mindful of creating a balance. Next, the practitioner documents all raw data related to each area. The raw data comes from a variety of sources such as observations, occupational profiles, analysis of performance evaluations, conversations with significant others, etc. Describe this raw data in detail and without judgment. Finally, after reflecting on each area, strengths, challenges and raw data, the practitioner offers a perspective or interpretation on what it all means to the specific person's story.

Does It Appear That You Are Repeating the Same Information About the Person's Story?: A-HA Moment

Does it appear you are writing similar information about the person on all of these clinical reasoning guidesheets? That is because you are! A person's story and goals stay the same. It does not matter what guidelines for action, occupational profile or documentation format is used during the intervention plan. The practitioner must determine how to create change with the person remaining as the central figure of the plan.

Are you having difficulty completing these clinical reasoning guidesheets? Consider going back to the person for a more in-depth understanding of the person's story. This clinical reasoning model will not work if the practitioner remains superficial and skims the surface of the person's story.

MMCR: Integrating These Four Ingredients for Effective Documentation

There are different styles of documentation formats (i.e., Subjective, Objective, Assessment and Plan [SOAP note] (Gateley & Borcherding, 2017); Data, Assessment and Plan (DAP note) (Cameron & Turtle-Song, 2002; Mahmoud, 2019) and communication methods (paper entries, electronic, narratives, fill in the blank). Similar to these styles, incorporating a person's strengths, challenges, raw data and interpretations into documentation is not unique to this clinical reasoning model. How the practitioner incorporates these ingredients differs from other formats, however.

Most evaluation summary formats separate the raw data and the interpretations into separate sections. First, the practitioner presents the objective evaluation findings and then offers subjective interpretations about those findings. Instead, consider integrating a person's strengths, challenges, raw data and interpretations related to the specific top-middle-bottom occupational performance issues altogether in one section. Substantiate interpretation with relevant raw data statements while presenting both the strengths and challenges.

MMCR: Documenting an Evaluation Summary Using the POP Acronym

Consider three basic parts to the evaluation summary, using the acronym POP to make it easier to recall and organize.

Person
Occupational Performance Issues
Plan

Evaluation Summary: Person

This first section of the evaluation summary provides relevant information about the person's situation so the reader can see the bigger picture. This will provide clarity for the reader to follow the specific evaluation results described in the next section in the evaluation summary. The practitioner strategically selects important background information to understand how the evaluation findings align with the person's story.

It may include detailed information about:

- Dates and reasons for the occupational therapy services referral
- Start and end date of the initial evaluation data collection
- Brief description of the type of evaluation(s) used (occupational profile and analysis of performance)
- Brief description of the person, including relevant information such as age, education, ethnic identity, diagnosis, health considerations, medications, race, religion, sexual orientation, spirituality and socioeconomic status
- Important events leading up to the referral for occupational therapy services
- Person's identified goals

Refer back to Appendix 1: "The MMCR Guide to Understanding a Person's Story (Triangle)" clinical reasoning guidesheet. The Person section has many of these unique characteristics identified in this section of the evaluation summary.

Evaluation Summary: Occupational Performance Issues

This next section of the evaluation summary highlights the person's unique life story obtained from the top- (occupational profile) and bottom-oriented (analysis of performance) evaluations. All strengths, challenges, raw data and interpretations emphasizing the top-middle-bottom occupational performance issues are included in this section of the evaluation summary.

When creating this part of the evaluation summary, use the information from Appendix 5 for a clinical reasoning guidesheet entitled "MMCR Guide to Evaluation Summaries." This guides the practitioner to compartmentalize relevant strengths, challenges, raw data and interpretations from the evaluation findings. Once this information is deconstructed and analyzed separately, the practitioner synthesizes the information, forming the foundation of the evaluation summary. All information presented in this section directly funnels into the intervention plan.

Note: The more time a practitioner spends on this clinical reasoning guidesheet, the easier it will be to "lift" this information into the actual evaluation summary.

Evaluation Summary: Plan

Now that the practitioner has described relevant information about the person's situation and provided specific evaluation results, it is time to document an action plan, including both long-term and short-term goals. Prior to creating these goals, the practitioner has already mentally formulated a potential intervention plan, making this process easier. Goal creation is a collaborative process that includes specific people, groups or populations involved such as:

- The person served
- Family members and/or significant others
- Religious, work or school group personnel
- The occupational therapy practitioner and other members of the interprofessional team
- Regulatory agencies

Voices of the Practitioners: How I Create the Goals for My Intervention Plan

I definitely let the client guide what the goals are so I can prioritize what is important. I have the person identify the strengths, barriers and the top three areas for me they want to focus on. (Kristen)

I usually ask the parents what their top three or four goals are for their child and what's most meaningful to them as caregivers. This is powerful because we know when the person's buying into it and it's motivating to them then they are likely to participate. (Casey)

I follow my process of understanding the person, environment and occupation. The goals change based on who the client is, but the process never changes. (Morgan)

Prior to creating goals, refer back to Appendix 3: "MMCR Overview Guide to Intervention Planning" and Appendix 4: "MMCR Planning Guide to Address Specific Sections of the Overall Intervention Plan" clinical reasoning guidesheets. Be mindful of the following information:

- What are the pros and cons of occupational therapy services delivered at this practice area location?
- How long do I have to work with this person, and what can be accomplished in this time frame?
- How many hours do I have to work with the person during each beginning-middle-ending section of intervention?
- What frame of reference and/or practice model influenced my intervention plan?
- What is the central idea of each beginning-middle-ending section?
- Am I focusing on creating a person's self-awareness or skill building in each section?
- What teaching-learning principles will promote change?

Summary

Effective documentation should be balanced by highlighting a person's strengths and challenges, backed up with detailed objective statements along with the suggested meaning of this information from an occupational therapy perspective. The MMCR Guide to Evaluation Summaries clinical reasoning guidesheet provides a blueprint for occupational therapy practitioners to determine that all four of these ingredients are incorporated around the top-middle-bottom occupational performance issues.

Once this step is completed, the practitioner is now able to use the POP acronym to write an evaluation summary highlighting the first set of occupational performance issues. In the first section, the practitioner describes the person (P) in terms of relevant background information, evaluations selected and/or identified goals. The next section (O) focuses on the identified occupational performance issues relevant to the person's story. This section incorporates the person's strengths, challenges, raw data and interpretations previously identified on the MMCR Guide to Evaluation Summaries clinical reasoning guidesheet. Finally, the evaluation summary ends with the plan (P) that provides the long-term and short-term goals to be achieved.

References

Cameron, S., & Turtle-Song, I. (2002). Learning to write case notes using the SOAP format. *Journal of Counseling and Development, 80*(3), 286–292. https://doi.org/10.1002/j.1556-6676.2002.tb00193.x

Gateley, C. A., & Borcherding, S. (2017). *Documentation manual for occupational therapy: Writing SOAP notes* (4th ed.). Slack Incorporated.

Kohlman, L., & Robnett, R. (2016). *KELS: Kohlman evaluation of living skills*. AOTA Press.

Mahmoud, S. H. (2019). *Patient assessment in clinical pharmacy: A comprehensive guide*. Springer International Publishing.

14 Documentation Continued

Goal Creation, Progress Notes, and Discharge Summaries

Laurie Knis-Matthews and Ashley N. Fuentes

Case Examples to Examine Goal Creation: Introducing Suzie and Joan

Suzie and Joan are two women who have difficulty regulating their emotions related to anger. Admitted to an inpatient psychiatric unit, Suzie is a 20-year-old woman living with her mother in a two-room apartment. Through observations, Suzie spits, clenches her fists, and raises her voice when her anger is escalating but is not aware of these behaviors until they are uncontrollable. Since the COVID-19 pandemic, Suzie is unable to participate in the day program she has attended for ten years and stays inside most of the day. For exercise and fresh air, Suzie's mom insists they walk around the neighborhood block daily. The adjustment to this new walking routine creates tension in the household and often escalates to the point where Suzie begins hitting her mother.

Joan entered outpatient services after completing a court-ordered drug rehabilitation program. During the occupational profile, Joan spoke about her increased dependency on cocaine. She is aware that she uses cocaine when getting angry, especially within specific work situations. Joan's boss in the shoe department at the discount department store constantly made sexual comments to her during work. Joan attempts to deescalate her angry feelings by snorting cocaine during work hours, but this method of de-escalation is becoming more habitual and creating further tensions with co-workers. Although the immediate boss was fired, Joan is angry with her co-workers for not helping her deal with the situation. She reports continued snorting cocaine daily during work to keep her anger in check. However, Joan is often late for work and irritable when working with the customers in the shoe department. These actions are habitual, and she reports being unable to change this behavior.

MMCR: Creating Long-Term Goals

A long-term goal represents a task that a person intends to accomplish in the future, requiring extended time and planning. The practitioner formulates the long-term goals in conjunction with a person's overall intervention plan, delineating the parameters for overall anticipated progress. The short-term goals provide blueprints for this overall achievement.

However, creating long-term goals is not easy. In the example that follows, the long-term goal addresses a child's age-appropriate scribbling but does not provide any context for why the child needs this skill. The two short-term goals do not align with the proposed long-term goal. The child improving their range of motion or stacking blocks does not necessarily generalize over to better scribbling.

Long-Term Goal 1: Child will scribble in one year.
Short-Term Goal 1: Child will stack a ten-block tower independently.
Short-Term Goal 2: Child will improve upper extremity range of motion to 180 degrees.

DOI: 10.4324/9781003392408-17

Following the MMCR, all long-term goals include and connect the identified top-middle-bottom occupational performance issue(s). In addition to including the bottom occupational performance issue(s) in the long-term goal, it is aligned with the short-term goals. Including the person's top and middle occupational performance issue(s) automatically makes it more client-centered and individualized. Long-term goals do not need to be measurable but provide a general description of what the person is trying to accomplish for the duration of the intervention plan. Using words such as increase, develop, improvement, or implement provides interested parties with general information about the direction of the long-term goal but does not identify the exact measurement of success.

Examples of long-term goals following the MMCR:

Suzie will manage her anger to decrease physical outbursts toward her mom during daily walks around the neighborhood block.

This example demonstrates a connection between anger (bottom), daily walks with her mom (middle) and returning to their apartment (top).

Joan will utilize healthy alternatives to using cocaine when managing her angry feelings toward her co-workers while working in the shoe department at the discount department store.

This example provides a connection between finding healthy alternatives to cocaine use (bottom) and managing her angry feelings toward her current co-workers (middle) while working in the shoe department at the discount department store (top).

MMCR: Creating Short-Term Goals

While there might be fewer identified long-term goals written on the evaluation summary, there tend to be multiple short-term goals. A short-term goal represents one task that a person intends to accomplish in the near future and is often viewed as the building block towards reaching the long-term goals. Achieving short-term goals varies greatly and can be accomplished in hours, days, months or years. Documented short-term goals encourage the practitioner and person served to pause and reflect on the intervention progress. Are we on the right path toward change? Are we moving at a good pace for the planned intervention hours? Has the person served changed their top and/or middle goals?

There is much variability in short-term goal formation from different practitioners and in different settings, but there are some key components pertinent to the occupational therapy profession.

Typical components of a short-term goal:

- State all terms clearly and must be measurable (so others can concretely determine if achieved or not).
- Always provide a connection to function so it is specific to the person's story.
- Identify how much (verbal, visual, gestural and/or physical) cueing is necessary for success.
- Include a time frame for goal achievement.

Example of a possible short-term goal set at the beginning of Suzie's intervention plan:

Suzie will identify two warning signs of escalating anger in order to prevent hitting her mother while going on daily neighborhood walks with three verbal prompts from others within three days.

Since Suzie does not have awareness of her escalating anger, intervention begins here. For this awareness to be measurable for a goal, she needs to identify, state or verbalize what is happening to her physically and mentally when getting angry. This is one of the earliest building blocks to prevent her from hitting her mother. By the end of the first three days, the practitioner suspects that Suzie can identify her feelings of escalation with some prompting from staff and eventually her mother, such as tell me your anger level now, your voice is getting louder, are you becoming angry? This awareness will then provide an opportunity to move forward to implement the most relevant ways for Suzie to calm herself when preparing to go on daily walks with her mother before returning home.

Example of a possible short-term goal set at the end of Joan's intervention plan:

Joan will demonstrate one healthy way to manage her angry feelings toward her co-workers while working in the shoe department at the discount department store with one verbal prompt from others within six months.

Meanwhile Joan has the awareness that she uses cocaine, especially when initially angry at her former boss during work. She is aware this anger is directed toward her co-workers, but she is unable to implement skills to change this ongoing behavior with any consistency. Since Joan already has the awareness, it is important to help her develop those skills to create change for resolution.

Intervention focuses on eliminating unhealthy habits (using cocaine when feeling angry) and creating new healthy replacement ones. This will require much education, trial and error of various approaches and practice. In this goal, the measurable word "demonstrate" shows action or "doing" in this part of the change process. It can be more challenging to "do" rather than "verbalize", so the practitioner anticipates it will take longer to accomplish.

MMCR Guidelines to Formulate a Short-Term Goal

Now it is time to examine the five components of a short-term goal. While this appears to be a fill-in exercise, there is much thought and clinical reasoning in all goal creation. Please see Figure 14.1 (also found in Appendix 6) for use of this clinical reasoning guidesheet entitled, "MMCR Guidelines to Formulate a Short-Term Goal".

MMCR Guidelines to Formulate a Short-Term Goal

1. _____ **will**

   (Person's name)

2. _____ **in order to**

   (measurable, comes from bottom occupational performance issues)

3. _____ **with**

   (functional and specific, comes from top or middle occupational performance issue)

4. _____ **in**

   (measurement, how much cuing, prompting or physical assistance)

5. _____

   (time frame for achievement)

Figure 14.1 Clinical Reasoning Guidesheet: MMCR Guidelines to Formulate a Short-Term Goal.

> **Voices of the Practitioners: Considerations When Creating Individualized Goals**
>
> I prefer to use their name with the goal. A lot of people will say student or patient or client or just their initials. I like using the actual name. That's something that I think is not something I've seen across the board. (Jackie)
>
> I keep the person in mind more than the skill in mind. I find it's more individualized that way and I'm not looking at just the little components that need to go in there. The goal is not realistic if it is not within the person's goals and what they want. (Rebecca)

Short-Term Goal Component #1

Suzie will identify two warning signs of escalating anger in order to prevent hitting her mother while going on daily neighborhood walks with three verbal prompts from others within three days.

Joan will demonstrate one healthy way to manage her angry feelings toward her co-workers while working in the shoe department at the discount department store with one verbal prompt from others within six months.

Identify the person by their actual name. Go against the norm and do not write "patient", "client" or "consumer". For the most part, people want to be called by their actual names, giving them a sense of belonging, identity and normalcy. Words such as patient, child, client and consumer are labels that remove the specific individual further from the intervention process.

Short-Term Goal Component #2

Suzie will *identify two warning signs of escalating anger* in order to prevent hitting her mother while going on daily neighborhood walks with three verbal prompts from others within three days.

Joan will *demonstrate one healthy way to manage her angry feelings* toward her co-workers while working in the shoe department at the discount department store with one visual prompt from others within six months.

This represents the measurable component of the goal. Re-examine the person's bottom occupational performance issue and now write it in measurable terms. Be mindful if the person served or caregiver is developing an awareness of a skill or building skills by demonstrating actions. Both of these women have similar bottoms of emotional regulation issues related to anger. With closer inspection, Suzie and Joan have different stories related to their anger and are in different phases of the change process, and the goals reflect this.

Listed next are some examples of words that can be used to measure progress in a short-term goal. Words such as identify, report and state fall in the category of self-awareness. Words such as illustrate, utilize and implement fall in the category of skill building.

Clear words that can be measurable in a short-term goal:

- Identify
- Report
- State
- Demonstrate
- Illustrate
- Utilize
- Implement

The words listed next are words that are unclear and not measurable when used to formulate a short-term goal. For example, using the word "understand" in a short-term goal is unclear to the reader. How does a person know when someone understands something? The practitioner typically looks for the person to say something (state, report) or do something (demonstrate or implement). Occupational therapy practitioners may write a goal to improve a person's intelligence, but this is not even a part of our domain of concern.

Unclear words that are not measurable in a short-term goal:

- Understand
- Knowledge
- Intelligence
- Increase

Examples of goals using unclear words that are not measurable:

Patient *will tolerate* having their hair brushed by a parent.
Patient *will show* reduced swelling in wrist.
Patient *will increase* lateral pinch strength in 2 weeks.
The patient *will complete* toilet transfers with supervision to begin his day of reading the news.

Voices of the Practitioners: How to Individualize Short-Term Goals

Goals are specific but the amount of specificity can vary. It is important to relate it to the "why". If there is not a connection to the why part then it shouldn't be in there. (Rebecca)

I always end my goal with "in order to". I feel like that "in order to" is the connection to the functional part, like that performance part. (Kristen)

Short-Term Goal Component #3

Suzie will identify two warning signs of escalating anger in order to *prevent hitting her mother while going on daily neighborhood walks* with three verbal prompts from others within three days.

Joan will demonstrate one healthy way to manage her angry feelings toward *her co-workers while working in the shoe department at the discount department store* with one visual prompt from others within six months.

This represents the functional component of a short-term goal. Aligning with the intervention plan, it comes from your middle and/or top occupational performance issues. The functional component is the key aspect of goal writing that assists the practitioner to individualize the goals based on the person's unique story that eventually connects with occupation-based interventions. This part of the goal highlights a person's uniqueness, so it should be specific to their story. By including this component in the goal, it is no longer interchangeable with other people.

The Functional Component of the Short-Term Goal Distinguishes Our Profession From Others: A-HA Moment

The ability to incorporate functional aspects into goal writing is an asset to the occupational therapy profession and a distinguishing factor from our interprofessional partners.

For example, reflect on this goal: Muhammad will identify three positive qualities about himself with three verbal prompts from others within five days.

While this goal is measurable, identifies the amount of cuing and provides a time frame, it is still not complete. The goal written in this format may lend itself to a practitioner simply asking Muhammad to identify any three positive qualities about himself for successful achievement of this goal. In fact, anyone (aide, family member, non-licensed professional or even a mail carrier) can ask Muhammad to identify three positive qualities about himself for successful goal achievement.

The functional component explains why this person needs to identify positive qualities about themselves and eventually how these positive qualities are relevant to the person's story. Does Muhammad need to identify positive qualities about himself to share this information during an upcoming job interview? Perhaps the qualities will help him to feel comfortable initiating a conversation with a new friend at the support group meeting. Understanding (and including) the reasons why Muhammad needs to identify positive qualities about himself directs the entire intervention plan toward an individualized approach.

Voices of the Practitioners: Adding Levels of Assistance to My Short-Term Goals

I really do like adding assistance levels like min, mod, max into my goals. Most therapists can understand what the percentage means. However, other therapists say "those words tell me nothing" so I get both sides of it. I also don't think it should just be written as "the client is max assist". You have to say what is the functional part of the goal. Is there a time limit? What is the purpose of this? (Jackie)

I write my goals in that way so it's very concrete and the person can understand it. I always ask how much help do you think you need with this? At the end of the day, I don't want a kid to be able to ride his bike 80 percent of the time like that means he's crashing and he can't do it. Sometimes the end goal has to be independence. (Casey)

Short-Term Goal Component #4

Suzie will identify two warning signs of escalating anger in order to prevent hitting her mother while going on daily neighborhood walks *with three verbal prompts* from others within three days.

Joan will demonstrate one healthy way to manage her angry feelings toward her co-workers while working in the shoe department at the discount department store *with one visual prompt* from others within 6 months.

Rarely do we expect people to be fully independent in a task. Reflect on how many daily reminders people set for themselves or are set by other people each day. With trends toward short-intervention durations, it is even more challenging for a person to leave services fully independent in tasks. Does the person served require verbal prompting, a visual reminder or physical assistance to be successful in a task upon discharge from occupational therapy services? A person can be very successful in life, even with some cuing or assistance from others.

Providing four visual cues is a lot different than one visual cue or completing a task independently. Reflect on the frequency and type of cuing needed. The amount of cuing represents where the person will be upon successful completion of this goal. It is important to provide cuing only when needed. For example, Suzie only has three days to make progress toward the beginning section of the overall intervention plan. It is not a lot of time, so the practitioner needs to move faster down the continuum for intervention to the "doing" part, so she does not continue hitting her mother when she returns home.

The word "other", rather than occupational therapy practitioner, was specifically used in this goal to expand who can provide this cuing. In addition to the staff members working with Suzie, it is more important that Suzie's mother use similar cuing to help her become aware of escalating anger while walking when she returns home.

Short-Term Goal Component #5

Suzie will identify two warning signs of escalating anger in order to prevent hitting her mother while going on daily neighborhood walks with three verbal prompts from others within *3 days*.

Joan will demonstrate one healthy way to manage her angry feelings toward her co-workers while working in the shoe department at the discount department store with one visual prompt from others within *six months*.

Time frames do matter. When completing this component of the short-term goal, consider how much time there is for each beginning-middle-ending section of the intervention plan. How long does the person have to accomplish a task? A few months? Maybe years? Even in the same practice area location, people participate in occupational therapy services for different amounts of time. Reflect back on decisions made during the intervention planning process, as the time frame will mirror the beginning-middle-ending sections.

Align All Five Components of the Goal Together

Look closely for consistency among the measurable part (#2), amount of cuing (#4) and time frame (#5) as a whole. All of these components need to line up together. For example, is it realistic for a person to be aware and then demonstrate a skill independently in four days? Does a person need six months to create awareness, or can this be accomplished in a shorter time?

Suzie will *identify two warning signs of escalating anger* in order to prevent hitting her mother while going on daily neighborhood walks *with three verbal prompts from others* within *3 days*.

Joan will *demonstrate one healthy way to manage her angry feelings* toward her co-workers while working in the shoe department at the discount department store *with one visual prompt* from others within *six months*.

A Word About Including Intervention Methods and Evaluations in the Goal: Don't Do It

These three goal examples highlight the use of methods and evaluations as a marker for successful achievement.

Patient will have a *normal nine-hole peg test score*.
Patient will *use a memory book* to improve executive functioning.
Patient will complete age-appropriate *mazes and visual motor activities*.

No person seeking services has ever said, "I want a normal nine-hole peg test score by discharge". Initial evaluations formulate a baseline measure of where the person is starting at in this change process. While reevaluations compare and contrast the change made from the initial evaluations as a result of occupational therapy intervention, this information is not part of a person's goal. Rather, reflect back to the person's top-middle-bottom occupational performance issues to capture the bigger picture.

Discussed in previous chapters, practitioners use specific strategies or methods to assist the person to move through the change process. Method selection forms the basis of the intervention plan. While methods are the catalyst for successful outcomes during intervention, it is not directly part of the short-term goal. Occupational therapy practitioners select and utilize relevant methods and strategies during intervention to assist the person served to achieve their personal goals. More often, it requires much brainstorming, trial and error and practice to identify the exact strategy, skill or task that will work for each individual person.

For example, Joan has been using cocaine as a way to manage angry feelings toward her co-workers and is searching for a healthy alternative. The practitioner intends to introduce different ways for Joan to try calming herself down. Based on previous success with other people, the practitioner initially plans to introduce deep breathing exercises. The practitioner also plans to include Joan in daily relaxation groups to connect with other group members who are looking for healthy alternatives to drug use. Assuming this will be the proposed intervention plan, the practitioner writes the following goals:

Goal example using a specific method #1: Joan will *perform deep breathing exercises for two minutes* to manage her angry feelings toward her co-workers in the shoe department at the discount department store with one visual prompt from others within six months.

Goal example using a specific method #2: Joan will *attend a relaxation group five out of ten times* to manage her angry feelings toward co-workers in the shoe department at the discount department store with one verbal prompt from others within six months.

However, by identifying these methods, the practitioner has already determined which healthy alternatives will be best for Joan. After trying out deep breathing exercises for a few days, Joan does not feel this technique helps to calm her angry feelings fast enough. She enjoys the relaxation groups but finds it more of a social opportunity, as this group will end upon discharge from services.

Instead, during the trial-and-error phase of the intervention plan, Joan enjoyed reciting a carefully crafted positive affirmation and found it to be most helpful to perform in her busy work environment of the shoe department. This technique is effective to manage her angry feelings until she gets a work break and can call her sponsor. Highlighting deep breathing or the relaxation group in the goal is tricky because it emphasizes one or two specific methods. If the goal instead highlights general healthy ways to manage her anger, then the goal is achievable even if Joan eventually prefers an unexpected positive affirmation technique.

Rewritten goal example without using a specific method: Joan will *demonstrate one healthy way to manage her angry feelings* toward her co-workers in the shoe department at the discount department store with one visual prompt from others within six months.

TRY IT: Writing Short-Term Goals Using All Five Components

Using the MMCR Guidelines to Formulate a Short-Term Goal clinical reasoning guidesheet, rewrite the poorly written goals. Identify the parts missing from each.

Patient will have improved sensation to 2.61 Semmes Weinstein monofilament.
Child will tolerate therapist input for desensitization.
Patient will increase grip strength by 5 pounds.

Patient will be able to lift a 10-pound bag of groceries.
Patient will stand without needing a break 2 times.
Consumer will improve self-esteem.
Patient will stop hearing voices in order to go back to work.
Therapist will provide the patient with a schedule of daily events to enhance memory.
Client will identify two decisions and solve two problems in lifestyle in order to improve functional living skills with three verbal prompts from OTR in two weeks.
Patient will come to group on time every day while in the hospital by 4/30/2023.

Considerations When Creating Short-Term Goals: A-HA Moment

Is the goal written in plain language with minimal occupational therapy jargon?
Do all the short-term goals form the building blocks to the long-term goal?
Does the goal focus on the top-middle-bottom occupational performance issues rather than methods or evaluations?
Does each short-term goal include all five components?
Is there alignment between goal components #2, #4 and #5?
Is goal component #2 measurable while highlighting the bottom occupational performance issues with more general wording?
Does goal component #3 emphasize a specific middle or top occupational performance issue?

Using the Same Clinical Reasoning Structure for Other Forms of Documentation

A person's documentation trail should be internally consistent stemming from the initial evaluation summary. Once the initial top-middle-bottom(s) is set in the evaluation summary, then the practitioner monitors progress toward these occupational performance issues throughout the intervention process. The basic four ingredients (strengths, challenges, raw data and interpretations) are included in other forms of documentation such as progress notes and discharge summaries.

Progress Notes

Progress notes are documented opportunities for the practitioner to review each beginning-middle-ending section of the continuum for intervention to determine progress made within each time frame. It is also a good reflection tool to change course if goals are unsuccessful. At times, the person served may not be motivated to continue with previous set goals, and this will alter the intervention path. Outside influences may also influence the success of a goal such as length of stay, regulatory agencies, institutional policies, etc.

The practitioner documents progress notes periodically along the continuum for intervention. These notes reflect on progress toward the top-middle-bottom occupational performance issues initially identified in the evaluation summary and now spiraled across the continuum. As the practitioner has mentally conceptualized how intervention will proceed, progress notes are the "stop and see" measure to track progress made after each beginning-middle-ending intervention section.

Evaluation summary _____x_____/**PN**_____/**PN**_____/**PN** & discharge summary

*PN stands for progress note.

The progress note (PN) typically follows the vertical line when conceptualizing a person's intervention plan. This cues the practitioner to pause, reevaluate and proceed accordingly with the plan. Documenting this progress coincides with the short-term goal time frames identified on the evaluation summary report and eventually will align with other documentation such as daily notes and discharge summaries. The "X" symbolizes any daily progress notes completed to identify smaller increments of progress along the beginning-middle-ending intervention section along the continuum for intervention.

Discharge Summaries

Evaluation summary _____x_____/PN_____/PN_____/PN & **discharge summary**

*PN stands for progress note.

Occupational therapy practitioners must reflect on a person's transition to the next location. Sometimes this transition preparation occurs very quickly, while other times it is a prolonged process. Either way, discharge summaries are a type of documentation created when the person is nearing the end of the continuum for intervention. Using the same basic four ingredients (strengths, challenges, raw data and interpretation), the practitioner provides a general overview of the progress made toward the selected top-middle-bottom occupational performance issue(s), what may still need to be addressed in the next practice location and an action plan of recommendations to continued growth and mastery.

How Practitioners Unintentionally Deter Goal Progress: A-HA Moment

During the discharge summary, the practitioner reflects on and documents the overall progress. There are situations where unfulfilled goals are the result of the practitioner and not the person served.

Even the most well-written long-term and short-term goals will not be achievable if the practitioner's intervention plan does not directly align with the person's top-middle-bottom occupational performance issue(s). A person cannot make necessary changes unless the practitioner directly addresses relevant tasks.

There is a greater risk of setting unachievable goals if the practitioner documents the evaluation summary, including long-term and short-term goals, without previously conceptualizing the intervention plan. Without a well-thought-out intervention plan, the practitioner is creating goals without strategy or direction.

Look closely for consistency among the measurable part (#2), amount of cuing (#4) and time frame (#5) as a whole. All of these components of the short-term goals line up together; otherwise, the practitioner may overshoot or undershoot the potential progress made during the continuum for intervention.

Strategically select the best methods and teaching-learning principles for each beginning-middle-ending section of the overall intervention plan. This will minimize the amount of non-purposeful activities implemented during the intervention plan that ultimately impacts on goal achievement.

Summary

Long-term and short-term goals are an important part of the documentation process, as they provide an opportunity to identify what is important to the person served and encourage practitioners to periodically pause and reflect on the amount of progress made throughout the duration of the intervention plan. When developing a plan following the POP acronym, long- and short-term goals align with the person's top-middle-bottom occupational performance issue(s). A long-term goal represents a task that a person intends to accomplish in the future, requiring extended time and planning

Short-term goals are written with more specific language to identify the building blocks needed while making progress toward the longer-term goal. Following the MMCR Guidelines to Formulate a Short-Term Goal clinical reasoning guidesheet, there are five basic components relevant to short-term goals The five components include identifying people by their names, reconceptualizing the bottom occupational performance issue to make it measurable, adding a functional component specific to their story, including the level of assistance and targeting a time frame for goal achievement. Aside from evaluation summaries, other forms of documentation may include progress notes and/or discharge summaries including a person's strengths, challenges, raw data and interpretations.

Section 4

Case Examples

15 Case Example

Using the MMCR in an Outpatient Hand Therapy Clinic Over 8 Weeks of Intervention

Paige Garramone, Pauline Gasparro, and Shaniqua Bradley

Introducing Amal

Amal sustained a right distal radius fracture while working a Friday evening shift at the restaurant 2 weeks ago. She was taking a pick-up order out to a customer's car when she slipped on the ice. Amal was holding the bag of food in her left hand and reached her right arm out as she was falling, resulting in a fall on her right hand. Later that night, one of her co-workers drove her to the emergency room, where she had x-rays done that showed a comminuted Colles' fracture (see Box 15.1) of her right wrist.

Box 15.1

What Is a Colles' Fracture?

A Colles' fracture occurs when a person falls with an outstretched hand, resulting in a dorsal displacement of the distal radius (Hoppenfeld & Murthy, 2000).

Due to the extent of her fracture, she required surgery to stabilize it with an open reduction and internal fixation (ORIF), as a reduction of the fracture would not be sufficient. Amal stayed the night in the hospital to have surgery the next morning with the on-call hand surgeon. A workers compensation case was filed the night of the injury because it occurred on work property during her shift.

Past Medical History Form

Amal is a single, 20-year-old, left-handed-dominant female. Her past medical history includes an appendectomy when she was 12 years old. She currently takes a multivitamin daily.

Hand Surgeon's Note From Last Office Visit

Amal underwent surgery to stabilize the fracture with an ORIF. She was placed in a temporary postsurgical cast until her follow-up appointment with the hand surgeon later that week. At her doctor's visit, she was given a prefabricated wrist brace to keep her wrist in a neutral position. Table 15.1 is an example of what Amal's occupational therapy prescription from her hand surgeon may look like.

DOI: 10.4324/9781003392408-19

Table 15.1 Sample Occupational Therapy Prescription From Amal's Hand Surgeon

Patient Name	Amal K.
Sex–DOB–Age	F-03/15/2001–20 years old
Diagnosis	Closed Colles' Fracture ICD—10: S52.531D
Order	Certified Hand Therapist Referral: 3× per week × 4 weeks. Please begin therapy 2 weeks postoperation.
Notes	Please first address A/AAROM, progress to PROM. Can utilize modalities as needed. Address edema control, scar tissue remodeling. Prescribe a home exercise program.

Surgeon's Postoperative Protocol

The hand surgeon provided a postoperative protocol for the occupational therapy practitioner to follow. From weeks 0–1, Amal will focus on keeping her arm elevated and moving her fingers and thumb within the brace. Weeks 2–4, formal occupational therapy intervention will begin, where the focus will be on active range of motion of the wrist and forearm and passive motion of the digits and thumb. Weeks 5–7, the practitioner can begin passive stretches to the wrist and forearm. Gentle weight bearing and grip/pinch strengthening can begin at 6 weeks postoperation. Starting at week 8 postoperation, strengthening of the wrist and forearm may begin. After 12 weeks postoperation, Amal can perform all activities as tolerated. Throughout, the practitioner will address edema, pain, muscle tightness, and scar tissue adherence.

Occupational Profile

Amal is a single, 20-year-old female who immigrated to the United States from Beirut, Lebanon, when she was 15 years old with her mother, father, younger sister and maternal grandmother. Amal's sister, Nardine, who is 2 years younger, lives with cystic fibrosis. Her family made the decision to immigrate to the United States for Nardine's medical care, as she was in need of a new medication not offered in Lebanon. Since immigrating 5 years ago, Nardine has been doing well on her current medication and therapeutic intervention.

Amal's family settled in Dearborn, Michigan, as there is a large population of people from the Middle East in this area, and her aunt and uncle live just a short drive away. They rent half of a two-family home that has two bedrooms, one of which Amal and Nardine share. Amal and her sister have a good relationship. Nardine likes to be independent and do things for herself; however, she knows Amal is always there to take her to medical appointments, helping her remember to take her medication and assisting with her home therapy regimen. Their grandmother, known as Teta, moved in with Amal's aunt and uncle after they immigrated to Michigan.

All members of Amal's family are fluent in Arabic and English. While in Lebanon, Amal and Nardine attended school that taught their classes in English. This started in kindergarten and continued as they progressed through grade levels. Their ability to speak fluent English made Amal and her family more comfortable with their move to the United States. Since coming to the United States, Amal and her family take turns accompanying Teta to many of her doctor appointments to help translate important medical information.

Amal's paternal family still lives in Lebanon who they keep in touch with via WhatsApp. Amal's father owned a grocery store while living in Lebanon. He currently works full-time at a home improvement retail store to receive medical benefits for the family. Amal's mother works part-time at the bank on the corner of their block. At age 17, Amal began working as a waitress at a local Lebanese restaurant within walking distance of her home to start saving money for college. The family shares one car; her father usually drives the car to work every day, but otherwise it is available for use by Amal and her mother. Amal has continued to work at the restaurant to pay for school and is now saving up money for her own car and to have extra pocket money.

Amal frequents her aunt and uncle's house to spend time with her female cousins and her Teta making Lebanese food (see Box 15.2). They particularly love listening to music by Nancy Ajram and dancing in the kitchen while preparing food for family dinners (see Box 15.3).

Box 15.2

Lebanese Food

People from Lebanon value preparing and sharing meals together with their family. Some traditional Lebanese foods often made for family gatherings include:

Warak Enab: stuffed grape leaves with rice and ground meat
Tabouli: parsley, tomato and bulgar wheat salad
Kibbeh: ground beef or lamb with bulgar wheat
Baklava: phyllo dough filled with nuts and sweetened with sugar syrup
Ma'amoul: rose water cookie filled with dates or pistachios
                                    (L.W. Eskander, personal communication, March 15, 2021).

Box 15.3

A traditional Lebanese dance is called the **dabke**. This is a fast-paced line dance often done at weddings.
                                    (L.W. Eskander, personal communication, March 15, 2021).

Spending time cooking with Teta and her cousins is important to Amal as she does not want to lose the family traditions that they have always enjoyed growing up in Lebanon. Amal also enjoys teaching Teta the English language during her visits. Amal's extended family gets together every Sunday for family dinners at her aunt's house.

Amal's parents have worked hard to provide a better life for their family and opportunities for their children and highly value the importance of a higher education. Amal has always felt that it was expected of her to attend college. Her career aspirations have been influenced by both her parents urging her to pursue a medical career and by Nardine's journey with cystic fibrosis. Her goal is to transfer to a 4-year college and finish with a degree in chemistry and later apply to pharmacy school. Amal has been taking courses at her local community college part-time so that she can continue working to save money for school, books, a car and pocket money.

When Amal immigrated to Michigan in her sophomore year of high school, she was nervous about making friends in her new school. Amal met Joyce in the cafeteria a few weeks into starting at her new high school. She was intrigued by the lunch Joyce was eating and approached her, asking about the dish. They began to bond over their love of their cultural foods and became close friends rather quickly. They later learned how similar their families and cultures were, and both cherish the family traditions they have grown up with (see Box 15.4).

Box 15.4

Some similarities between Lebanese and West African cultures include:

- Pursuing higher education
- Sharing meals together with family
- Strict parenting style
- Living in close proximity to family
- Taking care of elderly family members

(L.W. Eskander, personal communication, March 15, 2021;
E. Gyan, personal communication, March 31, 2021)

Joyce's family is from Ghana; however, she was born in the United States. Joyce often shares how she felt she was growing up with "two identities" as the culture and environment at home were very different compared to what she was seeing and learning at school.

Amal and Joyce have both always felt it was important to stay close to their families in case they were ever needed, so they decided to attend college locally. Although they both remain in the area, it is often difficult for them to hang out during the week since they are both very busy. Amal and Joyce typically hang out on the weekends and have been spending more time together the past couple of weeks since they are both on winter break from school.

On the weekends, Amal and Joyce enjoy going to each other's houses to watch sitcoms on Netflix, going shopping and eating dinner with each other's families. When Amal and Joyce go to the mall, they typically window shop, as they are both trying to save their money for school-related expenses. Back in high school, they developed an interest in yoga during their senior year. They never pursued actual classes, as they are expensive, and their parents would not approve since they are not open to the spirituality aspect of yoga. Both girls have tried to explain the benefits of yoga to their parents; however they did not want the girls investing their time in this activity. Since then, Amal and Joyce have been looking up yoga videos on YouTube to practice their skills and technique at Joyce's house when her parents are not home so they do not get in trouble.

Both Amal's and Joyce's parents try to assist with paying for college; however, the girls do not want to add any extra burden to their parents. Amal has been working for the past 3 years to help relieve some of the stress off of her parents and so she did not have to ask them for money to support her interests/hobbies. Amal typically works about 20 hours a week on nights and weekends to accommodate her class schedule. While on winter break, she picked up extra shifts at the restaurant, as she is very eager to purchase a car so she can drive herself to class. She is tired of taking the bus, especially during the winter months when she has to stand outside at the bus stop in the snow. Figure 15.1 provides an example of what Amal's completed Role Checklist (Scott, 2019) may look like.

While Amal identified three specific goals she would like to work toward, which included returning to work as a waitress, saving up money to purchase a car and transferring to a 4-year college, she identified returning to work as the most important area and the goal that needed to be addressed first. Amal's initial personal goal is to return to work as soon as possible, as she is hoping

Role Version 3 (RCv3)

1. For each role, indicate by circling either **YES** or **NO** (**not both**) depending on if you are performing this role. **PLEASE make sure you make one YES/NO selection for each role.**
2. For each role circled **YES** (currently doing), please indicate your level from very dissatisfied to very satisfied.
3. For each role circled **NO** (currently not doing), please indicate your interest in doing this role in the future.

STUDENT: Attending school on a **part-time or full time basis**	(YES)	Very Dissatisfied	Somewhat Dissatisfied	(Mostly Satisfied)	Very Satisfied
	NO	I would like to do this NOW	I would like to do this IN THE FUTURE		I am NOT INTERESTED
WORKER: *waitress→* Part-time or full-time **paid employment** *pharmacist →*	(YES)	Very (Dissatisfied)	Somewhat Dissatisfied	Mostly Satisfied	Very Satisfied
	(NO)	I would like to do this NOW	I would like to do this IN THE FUTURE		I am NOT INTERESTED
VOLUNTEER: Donating services, on a regular basis, to a hospital, school, community, & so forth	YES	Very Dissatisfied	Somewhat Dissatisfied	Mostly Satisfied	Very Satisfied
	(NO)	I would like to do this NOW	I would like to do this IN THE FUTURE		I am NOT (INTERESTED)
CARE GIVER: Responsibility, **at least once a week**, for the care of someone (ex. family, relative, or friend)	(YES)	Very Dissatisfied	Somewhat Dissatisfied	Mostly Satisfied	(Very Satisfied)
	NO	I would like to do this NOW	I would like to do this IN THE FUTURE		I am NOT INTERESTED
HOME MAINTAINER: Responsibility, **at least once a week**, for the upkeep of the home (ex. Cleaning, meal preparation, yard work)	YES	Very Dissatisfied	Somewhat Dissatisfied	Mostly Satisfied	Very Satisfied
	(NO)	I would like to do this NOW	I would like to do this IN THE FUTURE		I am NOT INTERESTED
FRIEND: Spending time or doing something, **on a regular basis**, with a friend.	(YES)	Very Dissatisfied	Somewhat Dissatisfied	Mostly Satisfied	(Very Satisfied)
	NO	I would like to do this NOW	I would like to do this IN THE FUTURE		I am NOT INTERESTED
FAMILY MEMBER: Spending time such as visiting, or sharing a meal, **on a regular basis**, with a family member	(YES)	Very Dissatisfied	Somewhat Dissatisfied	(Mostly Satisfied)	Very Satisfied
	NO	I would like to do this NOW	I would like to do this IN THE FUTURE		I am NOT INTERESTED
RELIGIOUS PARTICIPANT: Involvement, in groups or activities about one's religion	YES	Very Dissatisfied	Somewhat Dissatisfied	Mostly Satisfied	Very Satisfied
	(NO)	I would like to do this NOW	I would like to do this IN THE FUTURE		I am NOT (INTERESTED)
HOBBYIST/AMATEUR: Involvement, **on a regular basis**, in a hobby like woodworking, amateur activity, or sports	(YES)	Very Dissatisfied	(Somewhat Dissatisfied)	Mostly Satisfied	Very Satisfied
	NO	I would like to do this NOW	I would like to do this IN THE FUTURE		I am NOT INTERESTED
PARTICIPANT IN ORGANIZATIONS: Involvement, **on a regular basis**, in community or professional organizations	YES	Very Dissatisfied	Somewhat Dissatisfied	Mostly Satisfied	Very Satisfied
	(NO)	I would like to do this NOW	I would like to do this IN THE FUTURE		I am NOT (INTERESTED)

Figure 15.1 Amal's completed Role Checklist Version 3 (RCv3).

Source: Adapted with permission from the Board of Trustees of the University of Illinois.

to save up enough money to purchase a car by the end of her spring semester. Amal described wanting to take classes full-time after purchasing her car in order to shorten the amount of time it will take her to become a pharmacist. She is also concerned about her ability to take notes and keep up in class when winter break ends as a result of her recent injury.

Analysis of Performance

The Upper Extremity Functional Index (Stratford et al., 2001) can be used as a guide to help the practitioner assess which tasks Amal will have difficulty completing. These tasks may be meaningful for Amal to varying degrees, and each task listed may not be formally addressed in therapy. Figure 15.2 provides an example of what Amal's evaluation might look like.

The occupational therapy practitioner evaluates both affected and non-affected upper extremities; the unaffected side is measured to give the practitioner an idea of what Amal's normal measurements are. Range of motion of both right and left upper extremities was assessed using various sized goniometers (see Tables 15.2 and 15.3). The practitioner visually and physically assessed

UPPER EXTREMITY FUNCTIONAL INDEX

We are interested in knowing whether you are having any difficulty at all with the activities listed below <u>because of your upper limb</u> problem for which you are currently seeking attention. Please provide an answer for **each** activity.

Today, <u>do you</u> or <u>would you</u> have any difficulty at all with: (Circle one number on each line)

ACTIVITIES	Extreme Difficulty	Quite a bit of Difficulty	Moderate Difficulty	A Little bit of Difficulty	No Difficulty
a. Any of your usual work, housework or school activities	0	(1)	2	3	4
b. Your usual hobbies, recreational or sporting activities	(0)	1	2	3	4
c. Lifting a bag of groceries to waist level	0	1	(2)	3	4
d. Placing an object onto, or removing it from an overhead shelf	(0)	1	2	3	4
e. Washing your hair or scalp	0	1	(2)	3	4
f. Pushing up on your hands (e.g., from bathtub or chair)	(0)	1	2	3	4
g. Preparing food (e.g., peeling, cutting)	0	(1)	2	3	4
h. Driving	(0)	1	2	3	4
I. Vacuuming, sweeping, or raking	(0)	1	2	3	4
j. Dressing	0	1	(2)	3	4
k. Doing up buttons	0	1	2	(3)	4
l. Using tools or appliances	0	(1)	2	3	4
m. Opening doors	0	(1)	2	3	4
n. Cleaning	0	1	(2)	3	4
o. Tying or lacing shoes	0	1	2	(3)	4
p. Sleeping	0	1	2	(3)	4
q. Laundering clothes. (e.g., washing, ironing, folding)	0	1	(2)	3	4
r. Opening a jar	(0)	1	2	3	4
s. Throwing a ball	(0)	1	2	3	4
t. Carrying a small suitcase with your affected limb	(0)	1	2	3	4
Column Totals:	0	4	10	9	0

Score: __23__ / 80

Figure 15.2 Amal's completed Upper Extremity Functional Index (UEFI).

Source: © 1996 PW Stratford, reprinted with permission.

Amal's skin and scar, muscle and joint tightness (see Table 15.4). The practitioner also asked Amal about her pain level throughout the evaluation. Amal's pain was assessed through self-report following the practitioner providing Amal with the following range: 0 = no pain, 5 = makes you stop doing an activity, 10 = pain takes you to the hospital (see Table 15.5). Edema was measured using a measuring tape (see Table 15.6), and Amal's dexterity was tested by using the nine-hole peg test (see Table 15.7).

Table 15.2 Amal's Forearm and Wrist Range of Motion Measurements Using a Goniometer

Motion (normal range)	Right Side	Left Side
Forearm Pronation (80)	80	80
Forearm Supination (80)	20	80
Wrist Extension (60–70)	25	65
Wrist Flexion (60–80)	10	70
Wrist Radial Deviation (20)	5	20
Wrist Ulnar Deviation (30)	10	30

Table 15.3 Amal's Hand and Thumb Range of Motion Measurements Using a Goniometer

Digit/Joint	Motion	Right Side	Left Side
Index Finger—Small Finger	Flexion/extension	Within functional limits (WFL) *Able to fully open hand. Able to make loose fist; however, not a very tight fist.	Within normal limits *Able to fully open hand and make a tight fist.
Thumb MCP	Extension/Flexion	0/30	0/45
Thumb IP Joint	Extension/Flexion	0/45	+10/60
Thumb	Palmar Abduction	30	40
Thumb	Radial Abduction	30	40
Thumb	Opposition	To small finger distal interphalangeal (DIP) joint crease	To small finger distal palmar crease (DPC)

Table 15.4 Occupational Therapy Practitioner's Observations of Skin and Muscle Integrity

Area of Observation	Comment
Scar	4.5-cm longitudinal scar along the volar wrist. Sutures have been removed. There is some scabbing and slight redness along the scar. No sign of infection. Scar is severely adherent. Hypersensitive to the touch.
Skin	Skin appears healthy. Some flakiness likely due to the patient not washing her arm normally.
Intrinsic tightness	Minimal/moderate intrinsic tightness felt in right hand, left hand feels normal.
Extrinsic tightness	Right side: Severe extrinsic flexor and moderate extensor tightness felt. Left side: no tightness felt.

Table 15.5 Amal's Pain Rating on a Scale From 0 to 10

Pain at Rest	2/10
Pain with Movement	6/10
Worst Reported Pain	8/10
Location of Pain	Ulnar wrist, dorsal wrist along wrist crease, dorsal hand when making a fist

Table 15.6 Amal's Edema Measurements

Location	Right	Left
Wrist	18.2 cm	16.2 cm
Around Metacarpal Phalangeal Joints	19.5 cm	19.3 cm

Table 15.7 Amal's Time to Complete the Nine-Hole Peg Test Measuring Her Dexterity

Right Hand: 26 seconds	Left Hand: 17 seconds

Table 15.8 Amal's Sensation Score Using Semmes Weinstein Monofilaments (2.61 monofilament indicates normal sensation)

Area of Hand/Wrist/Forearm	Right Side	Left Side
Median Nerve Distribution	2.61	2.61
Ulnar Nerve Distribution	2.61	2.61
Radial Nerve Distribution	2.61	2.61

Table 15.9 Amal's Manual Muscle Testing Grades Completed at 7–8 Weeks Postoperation

	Right	Left
Wrist Flexion	4/5	5/5
Wrist Extension	4–/5	5/5
Wrist Radial Deviation	4+/5	5/5
Wrist Ulnar Deviation	4/5	5/5
Forearm Pronation	4–/5	5/5
Forearm Supination	4–/5	5/5

Table 15.10 Amal's Grip and Pinch Strength Measurements Completed at 5 Weeks Postoperation Using the Dynamometer and Pinch Meter

	Right	Left
Grip (Position II)	15	60
Using Dynamometer		
Lateral Pinch	10	16
Three-Point Pinch	9	15
Tip Pinch	5	10

Amal has a significant range of motion deficit in her non-dominant hand. These limited motions are wrist extension and flexion, radial and ulnar deviation, forearm supination, composite fist, thumb abduction and flexion (see Tables 15.2 and 15.3). Factors limiting her wrist/forearm range of motion include joint stiffness, extrinsic flexor and extensor tightness, swelling and pain and her adherent surgical scar (see Tables 15.4–15.6). Factors limiting thumb motion include webspace tightness, extrinsic flexor/extensor tightness and pain. Factors limiting composite fist include swelling, intrinsic and extrinsic muscle tightness and pain (see Tables 15.4, 15.3, and 15.4). She has pain in the ulnar wrist with forearm pronation and supination and pain in the dorsal wrist with both wrist flexion and extension (see Table 15.5). Her fine motor skills are slower than expected

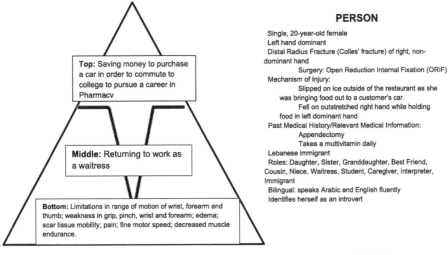

PERSON

Single, 20-year-old female
Left hand dominant
Distal Radius Fracture (Colles' fracture) of right, non-dominant hand
    Surgery: Open Reduction Internal Fixation (ORIF)
Mechanism of Injury:
    Slipped on ice outside of the restaurant as she was bringing food out to a customer's car.
    Fell on outstretched right hand while holding food in left dominant hand
Past Medical History/Relevant Medical Information:
    Appendectomy
    Takes a multivitamin daily
Lebanese immigrant
Roles: Daughter, Sister, Granddaughter, Best Friend, Cousin, Niece, Waitress, Student, Caregiver, Interpreter, Immigrant
Bilingual: speaks Arabic and English fluently
Identifies herself as an introvert

Top: Saving money to purchase a car in order to commute to college to pursue a career in Pharmacy

Middle: Returning to work as a waitress

Bottom: Limitations in range of motion of wrist, forearm and thumb; weakness in grip, pinch, wrist and forearm; edema; scar tissue mobility; pain; fine motor speed; decreased muscle endurance.

OCCUPATIONS

Occupations:
Family member - Sister, daughter, granddaughter, cousin, niece
    Amal helps her sister Nardine with her Cystic Fibrosis (takes her to medical appointments, helps her remember to take her medication and with her with home therapy)
    Cooking and baking with Teta and her cousins for family dinners while dancing in the kitchen to Arabic music. They make Lebanese food such as Warak Ennab, Tabouli, Kibbeh, Baklava, and Ma'amoul.
    Getting together for weekly family dinners every Sunday with extended family where they eat Lebanese food prepared by the cousins and Teta.
    Accompanying Teta to doctor's appointments to help with translating Arabic and English.
Best friend to Joyce
    Shopping - window shopping at the mall as they are both trying to save up money for school tuition and cars
    Having dinner at Joyce's parents' house and Amal's cousins' house with their families on the weekend. They often watch sitcoms on Netflix at each other's houses after family dinners
    Practicing yoga together at Joyce's house while her parents are at work. They follow yoga videos on YouTube.
Student
    Rides the city bus to school to attend local community college part-time while taking prerequisite classes. She has aspirations to attend a four-year college and ultimately become a pharmacist.
Waitress
    Waitress at the local Lebanese restaurant for the last three years in order to save money for college tuition/books as well as for a car. Recently picked up shifts to save more money now that she is on winter break from college. Walks to work from her family's home.

Activities:
    Cooking/Baking, Shopping, Watching television, Yoga, Part-time job as a Waitress, Rides bus to school

ENVIRONMENTS

Location: Emergency Room; Lebanese restaurant where she works that is walking distance from her home; Beirut, Lebanon; two-family house in Dearborn, Michigan; aunt's kitchen; car she uses to drive Teta to doctor's visits; local community college; bus stop and bus she takes to school

Physical: X-Rays, prefabricated wrist splint, customer's food she was carrying when she fell, shared family car, Middle Eastern foods, computer, textbooks and school supplies, ice, snow and cement where she fell, pad and pen to take orders at work, trays, dishes, apron and menus at the restaurant, snow when waiting for the bus for school

Temporal: Stayed the night in the hospital, surgery occurred the following morning; immigrated to the United States 5 years ago; family dinners every Sunday; does not enjoy waiting for the bus, especially in the winter months; hangs out with Joyce on the weekends; working as a waitress at the Lebanese restaurant for the past 3 years; works 20 hours per week at night and on the weekends to accommodate her class schedule, working extra shifts while on Winter Break

Social: Co-worker brought her to the Emergency Room; hand surgeon who performed the surgery; family members - Teta, mother, father, sister, Nardine, extended family (cousins, family in Lebanon); aunt, uncle and cousins also live in Michigan; Joyce - best friend

Virtual: Cell phone used for texting and WhatsApp, Arabic music, Netflix, Yoga videos on YouTube.

Figure 15.3 MMCR Guide to Understanding a Person's Story (Triangle)—Amal.

as per the nine-hole peg test (see Table 15.7). Her sensation is intact (see Table 15.8). Although not formally tested until later in Amal's rehabilitation due to postoperation precautions, it is expected that she has decreased grip, pinch and wrist strength (see Tables 15.9 and 15.10). Due to the deficits listed earlier, she has difficulty participating in many of her daily tasks.

Based on the information obtained from Amal's evaluations, Amal's long-term goal is to become a pharmacist within the next 5–6 years. In order to pursue pharmacy school, she needs to complete prerequisite courses at her local community college. Amal has to rely on public transportation to commute to classes, and she has been saving up money to purchase a car in order to make her commute easier. Having a car will also be beneficial when attending pharmacy school in the future as the commute may be farther than her current school. Amal has been picking up extra

Table 15.11 Analysis of Amal's Daily Tasks She Currently Has Difficulty Performing

Role	Tasks	Physical Requirements for tasks
Student	• Typing • Carrying books/bag	• Forearm pronation, radial/ulnar deviation, thumb abduction and extension, endurance • Forearm supination, grip strength, wrist strength, weight bearing
Worker	• Taking orders (holding order pad in right hand) • Tying work apron • Filling drinks • Holding tray of food • Passing out plates	• Forearm supination, grip strength, endurance • Wrist flexion and radial deviation, fine motor skills, pinch strength • Grip, wrist and forearm strength and endurance • Forearm supination, wrist extension, weight bearing, wrist strength and endurance • Grip and pinch strength, wrist and forearm strength and endurance

shifts at the Lebanese restaurant to save money, but due to her current injury, she is unable to work and therefore unable to continue saving money to purchase her car. Based on this information, the middle has been identified as returning to work as a waitress to resume saving money for her car. Amal's injury resulted in a distal radius fracture, impacting limited range of motion, weakness, decreased endurance, edema, scar tissue, pain and limited dexterity. These limitations in her right upper extremity have resulted in difficulty with performing various waitressing and student-related tasks. Table 15.11 provides some examples of tasks Amal currently has difficulty with and the physical requirements for these tasks.

Frame of Reference and/or Practice Model

Due to the nature of Amal's injury and the setting where she is receiving occupational therapy services for her distal radius fracture, the most fitting frame of reference to be used to guide the practitioner is the biomechanical frame of reference (see Figure 15.4). Using this frame of reference, the practitioner will take a bottom-up approach, looking specifically at how range of motion, strength and endurance impact Amal's ability to achieve her goals of returning to work to save money to purchase a car in order to pursue pharmacy school.

Overview Guide to Intervention Planning

Amal will be seen in an outpatient hand therapy clinic three times a week over the course of 8 weeks. Intervention will take place postoperation beginning at week 2 and ending at week 10. Typically, intervention for a distal radius fracture may be longer than 8 weeks; however, as this is a workers compensation case, 8 weeks is all that has been allowed by the insurance company.

There will be three phases of treatment, guided by the surgeon's postoperation protocol. During the first 3 weeks (week 2 to end of week 4 postoperation), intervention will focus on active and active assisted range of motion of the wrist and forearm, as well as passive range of motion to the hand (fingers and thumb). During this phase, the practitioner will also focus on pain and edema management. The hand surgeon has requested that Amal first return to work on a light-duty basis, specifically emphasizing that she is not to lift over 1 pound with her affected arm. Amal's job has offered for her to return as a hostess to fulfill the light-duty requirements. Therefore, Amal's first middle goal is to return to work as a waitress in order to pick up more shifts to save more money to purchase a car (see Figure 15.10).

Step 1: Frame of Reference (FOR)/Practice Model (PM):

Biomechanical Frame of Reference

Step 2: Words in a Box:

Remediation	Physical conditioning	Exercise	Kinematics	Torque

STRENGTH

RANGE OF MOTION
Active range of motion (AROM)
Passive range of motion (PROM)
Active assisted range of motion (AAROM)
Self-range of motion (SROM)

ENDURANCE

Passive stretching	Isotonic exercise	Resistance
Active stretching	Isometric exercise	Repetitions

Step 3: FOR/PM Party Paragraph:

The biomechanical frame of reference guides the practitioner to look at a person's range of motion (ROM), strength, and endurance and how they impact someone's participation in their daily tasks. Range of motion is the degree to which a joint move. There are four types of range of motion which include active range of motion (AROM), passive range of motion (PROM), active assisted range of motion (AAROM), and self-range of motion (SROM). Strength is the power of a muscular contraction and endurance is the ability to sustain muscular performance. Deficits in range of motion, strength and endurance may be restored, maintained or prevented through various methods such as physical agent modalities, movement, exercise, repetition and practice, stretching, positioning and splinting, graded activities, and altering the surrounding environment (Cole and Tufano, 2008; Fabrizio and Rafols, 2014; Whelan, 2014).

Step 4: Succinct summary of person's story emphasizing relevant occupational performance
∇ issues

Figure 15.4 MMCR Five-Step Guide to Infusing a Frame of Reference/Practice Model Into a Person's Evaluation Selection and Intervention Plan—Amal.

Amal, a current college student pursuing a career as a pharmacist (**top**), fell and sustained a distal radius fracture (DRF) of her non-dominant wrist while working as a waitress. As a result of this injury, she is experiencing limitations of hand, wrist, and forearm range of motion (**bottom**); strength deficits (**bottom**); and endurance deficits (**bottom**). These challenges are preventing her from participating in many daily tasks associated with her roles as a student, worker, caregiver, friend, and family member. She is currently unable to work as a waitress (**middle**) due to the above-mentioned limitations as many of her waitressing tasks require excellent ROM, strength and muscle endurance (**bottom**). Returning to this job is important to Amal in order to save money for a car to drive to school and pay for future pharmacy school expenses (**top**).

Step 5: Explanation of how the **FOR**/PM will directly influence the specific intervention plan:

Using the biomechanical frame of reference, the practitioner will address Amal's lack of range of motion, strength and endurance, which is a direct result of sustaining a distal radius fracture while working at the Lebanese restaurant.

As indicated by a distal radius fracture protocol, therapeutic intervention will first focus on restoring range of motion via active and active assisted range of motion. Improving her range of motion will allow Amal to perform activities with more ease, such as wiping down tables and taking orders at work, typing notes at school, meal preparation while cooking with her family, and driving her Teta to appointments.

Rehabilitation will then progress to passive range of motion and later focus on strengthening and endurance. Improving her strength and endurance will allow Amal to perform harder tasks on her joints and muscles, such as carrying trays and plates at work, books at school, weight bearing on her wrist during yoga, and rolling grape leaves while cooking with her family.

Figure 15.4 (Continued)

The second phase of intervention will focus on adding passive range of motion and gentle weight bearing to the wrist and forearm. Strengthening is still contraindicated during this phase. At this point, Amal will have returned to work as a hostess. Her next middle goal has now changed to returning to work as a full duty waitress in order to start making more tips and therefore resume saving money to purchase a car for commuting to school (see Figure 15.10).

The third phase of treatment can now incorporate strengthening, endurance training and full weight bearing. Amal will work toward obtaining an end range of motion as well. During this phase, Amal's immediate goal will be to build up enough muscle strength and endurance to be able to work more and longer waitressing shifts to save more money to purchase a car. Having a car will allow her to commute to college to eventually pursue a career in pharmacy (see Figure 15.10).

The second phase of intervention will focus on adding passive range of motion and gentle weight bearing to the wrist and forearm. Strengthening is still contraindicated during this phase. At this point, Amal will have returned to work as a hostess. Her next middle goal has now changed to returning to work as a full duty waitress in order to start making more tips and therefore resume saving money to purchase a car for commuting to school (see Figure 15.5).

The third phase of treatment can now incorporate strengthening, endurance training and full weight bearing. Amal will work toward obtaining an end range of motion as well. During this phase, Amal's immediate goal will be to build up enough muscle strength and endurance to be able to work more and longer waitressing shifts to save more money to purchase a car. Having a car will allow her to commute to college to eventually pursue a career in pharmacy (see Figure 15.5).

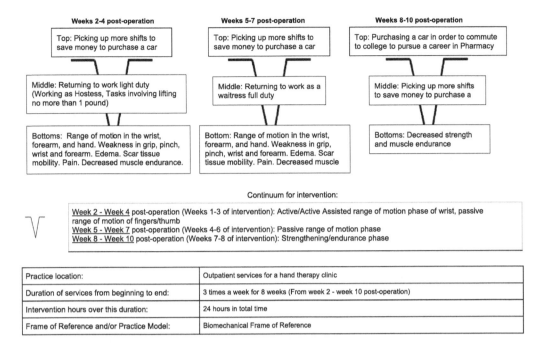

Figure 15.5 MMCR Overview Guide to Intervention Planning—Amal.

Planning Guide to Address Specific Sections of the Overall Intervention Plan

The beginning part of the overall intervention plan will focus on Amal returning to work as a hostess, as this was the light-duty position offered to her by her job. While working in the clinic, intervention will focus on respecting the protocol provided by the hand surgeon, such as focusing on active range of motion (AROM) and ensuring no strengthening at this time to allow the structures in Amal's wrist to heal. Specific job-related tasks, specifically hostessing skills, will be incorporated throughout intervention, which will be motivating for Amal and allow her to return to work at the restaurant light-duty by the end of this phase of intervention. Pain and edema will also be incorporated throughout intervention to assist Amal in managing these common postoperative issues while working a shift at the restaurant. Figure 15.6 provides a detailed explanation of what this part of the overall intervention plan may look like.

The middle part of the overall intervention plan will focus on Amal returning to work full-duty as a waitress, which will allow her to resume saving up money to purchase a car. While working in the clinic, intervention will now focus on transitioning from her light-duty position as a hostess to incorporating more challenging waitressing tasks. It is important to ensure continued adherence to her surgeon's postoperative protocol, including beginning passive range of motion (PROM) and gentle grip and pinch strengthening. As a result, Amal will begin engaging in waitressing tasks in the clinic that are unweighted and non-resistive at this time. Figure 15.7 provides a detailed explanation of what this middle part of the intervention plan may look like for Amal.

The end part of the overall intervention plan will focus on Amal increasing her strength and endurance in order to pick up additional waitressing shifts at the restaurant, which will be motivating to her as she is saving up money to purchase a car. Although Amal's top priority, which is saving money to purchase a car in order to commute to college to pursue a career, is not specifically being addressed at this time due to the 8-week duration of intervention, it will be discussed by Amal and the occupational therapy practitioner throughout this phase. While working in the clinic, intervention will now emphasize finalizing Amal's range of motion and strengthening her grip, wrist and forearm in order to allow Amal to successfully perform all waitress-related tasks

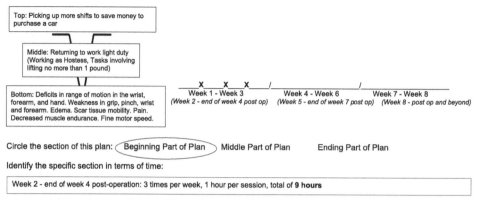

Circle the section of this plan: ⟨ Beginning Part of Plan ⟩   Middle Part of Plan   Ending Part of Plan

Identify the specific section in terms of time:

Week 2 - end of week 4 post-operation: 3 times per week, 1 hour per session, total of **9 hours**

Label and briefly describe the central idea of this specific section of the plan:

The practitioner will focus on specific job-related tasks required for Amal to return to the restaurant as a hostess (this is the light duty position that was offered to her by her job). The intervention will follow the specific post-op protocol provided by the surgeon. In this phase, the job-specific interventions will be focused on increasing the range of motion of her digits, thumb, wrist, and forearm through the use of occupation-based tasks. Some examples of tasks that will be simulated in the clinic are picking up and holding menus in her affected arm, practicing manipulating coins and bills for taking payments, and wrapping silverware in napkins. Pain and edema management will also be an important focus to help Amal deal with these common post-operative issues while working her shift.

How does this specific section connect to the overall intervention plan? Describe the ways these intervention ideas are related to ∇:

This connects to the overall intervention because addressing the above deficits will help her return to non-resistive, light duty tasks at the restaurant. Working as a hostess will be motivating for her because this is the first step to returning to full duty work as a waitress to be able to save enough money to purchase a car to commute to school. Although Amal is not currently able to work as a waitress, she is able to participate and successfully work as a hostess at the restaurant, which will likely be motivating for her as she will continue to make money to save up to purchase a car (top). At this time in treatment, she is not yet able to work as a waitress (middle) due to post-operative protocols, decreased range of motion, decreased strength, pain, endurance, and edema (bottom).

Describe the plan for creating awareness and/or skill building?

Early education (awareness) on her surgeon's post-operative protocols are important to establish boundaries for what Amal is and is not allowed to do at work and at home in order to avoid exacerbation of pain, edema and to protect the repaired fracture. This knowledge may also give her the confidence to begin moving her hand, wrist and forearm in a safe way even though it may feel scary and painful. Amal will be an active participant in identifying job-related tasks for being a hostess with the practitioner's help. The practitioner will educate Amal on the necessary skills required for each task (i.e. forearm supination, thumb flexibility, ability to make a full fist, and dexterity are required to handle cash/coins when taking payment from customers). This will be motivating for Amal to master these skills in order to return to her job. In this phase of Amal's recovery, pain, edema and lack of endurance will be very limiting both in therapy and at work. Amal will implement various techniques to reduce these symptoms during her treatment sessions. She can then carry these techniques over when starting her light duty position. Amal will observe the practitioner modeling the range of motion within various job-related tasks (i.e., supinating forearm to hold/carry menu, radial and ulnar deviation to answer the phone, finger flexion to grasp and hold wrapped silverware, etc.). She will then trial the various movements with her unaffected hand before attempting these tasks and activities with her injured hand. Amal will practice these exercises at home outside of treatment for increased repetition in order to increase her overall range of motion, which will allow her to be successful upon returning to work light-duty as a hostess.

Select specific methods used to promote change: (therapeutic use of occupations and activities, interventions to support occupations, education, training, advocacy, self-advocacy, group intervention and virtual interventions)

Occupations and activities: Hostess-related tasks that will address range of motion, dexterity, job-related endurance building (i.e., practicing picking up and holding menus in supinated position, wrapping silverware into napkins, holding various sizes of dowels to simulate gripping wrapped silverware, manipulating coins into cups to simulate taking payment).
Education and training: edema and pain management techniques (over the counter pain management, ice, use of gentle compression sleeve both at home and at work) to utilize while completing ADLs/IADLs and eventually at work as a hostess. Home exercises to assist in increasing range of motion through repetitions to allow her to successfully complete hostess-related tasks (and eventually waitress-related tasks). Post-operative protocol to give Amal a guideline for which tasks she will be allowed to perform at work and home. Scar management techniques to reduce hypersensitivity and improve wrist mobility.
Interventions to support occupations: *Physical Agent Modalities:* Use of moist heat to improve flexibility, use of ice to reduce swelling and pain. *Orthotics:* The surgeon will have provided Amal with a prefabricated wrist cock-up splint. The practitioner will emphasize the wearing schedule at home and eventually at work in order to protect the repair.

Identify and describe the specific teaching-learning principles to promote change

Modeling: The practitioner will first demonstrate range of motion exercises, edema management techniques, and job-related tasks.
Trial and error: Amal will then trial the motions, techniques and tasks modeled by the practitioner. Amal will trial and error various edema/pain management and job modification techniques both at home and when she returns to light duty position.
Education: Early education on her surgeon's postoperative protocol to establish boundaries of what activities are or aren't allowed. The practitioner will educate Amal on the necessary skills/motions related for job related tasks. She will also be educated on pain and edema management techniques.
Repetition/practice: This is an important part of the Biomechanical frame of reference and will be implemented within the clinic for range of motion and job-related tasks, as well as for home exercises. Due to Amal's pain and lack of endurance, she will not initially be able to complete multiple repetitions of each exercise; however, over time, as her pain and endurance improve, the number of repetitions she is able to complete will increase

Figure 15.6 MMCR Planning Guide to Address *Specific* Sections of the Overall Intervention Plan—Amal 1.

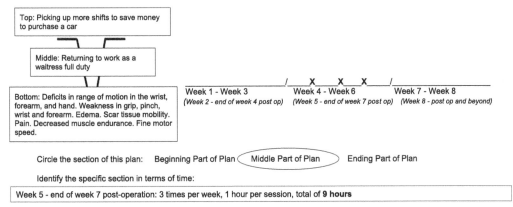

Top: Picking up more shifts to save money to purchase a car

Middle: Returning to work as a waitress full duty

Bottom: Deficits in range of motion in the wrist, forearm, and hand. Weakness in grip, pinch, wrist and forearm. Edema. Scar tissue mobility. Pain. Decreased muscle endurance. Fine motor speed.

	/ X X X /	
Week 1 - Week 3	Week 4 - Week 6	Week 7 - Week 8
(Week 2 - end of week 4 post op)	*(Week 5 - end of week 7 post op)*	*(Week 8 - post op and beyond)*

Circle the section of this plan: Beginning Part of Plan ⟨Middle Part of Plan⟩ Ending Part of Plan

Identify the specific section in terms of time:

Week 5 - end of week 7 post-operation: 3 times per week, 1 hour per session, total of **9 hours**

Label and briefly describe the central idea of this specific section of the plan:

The practitioner will focus on assisting Amal in transitioning from working as a hostess to beginning to take on more waitressing responsibilities, while adhering to the specific post-operative protocol provided by the surgeon (i.e., passive range of motion (PROM), begin gentle grip and pinch strengthening). In preparation for returning to work full-duty as a waitress, Amal will begin engaging in waitressing tasks that are unweighted and non-resistive. Some examples are 1. carrying an empty tray with her wrist in extension and forearm in supination, 2. wiping a table to address gentle weight bearing, wrist extension and radial/ulnar deviation, and 3. Tying an apron behind her back to work on forearm rotation, wrist flexion, and dexterity.

How does this specific section connect to the overall intervention plan? Describe the ways these intervention ideas are related to $\vee$:

Amal is now working as a hostess and has gained many of the skills required for hostess-related activities. Now that she has reached this goal, the middle has changed to returning full duty as a waitress (middle). In order to tap into her middle, which is motivating, the practitioner will incorporate various waitressing tasks into intervention at the clinic to work on end range of motion, gentle weight bearing, and gentle grip/pinch strengthening as described above (bottom). Amal will be motivated to practice these skills to return to work as a waitress so she can make tips again. This will allow her to save more money to purchase a car in the future (top).

Describe the plan for creating awareness and/or skill building?

Continued education (awareness) on post-operative protocols are important to establish boundaries for what Amal is and is not allowed to do at work and at home in order to avoid exacerbation of pain, edema and to protect the repaired fracture. Amal, with the help of the practitioner, will review and practice waitress-related tasks in order to rebuild the range of motion and skills required for being a waitress at the Lebanese restaurant. The practitioner will have Amal go through her typical day at work and practice the various tasks she will need to complete in the appropriate sequence as she would when attending to customers. These activities will be performed unweighted as her surgeon's post-operative protocol does not allow for strengthening of the wrist and forearm at this time and only allows for gentle weight bearing. As she continues to practice these job-related skills during intervention, these unweighted tasks will become easier and will set her up for success when she is able to try them with weight and resistance once cleared by her surgeon.

Select specific methods used to promote change: (therapeutic use of occupations and activities, interventions to support occupations, education, training, advocacy, self-advocacy, group intervention and virtual interventions)

Occupations and activities: Waitress-related tasks that will address end range of motion, job-related endurance building, gentle weight bearing and gentle grip/pinch strengthening. Some examples of this are: 1. Carrying an empty serving tray to work on forearm supination, digit and wrist extension, proprioception and stability, and gentle weight bearing. 2. Wiping a table to work on forearm pronation, wrist extension and weight bearing, radial and ulnar deviation. 3. Pouring cotton balls from a carafe into a cup to address gripping, forearm rotation, wrist flexion (*cotton balls used as this is unweighted and the practitioner wants her to practice the motion without breaking postoperative protocol*). 4. Tying apron behind her back to address forearm rotation, wrist flexion and radial deviation, and dexterity. ***Education:*** pain management techniques (for muscle soreness after a 4-hour waitressing shift) and energy conservation techniques (rest breaks as injured wrist will have reduced endurance for waitressing tasks). Upgrade home exercises to further challenge her range of motion (can incorporate some leisure interests for home exercises, such as rolling out dough while baking to address weight bearing, flexibility and grip strengthening). ***Interventions to support occupations:*** <u>*Physical Agent Modalities:*</u> Use of moist heat to improve flexibility, use of ice to reduce pain at the end of treatment sessions, at home, and at work as needed. <u>*Orthotics:*</u> The practitioner will decrease the wearing schedule requiring Amal to wear her splint only while working. ***Advocacy:*** <u>*Self-advocacy:*</u> The practitioner will encourage Amal to advocate for herself by requesting an additional employee to assist her as needed as she returns to working as a waitress.

Figure 15.7 MMCR Planning Guide to Address Specific Sections of the Overall Intervention Plan—Amal 2.

Identify and describe the specific teaching-learning principles to promote change:

> **Modeling:** The practitioner will model range of motion exercises, edema management techniques, and waitress-related tasks.
> **Trial and error:** Amal will then trial the motions, techniques and tasks modeled by the practitioner. Amal will trial and error various edema/pain management and job modification techniques both at home and when she returns to her waitressing position.
> **Education:** Continued education on surgeon's postoperative protocol to review boundaries of what activities are or aren't allowed. The practitioner will educate Amal on the necessary skills/motions related to waitress-related tasks. She will also continue to be educated on pain and edema management techniques.
> **Repetition/practice:** This is an important part of the Biomechanical frame of reference and will be implemented within the clinic for range of motion and job-related tasks, as well as for home exercises. Amal will continue to work on increasing the amount of repetitions of exercises she is able to do as she builds a tolerance and endurance to new passive exercises done in the clinic and at home for home exercises. Amal is now able to work a full four hour shift as a hostess as her endurance and pain have improved. The focus will now be on building enough endurance to work a four-hour waitress shift; this will be challenged by increasing sets and repetitions for job-related skills, in-clinic exercises, and home exercises.

Figure 15.7 (Continued)

independently. Per her surgeon's postoperative protocol, she is now able to engage in strengthening activities, which will incorporate grading waitressing tasks by increasing weight and resistance as tolerated, utilizing restaurant supplies in order to promote a more naturalistic environment within the clinic. At the conclusion of the 8 weeks of intervention, Amal will be provided with an extensive home exercise program to continue to work on her strength and endurance, as the insurance company has denied further visits due to the consistent progress Amal has made and her ability to return to work as a waitress. Figure 15.8 provides a detailed explanation of what the final part of the overall intervention plan may look like for Amal.

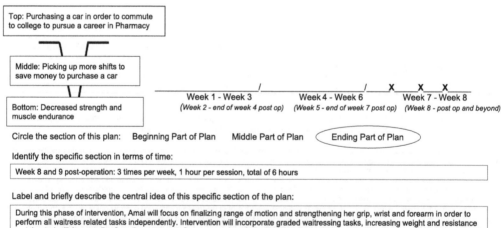

Circle the section of this plan: Beginning Part of Plan   Middle Part of Plan   ⟨ Ending Part of Plan ⟩

Identify the specific section in terms of time:

> Week 8 and 9 post-operation: 3 times per week, 1 hour per session, total of 6 hours

Label and briefly describe the central idea of this specific section of the plan:

> During this phase of intervention, Amal will focus on finalizing range of motion and strengthening her grip, wrist and forearm in order to perform all waitress related tasks independently. Intervention will incorporate graded waitressing tasks, increasing weight and resistance as tolerated utilizing supplies from the restaurant. Some examples of job-related tasks that will be utilized include carrying a serving tray with dishes and plates from the restaurant increasing weight and duration as tolerated, holding and pouring water from a carafe/pitcher and picking up and placing plates on the table with her affected hand.

How does this specific section connect to the overall intervention plan? Describe the ways these intervention ideas are related to ∇:

> Amal has been cleared by her surgeon to return to working as a waitress, however she currently needs assistance from other staff to carry food trays due to her limited strength and muscle endurance. Now that Amal will be returning to waitressing, her middle has changed to picking up additional shifts at the restaurant. Therefore, her treatment sessions will focus on building her strength and endurance in order to tolerate longer and more frequent shifts. As she is able to work multiple shifts within a week, she will then be able to save more money to purchase a car. Once she is able to purchase her car, she will have more freedom and flexibility to attend classes. The top will not be specifically addressed at this time, however it will be discussed by Amal and the practitioner throughout intervention.

Figure 15.8 MMCR Planning Guide to Address Specific Sections of the Overall Intervention Plan—Amal 3.

Describe the plan for creating awareness and/or skill building?

> Amal has been cleared for strengthening as tolerated in the clinic, but her surgeon has given her specific instruction to return to waitressing tasks with a five pound weight limit until her next doctor's appointment. Before her first day back to work, the practitioner will educate Amal on what a 5 pound weight limit means for her job (in example, what does 5 pounds look like in a water carafe and feel like on a serving tray) so she can then carry over this knowledge when working at the restaurant. Amal and the practitioner will review ways to modify heavy waitressing tasks to decrease the amount of stress on her wrist until she can perform the tasks as she did prior to injury. Two examples are 1. Using her forearm to stabilize the tray with a neutral wrist versus holding the tray only on her hand/wrist. 2. Using two hands to hold and pour water from the carafe. Amal will be instructed to trial the various techniques while working her shifts at the restaurant and provide a report of how her shift went at her next therapy session. Based on the information Amal provides, the various waitressing tasks and activities will be adapted and modified as needed and will direct the course of intervention. While in the clinic, Amal will continue to go through her typical day at work and practice the various tasks she will need to complete in the appropriate sequence as she would when attending to customers. These activities can now be performed weighted and the practitioner will gradually upgrade each task by increasing the weight and the duration and/or number of repetitions as tolerated over time during intervention to further develop these skills.

Select specific methods used to promote change: (therapeutic use of occupations and activities, interventions to support occupations, education, training, advocacy, self-advocacy, group intervention and virtual interventions)

> *Occupations and activities: Waitress-related tasks* practiced in the clinic, gradually increasing weight and number of repetitions to build strength and endurance. Some examples are: 1. Carrying tray with plates from the restaurant, gradually adding weight on top and increasing carrying time as tolerated. 2. Holding and pouring water from a carafe, beginning with a small amount of water and filling up to the top as tolerated. 3. Picking up and placing plates on table with affected hand, gradually adding weight as she gains grip/pinch and wrist/forearm strength. *Home exercises* incorporating her leisure interests to increase strength, weight bearing tolerance and endurance. One example is practicing graded yoga positions (wall planks transitioning to downward dog pose).
> *Education*: Energy conservation techniques (rest breaks as injured wrist will have reduced endurance for waitressing tasks) and proper body mechanics and ergonomics to decrease the amount of stress placed on her wrist joint. Upgrade home exercises to begin strengthening and increasing her muscle endurance (continue to incorporate leisure interests for home exercises as mentioned above). Educate Amal on her home exercise program upon discharge from therapy.
> *Interventions to support occupations: Physical Agent Modalities:* Ice to reduce pain at the end of treatment sessions, at home, and at work as needed.
> *Advocacy*: The practitioner advocated for more therapy sessions, however due to the steady progress Amal has made and her ability to return to work as a waitress, the request was denied. Therefore, the practitioner will discharge Amal with a home therapy program at the conclusion of Week 8.

Identify and describe the specific teaching-learning principles to promote change:

> *Self-directed learning:* Amal will now begin to carry over techniques taught to her in the clinic while working her shifts at the restaurant. During a shift, she will assess each task and evaluate/monitor her ability to perform the task. Based on her ability to perform the task, she, by herself, will implement a modification technique as needed in order to be successful at performing this task and independently complete a four hour waitressing shift. Amal will be discharged after 8 weeks of intervention and will likely need to continue to modify tasks for a little while longer until she obtains full range of motion and strength, which could take several months post-operation.
> *Modeling:* The practitioner will model strengthening and weight bearing exercises, pain management techniques, and job-related tasks.
> *Trial and error:* Amal will then trial the strengthening and weight bearing exercises, and body mechanic techniques for heavy waitressing tasks (such as holding a heavy tray, pouring heavy pitcher of water) modeled by the practitioner. Amal will then trial and error those techniques and will report back on whether they were successful or not.
> *Education*: The practitioner will educate Amal on what a 5 pound weight limit feels like for waitress-related tasks. She will get an updated home exercises program prior to discharge to continue practicing end range of motion, weight bearing, and strengthening.
> *Repetition/practice*: This is an important part of the Biomechanical frame of reference and will be implemented within the clinic for range of motion, strengthening, weight bearing and job-related tasks, as well as for home exercises.

Figure 15.8 (Continued)

Evaluation Summary Using the POP Acronym

P

Amal is a 20-year-old, left-hand-dominant female. She is currently a student at her local community college, and her dream is to become a pharmacist. Amal has been working as a waitress at her local Lebanese restaurant for 3 years in order to save enough money to purchase a car to make her commute to school easier and eventually commute to pharmacy school. Amal had been working extra shifts to save additional money while on winter break from school. Two weeks ago, Amal slipped and fell on the ice while taking a pick-up order out to a customer's car, injuring her right wrist. She was taken to the hospital where they did an x-ray and found a right comminuted distal radius fracture. Surgical intervention was required to stabilize the fracture with ORIF. She was placed in a cast 2 weeks ago and is now attending occupational therapy services to begin skilled rehabilitation according to the postoperative protocol in order to return to work. Amal's case is being managed by workers compensation due to this being a work injury.

The Role Checklist and Upper Extremity Functional Index were used to obtain Amal's occupational profile. The Role Checklist asked Amal about what roles she identifies with and how satisfied she is with her current ability to perform those roles. The Upper Extremity Functional Index asked Amal about specific tasks she needs to perform with her upper extremity and how difficult these tasks currently are based on her current status. The practitioner then used these evaluations to further probe and gather additional pertinent details and collaborated with Amal to develop her goals. Amal's main goal is to return to work in order to continue saving money for a car to commute to school to eventually become a pharmacist.

O

As a result of Amal's distal radius fracture, Amal presents with many physical impairments impacting functional use of her right non-dominant hand. She has decreased range of motion of the wrist, forearm and hand. She presents with increased pain and edema, decreased dexterity, and decreased strength and endurance. These deficits are impeding her participation in activities of daily living, school tasks, cooking and baking with her family, practicing yoga with her best friend and performing waitressing tasks. Amal's inability to work as a waitress at this time is particularly problematic, as it is a means to save money to purchase a car to pursue college classes and eventually become a pharmacist. Amal reports she is motivated to become a pharmacist; however, due to her recent injury, she is feeling frustrated and nervous that she will be unable to work and pick up extra shifts to save enough money for a car and for college.

Amal is in need of near full range of motion and good grip and wrist strength in order to perform waitressing tasks independently. Particular tasks that will be a challenge for Amal are holding a tray of food in her affected arm, passing out plates of food, filling drinks and tying her work apron. Upon returning to work, she will likely struggle with decreased endurance and will have to build up the tolerance to work a full shift and even more so to pick up extra shifts to continue saving for her car purchase. Amal will highly benefit from skilled occupational therapy services to address

Relevant areas to the person's evaluation findings	Strengths	Challenges	Raw Data	Interpretation
Fall at work causing right distal radius fracture		X	Amal reported that she sustained a right distal radius fracture while working a Friday evening shift at the restaurant two weeks ago. As she was taking a pick-up order out to a customer's car, she slipped on the ice reaching out her right arm to brace her fall. X-rays were taken that night at the emergency room that showed a comminuted Colles' fracture of her right wrist. Per the surgeon's note, Amal required an open reduction internal fixation (ORIF) as a reduction of the fracture would not be sufficient.	Even though Amal's injury impacted her non-dominant hand, there are many daily tasks requiring bilateral hand use and non-dominant hand use that are vital for work, school, home and leisure activities. Surgery will stabilize the fracture, but will subsequently cause scarring, swelling and increased pain. Amal will then have to learn to manage these symptoms as they will initially impact her ability to participate in the simplest of tasks, particularly work tasks. Simple tasks, such as returning to hostess activities, will be challenging.
			A Worker's Compensation case was filed the night of the injury since her injury occurred on work property during her shift.	When and how much therapy will be determined by the worker's compensation insurance company. This can possibly limit her ability to attend therapy sessions and obtain range of motion and strength measurements comparable to her prior level of function.
			The hand surgeon provided his specific postoperative protocol for the therapist to follow throughout intervention.	The postoperative protocol is important to guide the therapist in creating appropriate treatment interventions based on where she is in her recovery. This will also determine what tasks she will be able to do at work.

Figure 15.9   MMCR Guide to Evaluation Summaries—Amal.

Student pursuing career as a pharmacist	X	X	Amal identified performing the role of a worker on the Role Checklist, specifically working as a pharmacist in the future. Amal explained that her parents value the importance of a higher education. She reports that it was expected of her to attend college. Her career aspirations have been influenced both by her parents' insistence to pursue a medical career and by Nardine's journey with Cystic Fibrosis. Amal's goal is to transfer to a four year college and finish with a degree in Chemistry, and later apply to pharmacy school. Amal reports having "quite a bit of difficulty" completing her usual school activities at this time, such as typing and carrying her books/bag. Amal described wanting to take classes full-time after purchasing her car in order to shorten the amount of time it will take her to become a pharmacist.	STRENGTH: Amal appears to be excited and motivated to pursue a career as a pharmacist as she has always been interested in caring for Nardine with Cystic Fibrosis. This is likely a strength for Amal as she aspires to transfer to a four year college and pursue a degree in pharmacy. Amal has always felt the expectation from her parents to pursue higher education. CHALLENGE: Her recent injury has impacted her ability to achieve her goal of becoming a pharmacist as she cannot save money for a car, tuition and books. Completing various school-related activities such as typing her notes and carrying her school supplies are difficult, and may cause frustration and stress, likely decreasing her motivation to be fully invested in her schooling while recovering from her fracture.
Working as a waitress		X	Amal identified being a worker as a present and future role of hers via the Role Checklist. She reports currently working as a waitress and identified wanting to work as a pharmacist in the future. Amal has worked at the local Lebanese restaurant since she was 17 years old to help relieve some of the financial stress off of her parents. She typically works about 20 hours a week on nights and weekends to accommodate her class schedule. While on winter break, she picked up extra shifts at the restaurant. Amal is working to save enough money to purchase her own car so she can drive herself to class. Per the Upper Extremity Functional Index (UEFI), Amal reports having "quite a bit of difficulty" completing any of her usual work activities. Amal currently reports difficulty taking orders (holding order pad in right hand), tying her apron, pouring drinks, holding trays of food and passing out plates, therefore she is unable to work as a waitress at this time. Amal identified returning to work as a waitress as one of the specific goals she would like to work toward.	Working as a waitress is likely a challenge for Amal at this time as she is unable to work due to her recent injury. Amal is likely feeling uneasy about her inability to work and complete various work-related tasks. She has been very motivated and focused on working extra shifts over winter break in order to save up enough money to purchase a car, which she is now unable to do. Amal will likely want to return to work as soon as possible, which may help motivate her to complete various exercises and activities during therapy sessions that she initially may be hesitant to try due to fear of pain after her recent injury.
Saving money to purchase a car for transportation to school	X	X	The family shares one car; Amal's father usually drives the car to work every day, but otherwise it is available for use by Amal and her mother. Amal has continued to work at the restaurant to pay for school and is now saving up money for her own car. Amal has been taking courses part-time at her local community college, so that she can continue working to save money for school, books, a car, and pocket money. She currently takes the bus to class, however she stated she would like to start driving to class as it is very annoying waiting for the bus, especially in the winter months. Amal identified saving up money to purchase a car as one of the specific goals she would like to work toward.	STRENGTH: This is something she is motivated to do and has developed a plan in order to achieve this goal. Amal has been working since she was in high school to relieve her parents of any extra financial burden. She has always used the money she made while working as a waitress to support her interests and hobbies, however recently she decided she wanted to save up to purchase a car to make it easier to travel to and from school. CHALLENGE: She is currently relying on public transportation to get to and from class, therefore she must adapt her schedule to the bus schedule each day. As a result of her recent injury, saving money to purchase a car is also a challenge for Amal as she can no longer pick up extra shifts at work during winter break as she is currently unable to work as a waitress.
Enjoys cooking and baking with her family	X	X	Amal identified being a family member as a meaningful role she performs on the Role Checklist, which she is somewhat satisfied with. Amal shared that she has always enjoyed cooking and preparing desserts with her cousins and their Teta. Amal reports that Teta teaches her and her cousins Lebanese cooking, while Amal teaches Teta the English language during her visits. Amal's extended family gets together every Sunday for family dinners at her aunt's house. Amal currently reports difficulty cooking with Teta and her cousins. She states having difficulty washing and prepping ingredients, cutting/chopping, opening jars and bags and lifting pots and pans at this time.	STRENGTH: Amal appears to be proud of and value the time she spends with her family, specifically cooking and baking, which is likely a strength for Amal. This will motivate her to use her injured arm in cooking tasks which can further improve her motion and strength. Amal appears to have a very close relationship with Teta as she cherishes their time together and also teaches her English while they bake together with her cousins. CHALLENGE: As a result of her current injury, cooking and baking has likely now become more of a challenge due to her limited range of motion, weakness and increased pain and edema.

Figure 15.9 (Continued)

Practicing yoga with her best friend Joyce	X	X	Per the Upper Extremity Functional Index (UEFI), Amal reports having "extreme difficulty or unable to perform activity" for her usual hobbies, recreational or sporting activities, specifically reporting difficulty doing yoga at this time. Amal reports developing an interest in yoga during her senior year in high school. Amal and Joyce never pursued actual classes as they are expensive and their parents would not approve since they are not open to the spirituality aspect of yoga. Since then, Amal reports she and Joyce have been looking up yoga videos on Youtube to practice their skills and technique at Joyce's house when her parents are not home so they do not get in trouble.	**STRENGTH:** She will be motivated to return to this meaningful occupation with her friend, further encouraging her to improve her range of motion and strength to return to waitressing. Yoga can also be used as a home exercise tool to improve wrist extension and weight bearing in the later phase of therapy. Another strength is that yoga is a good coping mechanism for stress; Amal may be stressed due to her recent injury as she is worried about her recovery process and not being able to work to save money to purchase a car. **CHALLENGE:** It is a challenge because many yoga positions will be challenging and contraindicated in the early phases of therapy.
Decreased range of motion		X	**Range of Motion (using a goniometer)** <table><tr><td>**Motion** (normal range)</td><td>**Right**</td><td>**Left**</td></tr><tr><td>Forearm Pronation (80)</td><td>80</td><td>80</td></tr><tr><td>Forearm Supination (80)</td><td>20</td><td>80</td></tr><tr><td>Wrist Extension (60-70)</td><td>25</td><td>65</td></tr><tr><td>Wrist Flexion (60-80)</td><td>10</td><td>70</td></tr><tr><td>Wrist Radial Deviation (20)</td><td>5</td><td>20</td></tr><tr><td>Wrist Ulnar Deviation (30)</td><td>10</td><td>30</td></tr></table>	Amal's limited range of motion is an obstacle to participating in many of her activities related to her identified roles. She requires near full range of motion in her wrist and forearm to perform waitressing duties and her leisure activities such as yoga and baking. Amal needs full range of motion in order to return to work so that she can save enough money to purchase a car to commute to school.
Decreased strength		X	**Dynamometer and Pinch Meter (completed at 5 weeks post-operation)** <table><tr><td></td><td>**Right**</td><td>**Left**</td></tr><tr><td>Grip (Position II) *Using Dynamometer*</td><td>15</td><td>60</td></tr><tr><td>Lateral Pinch</td><td>10</td><td>16</td></tr><tr><td>3 Point Pinch</td><td>9</td><td>15</td></tr><tr><td>Tip Pinch</td><td>5</td><td>10</td></tr></table> **Manual Muscle Testing (completed at 7-8 weeks post-operation)** <table><tr><td></td><td>**Right**</td><td>**Left**</td></tr><tr><td>Wrist Flexion</td><td>4/5</td><td>5/5</td></tr><tr><td>Wrist Extension</td><td>4-/5</td><td>5/5</td></tr><tr><td>Wrist Radial Deviation</td><td>4+/5</td><td>5/5</td></tr><tr><td>Wrist Ulnar Deviation</td><td>4/5</td><td>5/5</td></tr><tr><td>Forearm Pronation</td><td>4-/5</td><td>5/5</td></tr><tr><td>Forearm Supination</td><td>4-/5</td><td>5/5</td></tr></table>	Amal's limited strength is an obstacle to participating in many of her activities related to her identified roles. It is also something that cannot be addressed until the end phase of treatment as per her surgeon's protocol. She requires at least a 4+/5 manual muscle test score to adequately perform many waitressing tasks, such as holding a tray of food and pouring water from a pitcher. Her grip strength is low and was likely around 55 pounds prior to her injury. Low grip strength will impact tasks such as holding a full pitcher of water. Improving her strength and muscle endurance will allow Amal to return to work full duty as a waitress to begin collecting tips to save money for a car.

Figure 15.9 (Continued)

the previously mentioned deficits in order to return to her waitressing job independently in order to save money for a car to pursue her scholastic career in pharmacy. Figure 15.9 provides a detailed guide of the relevant areas pertinent to Amal's evaluation findings and how this information was interpreted to create her evaluation summary.

P

Amal's Occupational Therapy Goals

Long-term goal (LTG): Amal will improve the functional use of her right upper extremity while working as a waitress to continue saving money to purchase a car to commute to pharmacy school in the future.

1. _____ Amal _____ **will**

   (Person's name)

2. | increase forearm supination to 50 degrees | **in order to**

   (measurable, comes from bottom occupational performance issues)

3. | hold menus with her right upper extremity | **with**

   (functional and specific, comes from top or middle occupational performance issue)

4. _____ no difficulty _____ **in**

   (measurement, how much cuing, prompting or physical assistance)

5. _____ 3 weeks _____

   (time frame for achievement)
   MMCR Guidelines to Formulate a Short-Term Goal – Amal

1. _____ Amal _____ **will**

   (Person's name)

2. | increase right grip strength to 30 pounds | **in order to**

   (measurable, comes from bottom occupational performance issues)

3. | hold a half-full pitcher of water | **with**

   (functional and specific, comes from top or middle occupational performance issue)

4. _____ minimal difficulty _____ **in**

   (measurement, how much cuing, prompting or physical assistance)

5. _____ 6 weeks _____

   (time frame for achievement)

Figure 15.10 MMCR Guidelines to Formulate a Short-Term Goal—Amal.

MMCR Guidelines to Formulate a Short-Term Goal – Amal

1. _____Amal_____ **will**

(Person's name)

2. | unilaterally hold a serving tray with 5 pounds of dishes | **in order to**

(measurable, comes from bottom occupational performance issues)

3. _____serve 3 meals at the restaurant_____ **with**

(functional and specific, comes from top or middle occupational performance issue)

4. _____independence and minimal pain_____ **in**

(measurement, how much cuing, prompting or physical assistance)

5. _____8 weeks_____

(time frame for achievement)

Figure 15.10 (Continued)

Short-term goal (STG)—Phase 1: Amal will increase right forearm supination to 50 degrees in order to hold menus in her affected arm without difficulty in 3 weeks.

Short-term goal (STG)—Phase 2: Amal will increase grip strength in her right hand to 30 pounds in order to hold a half-full pitcher of water with minimal difficulty in 6 weeks.

Short-term goal (STG)—Phase 3: Amal will unilaterally hold a serving tray with 5 pounds of dishes in order to serve three meals at the restaurant independently with minimal pain in 8 weeks.

Explanation of Goals

During each of the three phases of intervention, goals will reflect which challenges are being addressed at that time in relation to her work status. Figure 15.10 depicts the process and component parts utilized to create three potential short-term goals during each portion of Amal's overall intervention plan. Amal may not reach full range of motion and strength by the end of her intervention; however, she will continue working on achieving these goals through a home exercise program and during functional activities. Amal will likely return to full-duty work prior to discharge. By returning to full-duty work, she will be able to continue working toward her long-term goal to save money for a car and attend pharmacy school in the future.

References

Cole, M. B., & Tufano, R. (2008). Biomechanical and rehabilitative frames. In *Applied theories in occupational therapy: A practical approach* (pp. 165–172). Slack Incorporated.

Fabrizio, A., & Rafols, J. (2014). Optimizing abilities and capacities: Range of motion, strength, and endurance. In M. V. Radomski & C. A. Trombly Latham (Eds.), *Occupational therapy for physical dysfunction* (7th ed., pp. 589–613). Lippincott Williams & Wilkins.

Hoppenfeld, S., & Murthy, V. L. (2000). *Treatment and rehabilitation of fractures.* Lippincott Williams & Wilkins.

Scott, P. J. (2019). *Role checklist version 3: Participation and satisfaction (RCv3).* Model of Human Occupation Clearinghouse, Department of Occupational Therapy, University of Illinois at Chicago. https:\\moho-irm.uic.edu.

Stratford, P. W., Binkley, J. M., & Stratford, D. M. (2001). Development and initial validation of the upper extremity functional index. *Physiotherapy Canada, 53*(4), 259–267.

Whelan, L. R. (2014). Assessing abilities and capacities: Range of motion, strength, and endurance. In M. V. Radomski & C. A. Trombly Latham (Eds.), *Occupational therapy for physical dysfunction* (7th ed., pp. 144–241). Lippincott Williams & Wilkins.

16 Case Example

Using the MMCR to Guide a Seven-Day Intervention Plan in an Inpatient Acute Rehab Hospital

Christine A. Bodzioch, Marlee Murphy, Shaniqua Bradley, and Ashley N. Fuentes

Introducing Hannah

Hannah is a 25-year-old female who identifies as Persian Orthodox Jewish. She currently lives with her husband Jacob, who also identifies as Orthodox Jewish from an Israeli descent. Hannah and Jacob became first-time parents three months ago to their daughter Sarah. They also live with their four-year-old dog Toby.

Hannah and Jacob moved into a new home one year ago due to a work promotion Hannah received. They live in a single-level home in a small suburban northeast town in the mountain countryside. Prior to this move, both Hannah and Jacob were part of the same Orthodox community with a strong support system, surrounded by their family and close friends. Hannah reports that their families were mostly supportive of this endeavor. Hannah does display some hesitation at the idea and describes some strained relationships with her parents. Hannah reports that her parents had always envisioned that their children would raise their families in the same Orthodox community that Hannah was raised in. Hannah describes her mother as a "worrier" and reports that her mother has had a difficult time being so far away from Hannah and her granddaughter, especially during the pandemic with all the travel restrictions. Hannah reports that although she aims to focus on her own personal family, this does cause her some stress since she is so close with her family.

Onset of Current Medical Condition

One winter morning, Hannah described waking up feeling dizzy and a little "off". These symptoms did not subside, and new symptoms began to gradually emerge, including numbness and tingling along her entire right upper and lower extremities. Hannah also began to notice changes in fine motor control in her right hand when going about her daily routines. Her husband Jacob immediately contacted emergency medical services (EMS), and she was taken to the local hospital.

Medical Chart Review

Hannah is a 25-year-old female who arrived at the emergency department via EMS services accompanied by her husband Jacob. Hannah was admitted after initial observation and client report of symptoms. After further medical evaluation and imaging, it was determined that Hannah sustained a small acute infarct within the left posterior frontal lobe and parietal lobe. Due to the acute nature of the infarct, no surgical intervention or evacuation of bleed was warranted at this time. Hannah has a past medical history significant for a previous diagnosis of coronavirus disease 2019 (COVID-19), she is currently three months postpartum, and has a diagnosis of generalized anxiety disorder. She was evaluated by the acute care rehabilitation team and deemed an excellent

DOI: 10.4324/9781003392408-20

candidate for skilled inpatient therapy services. Hannah is scheduled for discharge and transfer to acute rehabilitation to further maximize her independence.

Overview of Acute Rehabilitation Stay

After a short stay in the acute care hospital for medical stabilization, Hannah was transferred to an inpatient acute rehabilitation setting to begin her recovery and journey back home. Hannah was seen by an occupational therapy practitioner the morning after her admission for a 90-minute evaluation which comprised an occupational profile via the Kawa Model evaluation (Iwama, 2006), an evaluation of activities of daily living via the Arnadottir OT-ADL Neurobehavioral Evaluation (A-ONE) (Árnadóttir, 1995), an evaluation of upper extremity motor control via the Wolf Motor Function Test (Figueiredo, 2021), range of motion, and manual muscle testing (Kendall et al., 1993). The evaluation process was completed across two sessions, including the initial evaluation and second treatment session, due to the length and depth of the evaluations utilized. Due to COVID-19 precautions, only one support person is permitted into hospital settings. Therefore, while Hannah is in rehab and after discharged to home, Jacob's sister and Hannah's parents will be present to help with childcare and household duties.

Hannah's Occupational Profile via the Kawa Model Results

Hannah's life flow has been impacted by a variety of things that she has identified during her interview. During this initial client interview, Hannah appears very worried and anxious. She is observed consistently rubbing her right arm/hand with her left, shifting her weight frequently in her chair, and tapping her foot on the floor. She is open to sharing her story, her challenges, and her strengths with the practitioner. She easily accepts the comfort and reassurance from her husband Jacob, whom she identifies as a part of her riverbank and has always been extremely supportive to her. Jacob has his arm around her back and is observed frequently rubbing her back, especially when sharing more difficult information. Hannah identified her sister-in-law as a positive support within her riverbank, as she is currently in town assisting with childcare. This level of support allows Hannah's river to continue to flow more smoothly, as childcare is one less thing she needs to worry about in the present moment.

Hannah reports that she works as an accountant. She describes this as a very high-demanding job which she identifies as one of her river rocks. This rock does not completely block the flow of her river, as water is still able to flow around this rock. Although it causes some disruptions in her river flow due to the stressful nature of her job, it provides her and her family with the financial security and freedom needed, especially with a new baby. Hannah states that Jacob also works full time in marketing. Hannah describes this recent move as ideal for her career advancement and offers them a new adventure. This can be seen as a part of her riverbank, as it supports their love for the outdoors. Hannah and Jacob both share a love for the outdoors, which she identifies as part of her driftwood, as this helps both of them refocus their energy after a long day of work to help guide their river flow and prepare for the next day. Hannah speaks with excitement as she describes this new home being within close proximity to nature and the outdoors. Hannah describes how her job makes up part of her life flow. She describes her work relationships as another aspect of her riverbank, providing support while at work, but they do not continue along her river. The stability of her job in the midst of the pandemic positively impacts her river as driftwood.

As Hannah's river continues, Hannah and Jacob described feelings of excitement at the start of 2020 being in a new place (part of her riverbank) and feeling as if they were about to fully start their lives together. Another rock Hannah identified in her life was a sense of frustration when the COVID-19 pandemic began and their expectations had gone to "the back burner". Hannah shares about their difficulty fully integrating into their new Orthodox community as a result of the pandemic. She highlights all the changes in rules and regulations that disrupted their typical routines associated with Shabbat, which created an obstacle in her life flow. Hannah reports that during Shabbat, one of her favorite parts is preparing the meals and sharing it with others (see Table 16.1.) She describes this meal as a pillar to community building and a means to create bonds and a support system within a community, which she views as a part of her riverbank. Without this presence, Hannah's riverbank is beginning to fall apart, and the flow of her river begins to quicken and become unsteady. This is causing a huge disruption in her daily activities and occupations.

Table 16.1 Key Orthodox Terms

Shabbat	• Shabbat, which is Hebrew for sabbath, is the seventh day of the Jewish week and is recognized as the day of rest and prayers (Jewish Virtual Library, 2008).
	• Shabbat, although associated with not performing any work, not utilizing any electronic devices, or driving, is a day eagerly anticipated by those individuals who observe. It is viewed as a means to rest and take a break from the busy day-to-day routines (Jewish Virtual Library, 2008).
Shabbat Rituals	• Shabbat begins at sundown on Friday evenings attending synagogue followed by a leisurely meal shared with family and/or friends (Jewish Virtual Library, 2008).
	• Shabbat meals begin with a prayer led by the man of the household. There is an additional prayer recited over two loaves of challah, which is a sweet bread formed in the shape of a braid (Jewish Virtual Library, 2008).
	• Meals are typically stewed or slow cooked due to cooking being prohibited during Shabbat (Jewish Virtual Library, 2008).
	• Saturday also begins with attending synagogue followed by sharing another meal with family and/or friends. Shabbat ends at sunset on Saturday (Jewish Virtual Library, 2008).

Hannah describes her weekday routines, including starting with a home workout, work, and ending the day taking her dog for a walk with Jacob. Hannah's routines are such a steady feature of her life and her life with Jacob, which makes them a big part of her riverbank. Her structure was necessary throughout the week, especially Wednesdays and Thursdays leading up to Shabbat. Hannah would spend longer hours on those evenings preparing meals for the weekend. This time and devotion to preparing meals prior was necessary, as the use of electricity and doing work of any kind are not permitted during Shabbat. Therefore, Hannah needs to have all of the meals prepared and ready to be warmed up on warming trays by Friday afternoon. She describes her weekends during and after her Shabbat routines and spending time in nature along the local hiking trails as also part of her driftwood, as this has positively influenced her life.

Shortly into the pandemic, Hannah reports that she and Jacob learned that they were expecting their first child, which would soon become a new addition to her riverbank. She describes the joy and excitement of this adventure as lightness in the midst of a dark year.

As Hannah's water of her river continues to flow, since life is constantly going, Hannah describes going to the doctor one day following onset of fever, chills, and a cough. She ultimately tested positive for COVID-19, which she identifies as a rock, as this added another challenge in her life and greater disruption to her river flow. Hannah describes getting COVID-19 as a large rock in her river. She quickly got better and realized her case was mild without need for any significant medical intervention. This rock began to break down into smaller rocks and ultimately pebbles. However, these pebbles are still present in her river flow and result in these mild ripples which appear as her brain fog, fatigue, and joint pain as she began to notice that her productivity at work would drop if she was not mindful to utilize her planner and make her daily to-do lists. Hannah also stated it was difficult to care for Sarah with all of her residual symptoms of fatigue and joint pain. Her daily walks and weekend hikes left her body feeling levels of fatigue she had not experienced in the past, which now created an obstacle in her life flow.

After her diagnosis of COVID-19, Hannah returned back to the office twice a week mid-summer and continued to work from home the other days of the week.

After the birth of Sarah, Hannah received 12 weeks maternity leave. The birth of her daughter and subsequent role shifts incited multidimensional changes and anxieties for Hannah. Hannah reported an internal struggle, which she identified as part of her driftwood, as this has negatively impacted her life. She identified this time as stress provoking and isolating, since her riverbanks were minimal due to the pandemic. Hannah reports she began to notice the things her mother warned her about such as being alone and away from family during a pivotal moment such as welcoming a child into the world. Hannah also began to experience increased anxieties related to having a newborn during the pandemic which she also stated was part of the driftwood in her river. Hannah reports that she began to feel an internal struggle between how she previously identified herself: hard working, goal driven, and independent (driftwood positively impacting her life) and where she now was: isolated and alone (driftwood negatively impacting her life). She reports that she often felt verbalizing these feelings out loud would make them real.

Hannah identifies her roles as a wife, mother, friend, family member, and accountant. She reports that her family (parents/sibling) and best friend are also huge parts of her life. Though they all live out of state, she still identifies them as part of her riverbank. Hannah also describes her personal characteristics (i.e., driftwood) as family oriented, religious, social, active, nature loving, hardworking, very goal oriented, and someone who has a difficult time with change.

As Hannah's river continues, she reports that another rock in her life will be upon discharge when she will help take care of Sarah (see Table 16.2). She reports that her sister-in-law will be staying with them after she is discharged, and her parents will be able to stay for a short time; however, Hannah wants to still be able to assist with childcare tasks. She reports that the other members in her community and synagogue have offered to support with meals. In terms of physical assistance, she will be able to have the assistance from her sister-in-law and parents.

Table 16.2 Hannah's Personal Goals

Personal goals as stated by Hannah
1. "To take care of Sarah and be her mom"
2. "Take care of my typical day-to-day routines; get myself dressed, take a shower, put on my headscarf, all those things"
3. "I want to be able to support my family and house again, to take care of things around the house and prepare a Shabbat meal"

Hannah reports that she anticipates Jacob will need to return to the office for work and does not want to add any additional stress to his life by requesting he stay home with her. One of Hannah's immediate challenges (i.e., rocks) she identifies is needing to manage her hair to be able to put on her wig, headscarf, or snood while going out into the community (see Table 16.3). She will often wear a headscarf or snood when going to pediatrician appointments, going for walks, or to the park

Table 16.3 Key Orthodox Terms 2

Head coverings: • Wigs • Headscarf • Snood	In the orthodox religion, women will not typically show their hair in public after their wedding. They will wear either a wig or a headscarf. This is referred to as a sheitel. This signifies that a woman is married (Salzberg, 2020).

with Sarah. She states that she will complete this routine while standing in front of her bathroom mirror. Hannah also described wearing her wig, headscarf, or snood as an important part of her identity and her roles as a wife and an Orthodox woman. She did mention that she has two wigs: one that she will wear daily during the week and one that she wears on the weekends, going to synagogue or events. Hannah describes that her wig is a major part of her daily routine. Hannah describes at home, her wig is kept on a stand in her walk-in closet, as she does not like to keep it near the sink for hygiene purposes. She explains that her typical routine around putting her wig or headscarf on includes brushing her hair, putting her natural hair into a ponytail, clipping her hair, then placement of the wig on her head. While her wig plays a role in her daily routine, Hannah stated she will not be wearing it while in a hospital setting. Hannah describes her use of a head scarf or snood during quick or casual interactions/outings and will be her primary head covering while in the hospital.

Hannah also identified additional rocks/areas of concern following her stroke: the anxiety returning to her role as a mother due to decreased use of her right upper extremity, mild balance deficits, difficulty efficiently engaging in her self-care skills, and an inability to drive (please refer to Figure 16.1 to review Hannah's Kawa River).

When looking at the end of Hannah's river, she explained that she sees this area as free from most rocks and driftwood that have been negatively impacting her. She stated that she sees this area as an opportunity to continue her role as a mother and being able to care for her newborn with the least amount of challenges and obstacles following her stroke and COVID-19 diagnosis (see Figure 16.1).

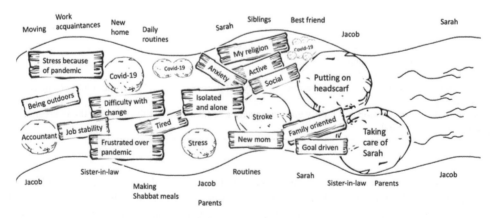

Figure 16.1 Hannah's Kawa. Created by Ashley N. Fuentes, OTD, OTR/L. Used with permission.

Analysis of Performance

ADL Evaluation via A-ONE (see Table 16.4)

Hannah engaged in her morning activities of daily living (ADL) routine within the confines of the rehabilitation setting. Upon admission, Hannah's husband brought her personal items for ADL sessions, including preferred clothing and toiletries. The bathroom within the room was utilized as well as the hospital-provided meals and meal tray. For the purposes of this evaluation, Hannah engaged in her grooming routine, dressing tasks, mobility tasks, and cognitive/communication skills.

Hannah's scores:

Dressing: 5/20
Grooming 5/24
Transfers/mobility: 15/20
Feeding: 8/16
Communication: 4/4

The results of this evaluation indicated the presence of premotor perseveration, difficulty with organization/sequencing, and motor deficits in her right upper extremity. Due to the presence of these neurobehavioral deficits, Hannah required considerable assistance in dressing, grooming, and feeding. She displayed the ability to safely navigate within her room without the use of an assistive device. She was observed with slower movements when walking within her hospital room and observed occasionally using environmental features (bed, countertop, etc.) to ensure stability when needed. These mild losses of balance occurred during less than 25% of the session.

An area of concern reported during the ADL evaluation was in regard to Hannah's ability to manage her headscarf. Hannah describes her headscarf as being a vital aspect of her identity and culture.

Table 16.4 Additional Information About the A-ONE

The A-ONE	• The Arnadottir OT-ADL Neurobehavioral Evaluation, which has been most recently referred to as the Occupation-Based ADL-Focused Neurobehavioral Evaluation, was utilized during Hannah's evaluation to determine performance in activities of daily living. This assessment is utilized in order to gain specific information about task performances, type, and severity of limitations (Árnadóttir, 1995).
	• Scoring for the A-ONE is completed via clinical observation and the determination to what degree various neurobehavioral impairments are impacting participation in ADL tasks.

Range of Motion

Hannah presents with full active range of motion in her unaffected left upper extremity. During testing of her affected right upper extremity, Hannah presents with full range of motion, however, with decreased fluidity of movement and observable lag in comparison to her left. There is no presence of hypertonicity.

Manual Muscle Testing

Left upper extremity (unaffected): 5/5 at all pivots
Right upper extremity (affected): 3+/5 at all pivots indicating full range of motion against gravity
    and ability to hold slight resistance at testing position

Wolf Motor Function Test

The Wolf Motor Function Test (WMFT) was utilized in order to assess and determine the quality of right upper extremity movement through completion of timed functional tasks (see Table 16.5). During testing, Hannah scored a 53. Her scores indicate mild deficits in right upper extremity motor control. The results indicate greater difficulty with refined fine motor movements as a greater degree of synergy observed during these testing components. Her greatest strengths appear proximally where her movements are close to normal; however, there is a presence of decreased fluidity.

Table 16.5 Additional Information About the Wolf Motor Function Test

The Wolf Motor Function Test (WMFT)	• This assessment was utilized in order to determine the quality of right upper extremity movement through completion of timed functional tasks • An individual is asked to perform a variety of functional movement patterns, and the quality of the movement is scored on a 0–5 scale based on efficiency and fluidity of movements (Figueiredo, 2021)

Hannah's Triangle Explanation

The middle and top are identified directly from Hannah's occupational profile to include her occupational performance issues, including management of her headscarf (middle), as she will need to be able to do this as she wants to be able to care for her daughter Sarah (top), including taking her to her pediatrician appointments and going to the park. Through Hannah's occupational profile and bottom evaluations performed utilizing the WMFT, A-ONE, and manual muscle test, the bottoms of the triangle were determined that will directly impact Hannah from performing the middle and top occupational performance issues independently mentioned earlier (see Figure 16.2).

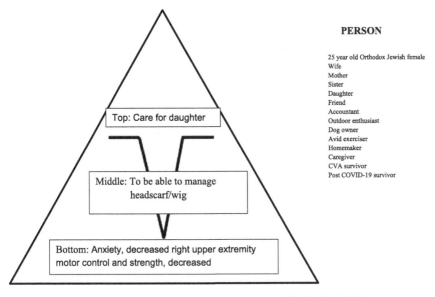

PERSON

25 year old Orthodox Jewish female
Wife
Mother
Sister
Daughter
Friend
Accountant
Outdoor enthusiast
Dog owner
Avid exerciser
Homemaker
Caregiver
CVA survivor
Post COVID-19 survivor

Top: Care for daughter

Middle: To be able to manage headscarf/wig

Bottom: Anxiety, decreased right upper extremity motor control and strength, decreased

OCCUPATIONS:

Occupations:
Putting on her headscarf, wig, or snood each morning while standing at her bathroom counter
Hair care including brushing her hair, putting hair in ponytail
Cooking in her kitchen at her kitchen island using her All Clad pans that were gifted to her from her aunt on her wedding day
Preparing Shabbat meals for her family each week using serving ware that has been passed down generations
Hiking with her family within their town carrying her favorite orange backpack filled with water and snacks
Breast feeding Sarah in her nursery rocking in her rocking chair, bottle feeding Sarah

Activities:
Going to work
Managing her home
Changing Sarah's diapers using Pampers Pure
Dressing Sarah
Giving Sarah a bath in their guest bathroom using Tubby Todd
Going to pediatrician appointments with Sarah
Cleaning, laundry
Travelling
Walking the dog around the loop in her neighborhood twice or to the town center
Going out to eat with husband
Going to the park with Sarah
Attending synagogue

ENVIRONMENTS

Location: Inpatient acute rehabilitation, single family home, local gym, accounting office, car, outdoor spaces (hiking trails, mountains, woods)

Physical: Head scarf, snood, two wigs, foam wig stand, hair brush, hair tie, hair clip, Pampers Pure diapers, Sarah's clothing, personal grooming supplies/toiletries, baby stroller, crib, baby carrier, changing table, Spectra breast pump, Aventi baby bottles, hiking boots, exercise clothing/shoes, exercise equipment (free weights, weight machines), Dyson cordless vacuum cleaner, All Clad pots/pans, family heirloom serving ware for Shabbat meals

Temporal: 90 minute OT sessions, 7 day length of stay in rehab facility, full time employment (40 hours a week), 30 minute commute twice a week, 3 months postpartum, 3 month old baby, moved 1 year ago, married for 16 months, 5 days post CVA, 3 months post COVID-19 diagnosis, 8 years working in accounting, Going to the gym in her town pre-covid at 5 AM, working out at home in their home office turned partial home gym 5 times a week

Social: Friends, coworkers, boss, Jacob, Sarah, religious group, parents, siblings

Virtual: working from home, using laptop computer with trackpad, using Zoom for video calls for work, texting/calling her friends/family, watching television, live streaming workout classes, social media to stay in touch with friends and get news (i.e., Facebook, Instagram)

Cultural: Follows practices of Orthodox Judaism, new motherhood, accounting/business world, health/wellness/exercise culture

Figure 16.2 MMCR Guide to Understanding a Person's Story (Triangle)—Hannah.

Frame of Reference/Practice Model

The Kawa Model serves as both an evaluation to gather information and a practice model to guide the intervention plan (see Figure 16.3). The motor learning frame of reference uses meaningful tasks of the person's choosing to assist with recovery (see Figure 16.4) (Gillen & Nislen, 2020). Both of these guidelines for action complement each other, as the Kawa was used to gather information about Hannah's story and the motor learning frame of reference guides the practitioner to assist Hannah to have an optimal recovery from her stroke while engaging in the tasks that are meaningful to her (i.e., managing her hair to be able to put on her headscarf, caring for her daughter).

Step 1: Frame of Reference (FOR)/**Practice Model (PM)**: The KAWA Model

Step 2: Words in a Box:

Social context	Personal assets and liabilities	Rocks	Personal Attributes
Cultural Context	River	Metaphor	Micro level	Values	Social role
Life flow and health	Water	Occupation	Macro level	Personality
Physical Environment	River walls and bottom (floor)		Spaces/channels
Life Circumstances	Social Environment	Driftwood	Person/environment relationship

Step 3: FOR/PM Party Paragraph:

The Kawa Model was developed by Dr. Michael Iwama. According to Iwama (2006), when the self is seen metaphorically as a river, all of the elements including self, society, and circumstances are constructed as elements of one; all things are connected and difficult to comprehend in isolation. Similar to a river, changes to one's aspect of their water course including the river sides and walls, driftwood and rocks, will end up affecting the entire river. The river is a metaphor for life and occupation is part of the flow of the water in the river. There can be no river without water flowing and without occupations, there can be no life. Through occupational therapy, this metaphorical representation is used to help enhance the person's life flow. The water symbolizes life and the water flow is shaped and bounded by the river walls and floor, and by rocks of various sizes. The floor symbolizes the family environment walls symbolize the social environment. Driftwood represents the person's personal attributes, values, character, personality, immaterial and material assets, living situation that can positively or negatively affect their circumstance and life flow. At times, these items can obstruct water flow, and in other instances, they can help to dislodge, or push through other factors that impede flow. Rocks of various sizes represent the person's life circumstances such as accidents, illnesses and other unexpected life events. There are also "spaces" between these areas that are the points through which the person's life energy (water) flows.

Step 4: Succinct summary of person's story emphasizing relevant occupational performance
        ∇ issues

Figure 16.3 MMCR Five-Step Guide to Infusing a Frame of Reference/Practice Model Into a Person's Evaluation Selection and Intervention Plan—Hannah's Kawa.

Hannah identifies herself as a hard working, goal driven, and independent woman. Hannah's culture is extremely important to her and plays a role in how she views herself as a woman and her roles and routines around Shabbat. Hannah enjoyed preparing meals and sharing it with others. She also embraces her role as new mother to her daughter Sarah. However, following a diagnosis of COVID-19 and recent stroke, Hannah is experiencing decreased right upper extremity motor control and strength (bottom), decreased organization and sequencing (bottom), and anxiety (bottom) impacting her ability to care for her daughter, perform her job, prepare Shabbat meals, take walks and going on weekend hikes with her family. Hannah would like to manage her hair care including brushing her hair, putting it into a ponytail, and clipping her hair into her head scarf or snood (middle). Being able to manage her hair and wear her headscarf will help her to participate in caring for Sarah, her newborn child when going to pediatrician appointments with her and going to the park or on walks together in order to fulfill her role of being a mother (top).

Step 5: Explanation of how the FOR/PM will directly influence the specific intervention plan:

The KAWA model will be utilized to guide Hannah's treatment intervention to address how her life (water/river) continues to flow. Her river is restricted by her problems and challenges (rocks) including her impairments impacted by having COVID-19 and a stroke including being able to put on her headscarf and being able to care for her newborn child. The KAWA model will help to reduce and remove the various elements that are currently impeding Hannah's river flow to allow it to flow more smoothly. The aim will be to manipulate Hannah's various rocks and reduce the obstacles by providing her strategies for managing her hair in order to be able to put on her headscarf which is important for her to be able to participate in outdoor activities including activities caring for her daughter. The open spaces in the river (ie. the areas between the rocks/driftwood where the water is still flowing) are areas for opportunity and/or improvement. As Hannah works on being able to manage her hair including strategies brushing her hair, learning techniques to put her hair in a ponytail, and managing the clip for her hair, the spaces in her river will become larger, which will allow for a better life flow/flow of the river. Also, as a result of learning the strategies and techniques for her hair care and management, the rocks may become smaller or even disappear as these may no longer be as great of challenges for her. These spaces also provide opportunities for enhancing life flow and providing new learning, which is where intervention takes place. The model will also utilize Hannah's driftwood including spending time outdoors, and her personal attributes to enhance her life flow and overcome her personal life circumstances of her stroke and COVID-19.

Figure 16.3 (Continued)

Step 1: Frame of Reference (FOR)/Practice Model (PM): Motor Learning Frame of Reference

Step 2: Words in a Box:

Motor Learning	Function-based	Person	Environment	Tasks
Purposeful movement	Client factors	Performance skills		
Meaningful Occupations	Varied Contexts	Variable Practice		
Whole Tasks	Activity Demands	ADLs	IADLs	Roles
Participation	Cognitive Systems	Psychosocial Systems	Task Analysis	

Step 3: Frame of reference and/or practice model party paragraph:

The motor learning frame of reference is considered to be a holistic approach to motor recovery pulling from theories of psychology, behavioral sciences, neurology and medicine (Cole & Tufano, 2019). Through this lens, motor recovery emerges as a result of multiple systems interacting within unique tasks and environmental contexts (Gillen, 2020). Using motor learning to guide intervention, that practicing variations of the same tasks within varied context is better than practicing the same task within the same context for upper extremity motor recovery. Therefore, engaging a person in a whole task versus components of a task is believed to create greater change.

The use of meaningful tasks of the person's own choosing is a vital aspect as it serves to facilitate greater motivation which in turn serves to improve the repetitive practice required for motor skill acquisition (Cole & Tufano, 2019). Therefore, practitioners develop a thorough occupational profile to fully understand the person's life story such as through the use of the Kawa model. Through a thorough understanding of the individual's life story, the practitioner then has a greater understanding of the person's meaningful occupations and is then able to collaborate with the person to select meaningful tasks to facilitate recovery.

Step 4: Succinct summary of person's story emphasizing relevant occupational performance
     ∇   issues

Figure 16.4 MMCR Five-Step Guide to Infusing a Frame of Reference/Practice Model Into a Person's Evaluation Selection and Intervention Plan: Hannah's Motor Learning FOR.

Hannah has identified she is a hard working, goal driven, and independent woman. Hannah's culture is extremely important to her, however since the COVID-19 pandemic began, there were rules and regulation changes that disrupted Shabbat. Hannah enjoyed preparing meals and sharing it with others. She also embraces her role as new mother to her daughter Sarah. However, following her diagnosis of COVID-19 and having a stroke, Hannah is experiencing decreased right upper extremity motor control and strength (bottom), decreased organization and sequencing (bottom), and anxiety (bottom) impacting her ability to perform her everyday tasks including caring for her daughter, preparing Shabbat meals, and managing her hair care routines. Hannah would like to now be able to manage her hair including brushing her hair, being able to put her hair in a ponytail and clip her hair to her head in order to be able to put on her head scarf or snood (middle). Being able to manage her hair and wear her headscarf will help her to participate in caring for Sarah, her newborn child when going to pediatrician appointments with her and going to the park or on walks together in order to fulfill her role of being a mother (top).

Step 5: Explanation of how the frame of reference and/or practice model will directly influence the specific intervention plan:

The motor learning frame of reference will be utilized to guide Hannah's intervention to address her decreased right upper extremity motor control and strength (bottoms). Through the lens of motor learning, meaningful tasks of Hannah's own choosing will be utilized to guide intervention sessions. This can be seen through addressing functional movement patterns in order for Hannah to be able to incorporate and use her affected right upper extremity to be able to brush her hair, put her hair in a ponytail, and be able to put on her headscarf.

Figure 16.4 (Continued)

Intervention Planning

First Phase: Inpatient Rehabilitation

As you can see by each of the occupational performance issues, the top/middle/bottom, Hannah's lived experiences and her recovery are evolving and can be seen through the changing aspects of her life (see Figure 16.10). As Hannah progresses through her recovery, she begins to experience shifts in her top, middle, and bottom and cannot be confined to just one. When Hannah enters the acute rehabilitation phase, as illustrated by the first occupational performance symbol, she has multiple bottoms while in the early phases of her recovery. While it appears that the next step would be to address putting on her wig, there is an important consideration. Although the wig plays an important role in her routine culturally, additional steps are first necessary to serve as steppingstones to achieve this. Due to the cultural significance and the value associated with the wig, Hannah will not bring her wig into an inpatient setting. Rather, she will be using alternative hair covering, including use of a headscarf or snood. Hannah's top goal is to return to caring for her daughter Sarah. This phase of her recovery will serve as preparation for ultimately putting on her wig once she gets back home. This aspect of her recovery will also address the necessary steps which come before putting on her headscarf such as brushing her hair and placing her hair into a ponytail. These components to her intervention plan are necessary for Hannah once she returns home, as a hair covering is required anytime she leaves her house, as she would like to bring Sarah to the pediatrician (top) or going to the park, for example.

It is important to note since this is only a seven-day stay in inpatient, the practitioner has to be aware of what immediately can be addressed in this short time. The practitioner needs to know that Hannah will probably not achieve independence of her goals during inpatient rehab because there is not enough time to fully practice. Therefore, her husband/family members will be included since they will be assisting her at home and upon discharge.

Transitioning to the Next Phase

It is important for the practitioner to also think about Hannah's other two occupational performance issues when transitioning to the next practice area (please refer to Figure 16.10). Hannah's interventions do not stop after the inpatient unit, and while the occupational therapy practitioners will not follow her throughout all the services, they need to be mindful of the progression of treatment.

Second and Third Phases: Outpatient Rehabilitation

When Hannah transitions from the inpatient level to the first phase of her outpatient recovery, there is a shift in her top/middle/bottom in the second occupational performance issue on the guidesheet. At this phase in her continuum, her middle has now shifted to identify a specific childcare task and her top remains the same, as these goals have not been achieved to Hannah's desired levels, although Hannah has made progress accomplishing putting on her wigs (please refer to Figure 16.5).

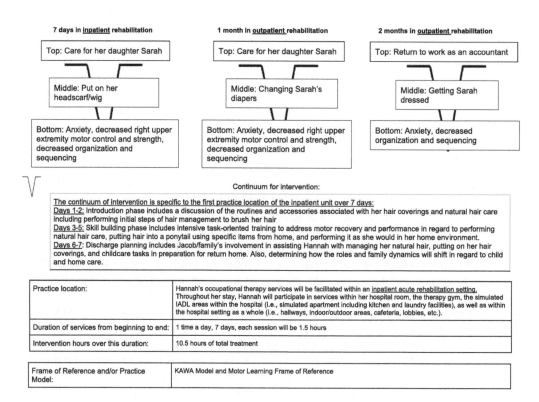

Figure 16.5 MMCR Overview Guide to Intervention Planning: Hannah.

During this phase, Hannah will continue to address her bottom/middle through a spiral up/down approach as well as begin to incorporate addressing her top through the interventions at this level of care. As Hannah progresses through outpatient rehab, she will begin to experience a shift in her top/middle/bottom as seen through improved mastery of skills and achieving goals. Hannah's final top/middle/bottom reflect these accomplishments as the number of bottoms have decreased. Her previous middle has now been accomplished; therefore, her previous top shifts downward and becomes her middle and a new top appears (returning to work as an accountant). As Hannah's recovery progresses, she may begin to notice or identify new goals and desires which impact her life. It is vital that the practitioner continuously communicate with the person to ensure client-centered care remains consistent throughout the continuum.

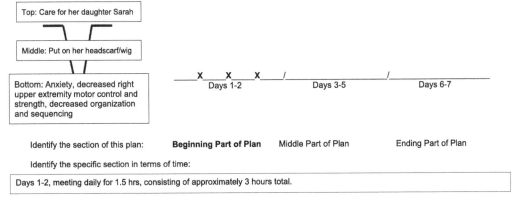

Identify the section of this plan: **Beginning Part of Plan**   Middle Part of Plan   Ending Part of Plan

Identify the specific section in terms of time:

Days 1-2, meeting daily for 1.5 hrs, consisting of approximately 3 hours total.

Label and briefly describe the central idea of this specific section of the plan:

Intervention will focus on discussing Hannah's specific hair care routine, cultural and daily aspects of wearing a head scarf including identifying appropriate accessories needed, home environment setup, and beginning to practice the movements and kinematics in order to brush her hair utilizing her right upper extremity.

How does this specific section connect to the overall intervention plan? Describe the ways these intervention ideas are related to ˅:

This connects to the overall intervention plan because it taps into Hannah's middle which is motivating to her. By discussing the cultural and daily aspects of wearing a headscarf/wig, hair routine, rearranging her hospital room to simulate her home environment, and strategizing a daily routine for Hannah while in rehab, this is helping her to organize and sequence what she will need in order to prepare for putting on her headscarf. While Hannah is not performing childcare tasks directly at this point, being able to wear a headscarf is important to her when doing outside activities with her daughter including doctor's appointments, going on walks, etc.

Describe the plan for creating awareness and/or skill building?

Hannah is motivated to put on her headscarf so this plan will primarily focus on building skills needed to complete this task. Hannah has been able to perform the steps to putting on her headscarf daily. However, she will now need to learn the skills necessary to be able to put on her headscarf in a different way following her stroke. It will be important to begin with the tasks needed to take care of her natural hair and manipulate accessories needed to be able to put on the headscarf.

Select specific methods used to promote change:(therapeutic use of occupations and activities, interventions to support occupations, education, training, advocacy, self-advocacy, group intervention and virtual interventions)

Education and therapeutic use of occupations and activities: This aspect of the intervention plan will teach Hannah strategies and identify the steps needed to be able to manage her hair and accessories in order to ultimately put on her head scarf through motor recovery and facilitate neuroplasticity. It will also help to foster optimal motor recovery of her right upper extremity which is required for the various tasks/steps including brushing her hair, putting her hair in a ponytail and clipping her hair to be able to wear the headscarf. A visual generation of the steps required for being able to put on her headscarf will be utilized to support her occupation and further improve her organization and sequencing skills.

Identify and describe the specific teaching-learning principles to promote change:

1. Identification of Hannah's learning style in order to ensure success during the remainder of the interventions, 2. Modeling proper right upper movement and kinematics needed to brush her hair, holding the hair brush 3.Organizing the physical environment to support Hannah's ability to learn and set her up for optimal success when transitioning back to her home environment including setting up the bathroom with all of the necessary equipment needed to put on her headscarf including the brush, hair ties, clip, headscarf

Figure 16.6 MMCR Planning Guide to Address Specific Sections of the Overall Intervention Plan—Beginning.

Specific Sections of the Overall Intervention Plan

Beginning

The first two days of intervention will focus on identification of Hannah's learning style, discussing cultural and daily aspects of wearing a headscarf, home environment setup, and daily routine setup while in rehab (see Figure 16.6). This process will include:

- Identify the steps needed to manage her hair, accessories for management, and putting on her headscarf and create a visual aid.
- Rearrange Hannah's hospital room to simulate her home environment as best as possible for the best learning to take place.
- Practice the movements and kinematics needed to brush her hair.

During this intervention plan, the practitioner will:

- Engage in therapeutic listening and utilize therapeutic use of self to determine Hannah's learning style and preferred learning methods.
- Learn Hannah's story associated with her headscarf and wigs, as well as understand her routines associated around her headscarf, snood, and wigs.
- The practitioner will collaborate with Hannah to create a visual aid for the steps needed to be able to put on her headscarf. This will also serve to decrease anxiety often associated with uncertainties of new learning.
- Identify any modifications to Hannah's accessories in order to utilize her right dominant hand to complete tasks (i.e., built up handle on her brush) and perform massed practice for the necessary movements required to brush her hair.

This aspect of the intervention plan revolves around Hannah's middle occupational performance issue, as this is motivating for her. Hannah values the ability to put on her headscarf, as this plays an important role in her culture and personal identity being an Orthodox woman. This is also a major part of her daily routine when leaving her home.

Another aspect of this intervention plan is to set up Hannah's hospital room to simulate her home environment. Placing a bedside table on the appropriate side of the bed can simulate the bassinet and the space required between getting out of bed and how she will need to care for Sarah while at home. The practitioner will also assist Hannah in creating a visual aid while in rehab to assist with her organizing and sequencing the steps required for putting on her headscarf, as well as to help decrease any anticipated anxiety.

Middle

The focus of the intervention is on assisting Hannah with practicing the steps required for all aspects of her hair care. This includes management of her natural hair and putting on her headscarf (see Figure 16.7). This process will include:

- Verbally breaking down the steps to put her natural hair up and put on her headscarf.
- Utilizing a visual schedule/checklist to determine the steps of tasks in order to address sequencing.
- Practice putting her natural hair up to ensure increased ease when donning the headscarf and ultimately the wig upon return home.
- Practice effective manipulation of the headscarf, including putting on/taking off of her head.

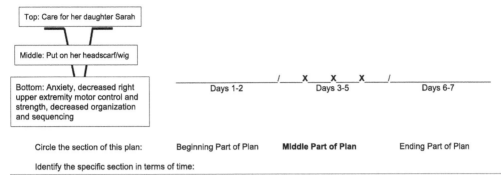

Circle the section of this plan: Beginning Part of Plan   **Middle Part of Plan**   Ending Part of Plan

Identify the specific section in terms of time:

Days 3-5, meeting daily for 1.5 hours. Approximately 4.5 hours total to address the middle portion of this intervention plan.

Label and briefly describe the central idea of this specific section of the plan:

The focus of the intervention plan is on assisting Hannah with practicing the steps necessary to manage her natural hair including brushing her hair, putting her hair in a ponytail, clipping her hair, and putting on her headscarf.

How does this specific section connect to the overall intervention plan? Describe the ways these intervention ideas are related to ∨ :

This aspect of the intervention plan continues to revolve around Hannah's middle occupational performance issue. Wearing and donning her headscarf are described as being vital aspects of her image and her routines as an Orthodox woman. By breaking down the steps of the task, she is addressing organization, sequencing, and fine motor aspects required for the task. Through the repetitive actions of reaching her affected and unaffected upper extremities overhead, she is addressing her decreased strength and motor control. The top occupational performance issue continues to be indirectly addressed as the neuromuscular re-education and motor planning being reinforced are critical for all aspects of carryover for childcare and parenting tasks. The practitioner will also discuss how this learning will transition home. Hannah will need to be mindful of her efficiency with completing the task. As putting on her headscarf becomes more habitual, it will take her less time and will impact the time needed for her daily routine to get ready for pediatrician appointments.

Describe the plan for creating awareness and/or skill building?

Hannah will work to break down the steps of putting her hair in a ponytail to work to mentally re-connect with the motor planning required for these movement patterns. She will incorporate adaptive devices suggested by the practitioner to assist with making the task easier (i.e., built up handle on brush, scrunchie, pre-tied head scarf). She will practice all aspects of hair care as a whole task to facilitate optimal motor recovery as outlined through the motor learning frame of reference

Select specific methods used to promote change:(therapeutic use of occupations and activities, interventions to support occupations, education, training, advocacy, self-advocacy, group intervention and virtual interventions)

Education will be provided on use of appropriate adaptive devices to utilize during the task of putting her hair in a ponytail and putting on her headscarf. Therapeutic use of occupations and activities will be used to practice putting her hair in a ponytail incorporating her right upper extremity and being able to manipulate the hair tie. A mirror can be utilized for visual feedback. Visual schedules will be utilized to break down each step of the task to provide a multi-sensory approach to re-learning as well as provide images of each item needed to assist with sequencing of the task.

Identify and describe the specific teaching-learning principles to promote change:

Repetition of practicing putting her hair in a ponytail, shaping proper kinematics of right upper extremity to put hair in ponytail, trial and error for sequencing and performing the task of putting her hair in a ponytail and putting on her headscarf, visual aid of steps to properly sequencing of being able to perform managing her hair.

Figure 16.7 MMCR Planning Guide to Address Specific Sections of the Overall Intervention Plan—Middle.

- Practice pinning her headscarf in place and trialing either hemi-techniques or bilateral techniques for completion of the task.
- Practice putting her headscarf on while standing at the sink as she does at home.

During this intervention plan, the occupational therapy practitioner will:

- Review hemi-techniques for hair care tasks as needed.
- Identify any modifications that may need to be made to Hannah's accessories in order to be able to utilize her right dominant hand to complete tasks.
- Massed practice of utilizing right upper extremity movements needed to be able to put on headscarf (brushing hair, putting hair in ponytail, etc.).

- Create and encourage use of home program tracker to facilitate carryover of skills addressed within treatment sessions outside of treatment sessions to promote recovery.

This aspect of the intervention plan continues to revolve around Hannah's middle, which is intrinsically motivating. As a result of her cerebrovascular accident (CVA), Hannah has difficulties with organization and sequencing. The use of breaking down the steps and utilizing a visual aid will serve as a compensatory strategy to these bottoms. Through the motor learning frame of reference, the use of whole meaningful tasks serves to foster motor recovery. As a result, Hannah will practice in repetition across intervention sessions managing her natural hair, managing and manipulating her headscarf, and being able to put it on and secure it in place. These functional tasks are serving to address her decreased neuromuscular control and strength.

Although the practitioner would possibly have Hannah practice washing her hair, this was not as important to her to be able to complete during her inpatient rehab. While Hannah's top is not directly addressed at this time, it is being indirectly addressed as previously stated due to the headscarf being required for childcare routines such as bringing Sarah to the pediatrician or taking her to the park and on walks. Addressing the underlying neuromuscular challenges will ultimately assist Hannah with specific activities and occupations, including changing diapers and dressing Sarah, as well as safely being able to transfer Sarah between environmental places (floor, car seat, bassinet, stroller, etc.).

Ending

The short focus of this intervention is on assisting Hannah with preparation for discharge home with her husband Jacob and daughter Sarah. This aspect of the intervention plan will include introduction to outpatient services, family training with Jacob, discussion of home modifications as needed, and preparing for any anticipated changes upon return home (see Figure 16.8). This process will include:

- Hands-on family training with Jacob to include management of Hannah's hair and putting on headscarf and home and community mobility.
- Preparation and anticipation of changes when she returns home along with self-advocacy training to facilitate delegation of household tasks.
- Anticipation of home modifications as needed to allow her to continue to be successful with her ADL and instrumental activities of daily living (IADL) tasks.
- Introduction to outpatient rehabilitation, including locating the outpatient clinic embedded within the larger hospital system.

During this intervention plan, the practitioner will:

- Facilitate a teach/reteach approach to family training sessions.
- Promote skill retention through the reteach method.
- Review hemi-techniques for participation in the tasks required to be able to put on her headscarf at home.
- Encourage and promote self-advocacy.

This aspect of the intervention plan involves both spirals from her bottom to middle, bottom to top, and middle to top. This addresses all aspects of her triangle as she begins to transition back home.

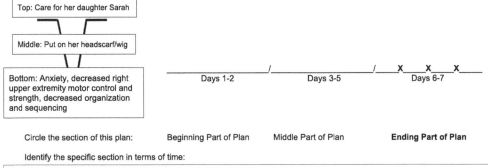

Top: Care for her daughter Sarah		
Middle: Put on her headscarf/wig		
Bottom: Anxiety, decreased right upper extremity motor control and strength, decreased organization and sequencing	Days 1-2 / Days 3-5 / X X X Days 6-7	

Circle the section of this plan: Beginning Part of Plan   Middle Part of Plan   **Ending Part of Plan**

Identify the specific section in terms of time:

Day 6-7, meeting daily for 1.5 hour sessions, approximately 3 hours

Label and briefly describe the central idea of this specific section of the plan:

Focus of intervention is on assisting Hannah with preparation for discharge home with her husband Jacob and daughter Sarah. This aspect of the plan will include introduction to outpatient services, family training with Jacob in order to be able to manage her hair, and being able to put on her headscarf to go to pediatrician appointments with her daughter and going on walks and to the park. Additionally, Hannah will prepare for any anticipated changes upon return home.

How does this specific section connect to the overall intervention plan? Describe the ways these intervention ideas are related to ∇ :

This aspect of the plan involves both spirals from her bottom to middle, bottom to top, and middle to top. This addresses all aspects of her triangle as she begins to transition back home. Hannah will be working to return back home and managing any associated anxieties which may pair with that. At this time, while Hannah has made great progress at this level of care, her opportunities for growth are still present therefore she may continue to require assistance from Jacob or other family members. Jacob will be an active participant in this phase of the intervention plan as he will be learning the most effective ways to assist Hannah at home physically, emotionally, and cognitively including being able to put on her headscarf. Through hands-on training and Hannah's direction, Jacob will learn how to assist her during the various steps leading up to and including putting on her headscarf. Hannah will also begin to familiarize herself with the outpatient clinic located within the larger hospital system she is currently staying. This will serve to alleviate any anticipatory anxiety with a new routine change.

Describe the plan for creating awareness and/or skill building?

During this phase, Hannah and Jacob will be working together to find a balance between independence and need for assistance to be able to put on her headscarf. During these sessions, the two of them will work to develop necessary strategies and approaches in order to find the counterbalance between fostering Hannah's independence and the ways in which Jacob can help her. Hannah will work to develop greater self-advocacy skills in order to delegate her care to Jacob to ensure that even during periods of assistance she still remains in control of her care. The two of them will collaborate together and utilize any modifications suggested and incorporated during treatment sessions that may assist with decreasing the level of care needed from Jacob or her family members and maximize independence from Hannah. She will also work to break down the steps of putting on a headscarf to address organization and sequencing challenges.

Select specific methods used to promote change:(therapeutic use of occupations and activities, interventions to support occupations, education, training, advocacy, self-advocacy, group intervention and virtual interventions)

During this phase of her intervention,, use of therapeutic activities (i.e., ADL and IADL skills) in order to accurately perform the steps of managing her hair and putting on her headscarf, education for properly performing the steps and how to incorporate Hannah's affected right upper extremity, family training with Jacob so that he as well as other family member will be able to learn how to assist Hannah, and self-advocacy will be utilized to promote change and prepare for discharge to the home setting.

Identify and describe the specific teaching-learning principles to promote change:

Modeling techniques for using and incorporating her right upper extremity when brushing her hair, putting her hair in a ponytail, clipping her hair, and putting her headscarf on, trial and error when sequencing the steps of the task correctly, teach back method to know that Hannah understands the proper steps in order to be able to put on her headscarf, reinforcement and positive feedback in order to motivate Hannah to be able to successfully complete the task

Figure 16.8 MMCR Planning Guide to Address Specific Sections of the Overall Intervention Plan—Ending.

Hannah will be working to return home and managing any associated anxieties which may arise with these coming changes. At this time, Hannah and Jacob will be working together to develop the necessary teamwork needed to manage personal and household routines after Hannah's CVA. Jacob's role is amplified during this phase, as he will be learning how to best support and facilitate Hannah's independence during her transition back home and how other family members can assist Hannah. Simultaneously, Hannah will be working to develop strong self-advocacy skills so that she can delegate and dictate her own care. This aspect of self-advocacy will allow Hannah to feel in control of situations or scenarios in which she may need to rely a little more on Jacob or other family members for assistance. This concept of delegation of care will also translate into IADL skills including household tasks in which Hannah and Jacob will learn which tasks Hannah feels confident she can take on and which she may require continued support for. Together, Hannah and Jacob will demonstrate understanding of learning through a teach-back method in which the therapist will teach followed by Hannah and Jacob reteaching the skills to one another to facilitate carryover and retention.

Evaluation Summary

Utilizing the "POP" acronym for person, occupational performance issues, and plan and information from the evaluation summary chart (see Figure 16.9), *the evaluation summary can be written as follows:*

P: Hannah is a 25-year-old female who identifies as Orthodox Jewish. She currently lives with her husband Jacob, who also identifies as Orthodox Jewish. Hannah and Jacob became first-time parents three months ago to their daughter Sarah. Hannah and Jacob moved one year ago to a single-level home in a small suburban northeast town in the mountain countryside.

Hannah recently sustained a small acute infarct within the left posterior frontal lobe and parietal lobe. No surgical intervention was required at the time of injury. Hannah has a past medical history significant for a previous diagnosis of COVID-19, she is currently three months postpartum, and has a diagnosis of generalized anxiety disorder. Prior to this admission, she was not currently on any medications. Hannah reported major life changes prior to the onset of her CVA, including moving away from her family, onset of the COVID-19 pandemic, and the birth of her first daughter. She reports that while these changes were both positive and negative, they increased her anxiety.

During this evaluation, the Kawa Model was utilized to guide the occupational profile. The Kawa is an evaluation tool utilized to gain an in-depth understanding of a person's life story. Through the lens of the Kawa Model, their life story is understood through the symbolism of a river and how various life events comprise the riverbank, rocks, and driftwood commonly found within a river. Additionally, the A-ONE was used to determine the impact of neurobehavioral challenges after her CVA, the WMFT test was utilized to determine quality of right upper extremity movement patterns, and manual muscle testing (MMT) and range of motion (ROM) testing were completed to determine overall strength and mobility.

O: Through her occupational profile, Hannah identified her primary goal is to return to caring for her daughter and return to her role as a mother. Through the Kawa Model, rocks represent circumstances that impact Hannah's life. She identifies challenges associated with this task such as her decreased motor control, strength, and ability to confidently complete the steps for all of the small tasks which make up this big role (decreased organization/sequencing). Driftwood represents Hannah's personal attributes and resources that can positively or negatively affect her circumstances. Part of Hannah's driftwood describes the important role her faith and her Orthodox culture play in her life. She reports that this is a priority in her life, and one aspect of this identity is the ability to put on her headscarf. She describes that wearing the headscarf is part of her identity when she goes out in the community, including bringing her daughter to pediatrician appointments, going on walks, going to the synagogue, going to the grocery store, etc. Similar to her desire to return to caring for her child, Hannah also describes the potential challenges/rocks to this as her control, coordination, and strength in her right upper extremity. She identifies herself as hardworking, goal driven, and independent, which are part of her driftwood and will assist Hannah in striving to achieve her goals.

Through completion of the A-ONE, Hannah's results indicated the presence of premotor perseveration, difficulty with organization/sequencing, and motor deficits in her right upper extremity. Due to the presence of these neurobehavioral deficits, Hannah required considerable assistance in dressing, grooming, and feeding. She displayed the ability to safely navigate within her room without the use of an assistive device. She was observed with slower movements when walking within her hospital room and observed occasionally using environmental features (bed, countertop, etc.) to ensure stability when needed. These mild losses of balance occurred less than 25% of the session.

Hannah's scores on the WMFT indicated mild deficits in right upper extremity motor control. Results indicate greater difficulty with refined fine motor movements as a greater degree of synergy observed during these testing components. Her greatest strengths appear proximally where her movements are close to normal; however, there is a presence of decreased fluidity. Furthermore, MMT and ROM testing indicated full ROM against gravity and ability to hold slight resistance at the testing position.

Relevant areas to the person's evaluation findings	Strengths	Challenges	Raw Data	Interpretation
Caring for newborn daughter Sarah	X	X	Hannah stated her role as a mother was very important to her. Following discharge, Jacob may be able to be home with Hannaha for a little while, however her sister-in-law will be staying with her, and her parents will be coming to stay for a short time to help with taking care of Sarah. Hannah does want to be able to take her daughter to pediatrician appointments and take her on walks and to the park.	Hannah's ultimate goal is to be able to care for her daughter and continue her role as a mother following her CVA. This will be challenging for her following her CVA. Being a first-time mom comes with many new roles and responsibilities which can become overwhelming to manage. Her family members/support system will be able to be there for her following discharge to assist with caretaking Sarah. In addition to the emotional challenges, Hannah also faces challenges with the physical aspect of her CVA including decreased right upper extremity motor control, strength, organization and sequencing.
Hardworking, goal driven, independent	X		Hannah describes herself as hard working, goal driven, and independent which she also identified as part of her driftwood.	Hannah will be challenged by decreased right upper extremity strength and motor control and impairments with organization and planning which will affect her ability to independently be able to manage her hair and put on her headscarf. Hannah having these characteristics will motivate and help her strive to achieve her goals of being able to put on her headscarf and care for daughter.

Figure 16.9 MMCR Guide to Evaluation Summaries: Hannah.

Putting her wig or headscarf on to bring her daughter to the pediatrician, go to the park or go to synagogue		X	Hannah stated this was important to her as an Orthodox woman. She stated, "Take care of my typical day to day routines; get myself dressed, take a shower, put on my headscarf, all those things." Hannah expressed that this is one of her rocks as she needs to be able to manage her hair when putting on her headscarf. When Manual muscle testing was completed, Hannah demonstrated 3+/5 strength in her right upper extremity which would impact her ability to complete this task.	This is a priority for Hannah as an Orthodox married woman. She needs to be able to complete this task in order to be able to bring her daughter to the pediatrician, go to the park or go to synagogue. Hannah's decreased strength and motor control currently impact the functional use of her right upper extremity. Furthermore, difficulties with organization/sequencing will impact the ability to efficiently complete this task independently.
Cooking Shabbat meals for her family	X	X	Hannah reports she would spend long hours preparing meals for her family on the Wednesdays and Thursdays leading up to Shabbat. Hannah reports that during Shabbat, one of her favorite parts is preparing the meals and sharing it with others. She describes this meal as a pillar to community building and a means to create bonds and a support system within a community which she views as a part of her river bank.	Hannah identified cooking a Shabbat meal as an important and meaningful occupation. This was a vital aspect of her life prior to her CVA. Hannah's decreased balance, decreased right upper extremity motor control, strength, decreased organization and sequencing will present as a challenge during completion of this task.
Decreased organization/sequencing		X	When completing the A-One evaluation, Hannah scored 5/20 for dressing, 5/24 for grooming, 15/20 for transfers/mobility, feeding 8/16, and Communication 4/4. Hannah also reports in her occupational profile continued brain fog since COVID-19 diagnosis.	Based on the A-one evaluation results, this indicated that Hannah has difficulty with organization/sequencing. This will indicate that Hannah has difficulty sequencing the steps of putting on her headscarf, preparing meals, and participating in childcare tasks including changing diapers, giving her daughter a bath, and completing tasks needed for her job.
Decreased right upper extremity motor control and strength		X	Through manual muscle testing, Hannah demonstrated 5/5 at all pivots for her non-affected left upper extremity and 3+/5 at all pivots in her affected right upper extremity. She also scored a 53 on the Wolf Motor Function Test.	Based on the results of manual muscle testing, Hannah has decreased strength in her dominant right upper extremity that indicates full range of motion against gravity and ability to hold slight resistance at testing position. Hannah will have difficulty using her right upper extremity when doing tasks including putting her wig on, caring for her daughter including changing her diaper, holding Sarah, and pushing her stroller.
Anxiety		X	Hannah has a past medical history significant for generalized anxiety disorder. Hannah reports that her anxiety stems from difficulty processing changing situations. Hannah reports that she has difficulty with life events are outside her control.	Following Hannah's stroke, she has decreased use of her right upper extremity, balance deficits, difficulty engaging in her self-care skills including putting on her headscarf and caring for her daughter as well as an inability to drive. There are various changes to her routine and schedule all causing increased anxiety for Hannah currently.

Figure 16.9 (Continued)

P

Long-term goal: Hannah will demonstrate increased right upper extremity function while putting on her headscarf in order to be able to go to pediatrician appointments with her daughter.

Short-term goal #1: Hannah will demonstrate increased right upper extremity strength by being able to brush her hair for at least 30 seconds in order to put on her head scarf to go to pediatrician appointments with her daughter with moderate assistance from family members in two days (see Figure 16.10).

1. Hannah **will**

(Person's name)

2. demonstrate increased right upper extremity strength by being able to brush her hair for at least 30 seconds **in order to**

(measurable, comes from bottom occupational performance issues)

3. to put on her head scarf to go to pediatrician appointments with her daughter **with**

(functional and specific, comes from top or middle occupational performance issue)

4. moderate assistance from family members **in**

(measurement, how much cuing, prompting or physical assistance)

5. two days

(time frame for achievement)

Figure 16.10 MMCR Guidelines to Formulate a Short-Term Goal—Hannah 1.

1. Hannah **will**

(Person's name)

2. utilize one adaptive device to put her hair in a ponytail bimanually **in order to**

(measurable, comes from bottom occupational performance issues)

3. to put on her head scarf to go to pediatrician appointments with her daughter **with**

(functional and specific, comes from top or middle occupational performance issue)

4. minimal assistance from her family members upon discharge **in**

(measurement, how much cuing, prompting or physical assistance)

5. 5 days

(time frame for achievement)

Figure 16.11 MMCR Guidelines to Formulate a Short-Term Goal—Hannah 2.

1. Hannah _____   **will**

(Person's name)

2. demonstrate accurate sequencing of putting   **in order to**
on her headscarf 2 out of 4 trials

(measurable, comes from bottom occupational performance issues)

3. be able to take her daughter to pediatrician   **with**
appointments

(functional and specific, comes from top or middle occupational performance issue)

4. minimal assistance from her family   **in**
members upon discharge

(measurement, how much cuing, prompting or physical assistance)

5. 7 days

(time frame for achievement)

Figure 16.12 MMCR Guidelines to Formulate a Short-Term Goal—Hannah 3.

Short-term goal #2: Hannah will utilize one adaptive device to put her hair in a ponytail bimanually in order to put on her head scarf to go to pediatrician appointments with her daughter with minimal assistance from her family members upon discharge in five days (see Figure 16.11).

Short-term goal #3: Hannah will demonstrate accurate sequencing of putting on her head scarf in two out of four trials in order to be able to take her daughter to pediatrician appointments with minimal assistance from her family members upon discharge in seven days (see Figure 16.12).

Hannah's Occupational Therapy Goals

Explanation of Goals

Given the length of Hannah's stay in acute inpatient rehab, it is realistic to think that she will not be completely independent with all of the tasks associated with putting on her headscarf. She will most likely require increased assistance from Jacob and her family, as noted in each goal. This also does not signify the end of her recovery, as she will transition to outpatient services.

References

Árnadóttir, G. (1995). *The brain and behavior: Assessing cortical dysfunction through activities of daily living (ADL)*. Mosby.

Figueiredo, S. (2021, March 5). Wolf motor function test (WMFT). *Stroke Engine*. strokengine.ca/en/assessments/wmft/

Gillen, G., & Nislen, D. (2020). *Stroke rehabilitation: A function-based approach* (5th ed.). Elsevier.

Iwama, M. K. (2006). *The Kawa model: Culturally relevant occupational therapy*. Elsevier.

Jewish Virtual Library. (2008). *Shabbat: What is Shabbat?* www.jewishvirtuallibrary.org/what-is-shabbat-jewish-sabbath

Kendall, F. P., McCreary, E. K., & Provance, P. G. (1993). *Muscles, testing, and function* (4th ed.). Lippincott Williams & Wilkins.

Salzberg, A. (2020, October 14). Hair coverings for married women. *My Jewish Learning*. www.myjewishlearning.com/article/hair-coverings-for-married-women/

17 Case Example

Using the MMCR to Guide a Six-Month Intervention Plan for an Adult With an Intellectual and Developmental Disability

Maureen Grainger, Thais K. Petrocelli, Shaniqua Bradley, and Ashley N. Fuentes

Introducing Jacque

Jacque is a 27-year-old who identifies as a Black Haitian American male. When given a choice, he prefers to be referred to by the pronouns "he, him, and his" (see Box 17.1).

Box 17.1

Sexual Identity

Sexual orientation, which includes sexual preference and sexual identity, and gender identity, are considered personal factors in the *Occupational Therapy Practice Framework*, fourth edition (AOTA, 2020) that reflect the essence of a person and are enduring and stable attributes. A person's sex is assigned at birth based on the experience of external anatomy (GLAAD, 2021). The broad umbrella term of "transgender" is used by persons who may not gender-identify as their assigned birth sex. A large spectrum of identities and labels can be used to express both sexual and gender identify outside of the more well-known binary terms of "male" and "female".

As an occupational therapy practitioner, it is essential to address and integrate all personal factors into assessment and treatment. It is important to facilitate a therapeutic milieu that allows a person to feel comfortable and safe in self-identifying their gender and preferred name and pronouns. It is essential to have an awareness of a person's gender and sexual identity in order to ensure the care you are providing is inclusive, client-centered, and reflective of that person's individual needs (APA, 2014).

Jacque attends a local adult day program serving adults with intellectual disabilities in the southeastern United States. Jacque graduated high school in a small, rural town before moving to a more suburban community, where he now lives in a group home for individuals with disabilities that provides 24-hour supervision. During a screening with an occupational therapy practitioner at the day program, Jacque expressed an interest in obtaining a job so that he can live more independently in the community. Jacque will be seen for occupational therapy (group and individual) five times a week for six months as part of the services at the day program.

Information Obtained From the Chart Review

Jacque has a paper chart at the day program that details his annual intervention plan, quarterly progress at the day program as well as other insurance documents, contact information, and medical

DOI: 10.4324/9781003392408-21

supplements. According to his chart, Jacque was diagnosed with mild cerebral palsy (CP) and intellectual disability disorder (IDD) at five years of age. He was also later diagnosed with major depressive disorder at age 14. Per this information, Jacque's legal guardian is his mother, and she makes all decisions in terms of his legal and medical care. His day program and care at this group home is funded by Medicare waivers through the Agency for Persons with Disability (APD) in each state (APD, n.d.), and he currently has all of his medical appointments scheduled through the agency.

Per Jacque's annual intervention plan, he is to attend the day program five days a week for six hours. During this time, he is enrolled in a variety of classes, including physical education, culinary arts, computer skills, and communications. At his last annual review, he voiced that he would like to return to work and had an interest in joining the "fun OT groups" because they do community trips. Other goals for Jacque over the next year include increasing independence with activities of daily living (ADLs) and general life skills tasks, increasing his ability to cope with stress, and increasing his ability to navigate on his own in a community setting.

The chart also contains an updated copy of his annual behavioral plan. Per the plan, Jacque is to be given cues for utilizing a variety of preferred coping skills by staff, which include offering deep breathing exercises, an opportunity to go for a walk, and/or a 1:1 time to chat with a preferred staff member. If he is unable to be redirected and becomes physically aggressive to the point that he is a danger to himself or others, the consequence may be seclusion or restraint.

Information Obtained From Jacque's Mother

The occupational therapy practitioner contacted Jacque's mother, Catherine, via phone to obtain further background information. Catherine is Jacque's legal guardian and was open to having Jacque work with the practitioner to gain more "freedom".

Family Background

Jacque does have a large extended family including two sisters and two half-brothers (paternal side), all of whom are older than Jacque and have children of their own. However, his siblings are scattered all over the southeastern United States, and Jacque often only sees them at major holidays.

Catherine is from the southeastern United States and comes from a Haitian American and African American family. Her parents have passed, and she is an only child. Jacque's father, Emmanuel, is originally from Haiti and immigrated to the United States at age 19. Currently his father is living with his large extended family, excluding those who still reside in Haiti. While he does stay in touch with Jacque, he is not an active participant in his care, as he is still upset that Jacque is living in a group home and not with family. Catherine stated that the father believes that family should be the only ones caring for Jacque and is embarrassed that Jacque is getting services through the community agency.

Box 17.2   Haitian American Cultural Norms

Haitian Americans are a very religious people, largely Catholic in religious affiliation, who rely on their large extended families, church congregations, and social communities for support during difficult times.

Haitian Americans have wide social connections, often coming from large families of eight or more children and often gathering with grandparents, aunts, uncles, and first, second, and third cousins. Haitian American holidays often revolve around food, with each member of the family contributing a dish. Common Haitian American foods include Haitian macaroni and cheese made with onions, peppers, condensed milk, and common Haitian spices; Haitian patties; rice and beans; and Haitian black rice, or *diri jon jon*.

Haitian Americans prefer holistic remedies to physical and mental problems, opting for prayer and herbal remedies rather than approaching a medical professional. Many Haitian Americans are distrustful of medical professionals who have been historically white, assuming that this person does not understand them or their deep cultural traditions.

Additionally, Haitian Americans do not possess a deep understanding of mental health or intellectual disability issues. A child with a diagnosis of a mental illness or intellectual disability is often regarded as the result of a failure on the part of one or both parents. Because of the stigma surrounding these diagnoses, parents with children affected by intellectual disability or mental illness prefer to avoid seeking medical help or other assistance through state-sponsored programs, as the parents would prefer to keep this perceived shame private.

(M. Francois, personal communication, April 1, 2021)

As part of his Haitian upbringing, Jacque's parents placed a strong emphasis on success in school and work (see Box 17.2). Though Jacque had difficulty keeping up with his coursework and fell behind in school, Jacque's father declined to involve support from the school or the state to address Jacque's difficulties paying attention during class and comprehending the increasingly complex material covered each year.

Involvement in State-Sponsored Programs

After graduation from high school at the age of 21, Jacque was enrolled in a county-supported vocational training program. He spent one year in this program. Jacque then participated briefly in a pre-vocational day program but did not feel like he fit in and left after only one month.

Box 17.3   Did You Know?

Home and community-based waivers (HCBWs) were established as part of the federal Medicaid program to allow persons who require long-term care services the ability to choose and receive services in the community versus an institution (Centers for Medicare & Medicaid Services, 2021). These services are varied in nature, depending on individual need, and can include funding for housing, nursing care, case management, and day program services. Day programs or day services, such as the one described in this chapter, are a coordinated program of services typically held five to six hours a day during the week in a community-based setting that address the various social, emotional, and physical needs of a person who requires additional supports and care for success in the community.

Each state operates their own types of Medicaid waiver programs for a variety of populations in need, including intellectual and developmentally disabled persons (Agency for Health Care Administration, 2021). Funding for such programs comes from a combination of both federal and state contributions and can vary depending on the person's state of residence. In the state of Florida, where Jacque resides, there are currently over 22,000 persons with developmental disabilities on the Medicaid waiver waitlist (University of South Florida, 2016).

While Catherine felt that Jacque needed further services, Jacque's father was still adamantly against involving social services or an outside agency to assist with managing Jacque's behavior and needs, just as he had been throughout Jacque's grade school and high school experiences. Please review Box 17.3 to learn more about home and community-based waivers.

Social History

Jacque was momentarily in a gang and was "used" by fellow gang members to do dangerous tasks such as run drugs because he wanted to be "accepted". Jacque was arrested two times while being involved in various gang activities but was subsequently released to his mother due to his cognitive issues and medical diagnosis.

Catherine had limited options for Jacque's care, as she was on the Medicare waiver waitlist for over two years to assist with more full-time support services for Jacque. She credits the court-appointed social worker with getting her the appropriate funding after waiting for so long and connecting her with the community agency who is currently providing services to Jacque. She states that her estranged husband and his family were unhappy with the outcome of him living in a group home, but she was happy Jacque was not at risk to go to jail again.

Conversations With Group Home Staff

Jacque lives in a 24-hour supervised group home with five other male peers. Jacque often requires verbal cues to initiate all ADLs and instrumental ASLs, including remembering to shower, comb his hair, and brush his teeth. In the group home he has an assigned "chore" but often needs staff reminders to complete the task. Jacque does enjoy these tasks but can get easily frustrated when he feels that his staff is "correcting him" too much. When he is frustrated, he will yell at people and become physically aggressive. Due to this behavior, staff do tend to "tread lightly" when prompting him and will often just do his chores for him. While he does have a behavior plan in place through the agency, staff prefer to not escalate him to that point.

Jacque is very social. He likes to interact and engage in lengthy conversations with his roommate, his housemates, and the staff. Jacque also enjoys sitting down for group meals and talking to his housemates. Although several of his housemates are non-verbal, he will often engage in one-sided conversations with them. At times Jacque needs reminders of boundaries, as he will sometimes interrupt staff or others.

Interview With Day Program Staff

Staff reports that Jacque is mostly friendly and likes to attend groups. He does require moderate cueing to complete one- to two-step tasks in a group, as he will get easily distracted by items in a classroom, activity outside of the windows, or side conversations with staff.

Jacque does not drive but would like to learn to take the local bus transportation so he can go out to eat and shop per staff. He previously had those privileges but got lost and frustrated and was escorted home by the local sheriff's office after he was seen yelling at others at the bus stop.

Jacque is able to identify when he gets frustrated and will try to take deep breaths when prompted to do so by day program staff. Jacque had one incident of self-injurious headbanging in the past three months, but staff members were able to redirect him, and they would like to continue to be able to do so.

Jacque enjoys attending the day program and interacting with peers. However, he often needs cueing in terms of boundaries when interacting with the opposite sex. He will often call someone his "girlfriend" even if they are not and will get upset when they dispute that fact. He has had several verbal arguments with his peers over his dating status, which ultimately has to be redirected by staff.

Occupational Profile (Top Evaluation)

Wellness Model Evaluation

In order to gain more information about Jacque's habits, routines, and self-perceptions, the occupational therapy practitioner at his day program encouraged Jacque to complete a Wellness Model Evaluation consisting of self-inventory checklists across the eight dimensions of wellness (Swarbrick, 2006) (see Box 17.4 and Figure 17.1).

Box 17.4

Eight Dimensions of Wellness

Under the Wellness Model (Swarbrick, 2006), wellness is conceptualized in eight dimensions: physical, occupational, environmental, financial, emotional, spiritual, social, and intellectual. According to the Wellness Model, these dimensions overlap such that changes made in any of the eight dimensions will result in improved wellness in other areas. This model emphasizes the client's view of his or her own wellness, using self-rated checklists to determine the level of wellness in each area.

Occupational Wellness

Jacque expresses a strong interest in the dimension of occupational wellness (Figures 17.2 and 17.3), explaining that his father Emmanuel taught him at a young age that "a good Haitian man works hard for his family". Jacque further explains that he wants to "make my family proud of me".

Jacque remembers joining a supported employment program after finishing high school, but he reports "feeling down" a lot of the time during this program. He recalls how the program made him feel like "I can't do anything good" and that "pissed me off a lot too".

Jacque remembers trying a pre-vocational program after leaving supported employment, but states "they gave me too many things to do". Jacque reports becoming frustrated with "having too many things in my head" at the same time and ultimately left the pre-vocational program soon after joining.

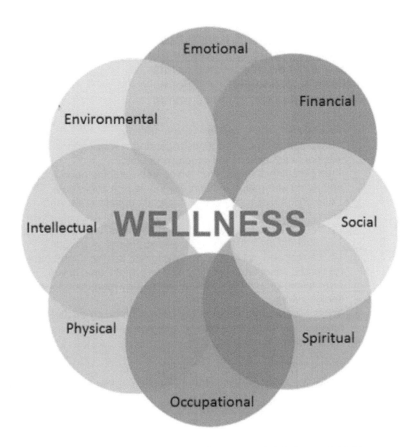

Figure 17.1 Depiction of the Eight Dimensions of Wellness (Swarbrick & Yudof, 2017).

Source: (Reprinted with permission from Collaborative Support Programs of New Jersey.)

<u>*Occupational Wellness*</u> involves participating in activities that provide meaning and purpose, including employment.

<u>Strengths</u>
These are the things I **do** well – my daily routines, habits, and valued life activities that build and maintain my occupational wellness:

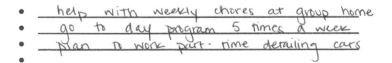

- <u>help with weekly chores at group home</u>
- <u>go to day program 5 times a week</u>
- <u>plan to work part-time detailing cars</u>
-

Figure 17.2 Wellness Self-Inventory for Occupational Wellness Domain, Part 1 (Swarbrick & Yudof, 2017).

Source: (Reprinted with permission from Collaborative Support Programs of New Jersey.)

I am Looking for Work (I plan to enter or return to the workforce or I hope to increase my work hours)

I almost always do this	= 2 points
Sometimes/occasionally	= 1 point
I very seldom do this	= 0 points

1. __1__ I am actively pursuing work and/or training.
2. __1__ I have considered my options regarding career change, getting additional education, self-employment, etc.
3. __0__ I am pursuing an organized job search, keeping good records, and doing something towards my job search every day.
4. __0__ I use online resources to look for work, update skills, and network with others regarding my job search.
5. __0__ I assertively market myself through personal networking.
6. __1__ I confidently describe my skills and strengths as a worker.
7. __0__ I have reached out to former colleagues, teachers, and other resources associated with my field or professional group.
8. __1__ I am aware of and use general community resources for people seeking work.
9. __2__ While I am waiting to get a job, I use my time productively to maintain my skills, support my community, etc.
10. __1__ I am hopeful in my job search.

Figure 17.3 Wellness Self-Inventory for Occupational Wellness Domain, Part 2 (Swarbrick & Yudof, 2017).

Source: (Reprinted with permission from Collaborative Support Programs of New Jersey.)

Jacque identified an interest in working at a car dealership and detailing cars so that he can "make a lot of money" and "get a real nice car" of his own. Jacque tells the occupational therapy practitioner that his favorite car is a Lamborghini, "orange like the poster I have in my room".

Jacque also stated an interest in using money from his job to "get my own place" and live on his own "like the guys from high school". However, he reported that he does not know how to get this job and is worried he might have to go back to pre-vocational or supported employment programs, which he identifies as being "too hard" for him.

He explained that his father often asks him when he plans to get a job during their biweekly phone calls. He said that if he had a job, "my dad would be proud of me" and that it would "feel good to work" and participate in something that made him "feel smart". When asked where he would like to work, Jacque stated that his dream was to work "on cars like they do in NASCAR". With additional prompting from the occupational therapy practitioner, Jacque further explained that he wanted to clean and detail cars, as he was not interested in mechanical work.

Spiritual Wellness

Jacque identified attending church regularly with his parents, praying for help with "things that are hard", and listening to gospel music as specific spiritual strengths. Jacque also explained that his *grann* (grandmother) on his dad's side "taught me to trust God more than anything else because God knows the way, and He will show me, too".

Jacque says that he gets much of his spiritual support and guidance from his mother and from the members of her church community at St. Joseph's Catholic Church. Jacque especially enjoys going to church in person at "St. Joe's" once a month when he visits his mother at home. Jacque says his favorite parts of his religious community are "how they help me with things, they take care of me, and all the good food we eat together". He remembers attending a congregation pot-luck after the Sunday service, where he explains his favorite foods are traditional Haitian mac and cheese and Haitian patties.

Social Wellness

Jacque was especially proud of how well he gets along with everyone in his group home and of his strong relationships with his mother, father, and his *grann*. Jacque reported he had lots of friends and cousins in Haiti, though he had only been to see them twice. Jacque expressed a desire to return to Haiti on another trip "once I get a job and get rich".

Jacque reported video chatting with his mom two or three times per week and speaking to his dad on the phone once every two weeks. Jacque also receives frequent text messages from his two sisters but has a harder time communicating via text and often only sends emojis.

After finishing high school and joining supported employment programs, Jacque briefly became part of a small local street gang of fewer than 20 members. Jacque mentions that he was looking for people who "get me" and felt part of a family with the gang's members. Jacque remembers that one of the members, Marcus, often gave him jobs to do, such as running special packages from one house to another. Jacque remembers being excited that Marcus would trust him with something so important and remembers that Marcus always "treated me normal, not like everybody else".

However, Jacque also remembers appearing before a county judge who told him that they were "bad people" that "they hurt me and my mom and dad when they asked me to do bad stuff". After only three months of membership, Jacque was forced to stop spending time with Marcus and the other gang members. The judge who heard Jacque's case recommended he start living and spending his day with people "more like me", which is how Jacque met his new group home and day program friends.

Physical Wellness

Jacque identified eating healthy and going to bed at bedtime as specific strengths in the domain of physical wellness. Jacque mentions that he really enjoys eating healthy meals provided at his day program and his group home, but states that "no one cooks like my mom and her friends".

When asked about exercise, Jacque says that his favorite activity in his day program is physical education where he can "work out like one of the guys". Jacque explains that his father, Emmanuel, taught him about taking care of his body when he was in his teens. Jacque remembers watching his father work out in the garage at home, where Emmanuel taught him "all about being a man, being strong".

Emotional Wellness

Jacque recognizes that he has a hard time dealing with criticisms from certain group home staff, stating "I get mad when they tell me too many things to do". Jacque explains that "Jason and Therese are the best", but does mention that some other group home staff members "piss me off". Jacque admitted to getting "angry" at group home staff, recalling often throwing objects or punching walls to "help me feel better". Jacque explained that while he enjoys completing weekly chores in his group home, he feels embarrassed "when I need too much help and they yell at me that I do it wrong".

When asked how he deals with getting "angry", Jacque stated, "they tell me to breathe and stuff". Jacque reported that deep breathing "kinda works sometimes", but indicated that he preferred using the treadmill at the day program to "get less angry". Jacque had difficulty identifying other strategies for dealing with his feelings of anger.

Intellectual, Financial, and Environmental Wellness

While completing self-inventories for each area of wellness, Jacque indicated that these areas were less important to him and that he is satisfied with his level of wellness in them. The practitioner administering these assessments educated Jacque on the overlap between each area of wellness and that changes in other dimensions of wellness may impact the previously listed dimensions. However, as Jacque did not indicate these areas as personally meaningful, the practitioner chose not to focus on this information when developing an occupational profile.

Analysis of Performance (Bottom Evaluation)

Social Profile Results

Using the Social Profile (Donohue, 2013), the occupational therapy practitioner at the day program observed a group Jacque was in to help determine group goals for him. The group observed was the culinary arts group that meets three times a week in the mornings. During this time, the group members tend to the garden and then make one- to two-step recipes using the fruits and vegetables from the garden under the direction of a culinary arts teacher and an occupational therapy student (OTS). During this specific group, Jacque and his group members picked green beans, cleaned them, and then roasted them in the oven.

Social Profile: Group Performance

While group members did display interactions that spanned the five areas of the social profile (parallel, associative, basic cooperative, supportive cooperative, and mature), much of the group average summaries indicate that the group was at an associative to basic cooperative level of social and group participation. Members are motivated by their self-interest in making and eating food as well as getting out of the building to tend to the garden. They were able to execute a work task in the interest of a goal and displayed motivation throughout. As a group, members would express ideas and act as group members; however, there are times that members needed cueing from staff to remember group rules and respect others' rights within the group.

Social Profile: Jacque's Role

Jacque was able to individually give words of affirmation when one of his group members did or said something correctly in the group but did struggle when prompted by the group leaders to engage in self-expression about how he feels about an activity. During the group wrap-up, his response to the day's activity was "that was good". Per the group teacher, this is his response to every activity or group she runs. Although Jacque was excited about picking the beans and making something to eat, he required verbal cues throughout from the occupational therapy student and teacher to attend to the gardening task and not wander away from the area to look in the windows of the building or at the activity going on in the facility parking lot. He was able to transition with the group from the garden to the kitchen prep area but did require both visual and verbal cues to follow the steps for cleaning the beans and for safety when preparing and putting the beans in the oven to cook.

COTE Scale Results

Jacque was observed utilizing the Comprehensive Occupational Therapy Evaluation (COTE; Shotwell & Allison, 2020) scale during an arts and crafts activity group where they were working on making collages about themselves. Jacque did well in the areas of appearance, attendance, and reality orientation and was cooperative with transitioning into the group, as Jacque "really likes" the arts and crafts group. He was social with the staff and his peers as well as the observing OT throughout the session.

Jacque required moderate cueing for group rules, which included not wandering around the room when distracted and taking turns during the sharing portion of the activity. He sought out praise for his work by asking the staff frequently "I'm doing good, aren't I?" and "I think I am good at this—what do you think?" (Figure 17.4).

Jacque needed moderate cueing for following the directions given by the teacher and support staff, as he was easily distracted by his environment throughout the task and needed assistance from staff to organize his materials. He was moderately frustrated and got upset when he could not find the exact pictures he wanted for his collage but was redirected back to the task by a staff member when he was given praise (Figure 17.5). Jacque had an overall COTE scale score of 68 at the time of this observation, with subscores of 17 in general behavior, 12 in interpersonal behaviors, and 39 in occupational behaviors.

A. Reality Orientation Addresses the patient's awareness of person, time, place, and situation. The behavior rating is based on the number of factors of which the patient is aware.	0- Complete awareness of person, place, time, and situation 1- General awareness but inconsistency in 1 area 2- Awareness of only 2 areas 3- Awareness in 1 area 4- Lack of awareness of person, place, time, and situation

Scale (Observed Impairment): 0 = Typical   1 = Minimal   2 = Mild   3 = Moderate   4 = Severe

Figure 17.4 COTE Scale, Part 1, Scoring for reality orientation.

Source: Adapted with permission from Sara Brayman.

P. Concentration/ Attention An important patient factor and can be measured by the patient's ability to sustain engagement in activities and occupations. This mental function is measured by the amount of time spent attending to the activity at hand.	0- No difficulty concentrating during session 1- Off task less than 25% of the time 2- Off task 50% of the time **3- Off task 75% of the time** **Inability to maintain concentration on** **task for more than one minute**

Scale (Observed Impairment): 0 = Typical   1 = Minimal   2 = Mild   3 = Moderate   4 = Severe

Figure 17.5 COTE Scale, Part 2, Scoring for concentration/attention.

Source: Adapted with permission from Sara Brayman.

Understanding Jacque's Story

In order to begin to formulate Jacque's goals for treatment, the complex interaction between person, occupations, and environments must be examined (Figure 17.6). As a person, an emphasis needs to be placed on Jacque being a young adult who desired to do what most of his same-aged peers would like to do—live independently and have his own money. He has a variety of occupations, but for this specific piece of treatment, the therapist will be focusing on his preferred occupation of getting a job. In terms of environment, Jacque's current status of living in a group home and attending a structured day program all need to be taken into account when looking at how to progress his interventions.

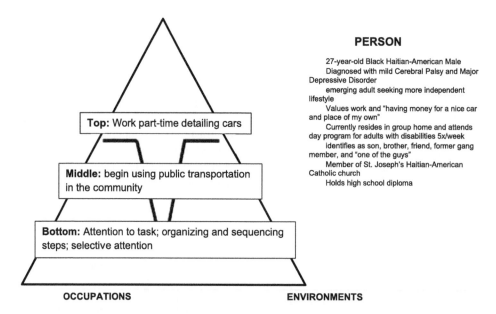

PERSON

27-year-old Black Haitian-American Male
Diagnosed with mild Cerebral Palsy and Major Depressive Disorder
emerging adult seeking more independent lifestyle
Values work and "having money for a nice car and place of my own"
Currently resides in group home and attends day program for adults with disabilities 5x/week
identifies as son, brother, friend, former gang member, and "one of the guys"
Member of St. Joseph's Haitian-American Catholic church
Holds high school diploma

Top: Work part-time detailing cars

Middle: begin using public transportation in the community

Bottom: Attention to task; organizing and sequencing steps; selective attention

OCCUPATIONS

Occupations:
Attending 10:30 am church service at St. Joseph's Haitian-American catholic church once per month with mom
Listening to Gospel, rap, and rock music on CD player in group home room to relax every night before bed
Watching football games every Sunday on couch in his parents' home with dad, watching NASCAR racing with dad on parents' couch, eating Haitian patties and drinking root beer; watching NASCAR on phone in group home bedroom
Videocalls mom every Mondays, Wednesdays, and Saturdays at dinner time to talk about his day
biweekly Friday night phone calls with his father to talk about sports and getting a job

Activities:
Staying in touch with family members
Groups at the day program
Exercising
Attending church potlucks
Playing games on smartphone during breaks at day program while sitting out in courtyard

ENVIRONMENTS

Location: bedroom in group home; group home in suburban neighborhood; courtyard, classrooms, gym, and cafeteria in day program; Haitian-American community church and parish center; couch in father's basement in front of TV

Physical: CD player; Gospel, rap, and rock CDs in stacks on desk in group home room; smartphone; desks in day program classrooms; group home van; weights and treadmill in day program gym; Bible given to Jacque by his mother; bed, desk, and closet in group home room; poster of Lamborghini in group home room; traditional Haitian food after church on Sundays; supplies for Arts and Crafts group; materials for cooking and gardening group

Temporal: lived at home for 23 years; involved with a gang after completing high school at age 21; living in a group home for the past 4 years; attended a supported employment program for 1 year; attended a pre-employment program for 1 month; has been attending a day program for the last 3.5 years; parents have been separated for past 3.5 years; attends church with family once per month; completes 1 of 3 rotating weekly chores at group home

Social: group home residents; day program participants; Haitian-American extended family on father's side; mom, dad, and two sisters; members of catholic church congregation; day program staff; group home staff;
members of gang whom Jacque refers to as his "brothers"

Virtual: Virtual: uses smartphone to videocall family members; uses smartphone to play games; uses smartphone to text family; listens to CDs using CD player; attends church virtually using smartphone

Cultural: Haitian-American culture places high value on family and connectedness; Jacque's Haitian-American family chooses not to acknowledge his disabilities; Jacque is expected to complete chores as part of group home; Jacque's father taught Jacque to value success in school and working as part of his Haitian cultural upbringing; Jacque's father encouraged Jacque to be "one of the guys" which led to his interest in football and working out in PE class; Jacque feels the pressure from the culture of the town where he grew up to be successful with a "nice car" and "lots of money" and "have my own apartment;" mother is currently his legal guardian which limits Jacque's ability to independently make decisions for himself in the way that his high school classmates can

Figure 17.6 MMCR Guide to Understanding a Person's Story (Triangle)—Jacque.

All of these factors influence the formation of the initial top, middle, and bottom portions of treatment. His values of working and earning money as well as his interest in cars directly relate to the formation of his top portion. In order to facilitate independence with attending a job as well as taking into account his past difficulties with navigating transportation, the middle portion will focus on learning to access and use public transportation near his current place of residence. Jacque's bottom portion of decreased attention to task and difficulty with sequencing will also be addressed as the therapist formulates viable adaptations and intervention techniques that will address his specific deficit areas while proving an intervention that is specifically meaningful and occupation based for Jacque.

Step 1: Frame of Reference (FOR)/**Practice Model (PM)**: Wellness in Eight Dimensions

Step 2: Words in a Box:

Wellness	Conscious, deliberate process	Choices for a satisfying lifestyle
Self-defined balance	Health promotion	Purpose in life
Empowerment	Healthy habits	Resilience and strength
Wellness journey		

8 Dimensions of Wellness:

Emotional	Social
Environmental	Physical
Financial	Spiritual
Intellectual	Occupational

Connectedness of dimensions
Active involvement in satisfying work and play
Personal responsibility for day to day choices

Step 3: FOR/**PM** Party Paragraph:

The Wellness Model was originally developed for those with mental illness that can be applied broadly to a wide variety of individuals and populations. This model focuses specifically on recovery, which is defined as a process of gaining or regaining physical, spiritual, mental, and emotional balance. Wellness exists in eight dimensions: emotional, environmental, financial, intellectual, social, physical, spiritual and occupational. This model supports an individual's ability to make meaningful change through the creation of healthy habits that will lead to a self-defined sense of well-being. Wellness is evaluated using self-inventories, which individuals can use to identify strengths and opportunities for growth in each dimension. The intervention process through this practice model views wellness as a journey in which individuals build resilience and strength through their ability to adapt to change and re-establish balance across the eight dimensions.

Step 4: Succinct summary of person's story emphasizing relevant occupational performance issues ⊻

Jacque is a 27-year-old male currently attending a day program for adults with an Intellectual Disability Disorder. During the occupational profile, Jacque expressed an interest in a job detailing cars at a local dealership (top). Jacque has previously

Figure 17.7 MMCR Five-Step Guide to Infusing a Frame of Reference/Practice Model Into a Person's Evaluation Selection and Intervention Plan—Jacque's Wellness in Eight Dimensions.

attended county-sponsored programs to support his ability to work in the community, but he quickly became overwhelmed with the amount of new information. Jacque has difficulty attending to tasks, particularly if new information is provided, and becomes frustrated when he is unable to follow written instructions provided to complete the task (bottoms). Jacque reports that a job in the community would give him a sense of freedom he does not currently have. Jacque has chosen to participate in services that will support his overall goal of working part-time in a local car dealership detailing cars (middle).

Step 5: Explanation of how the FOR/PM will directly influence the specific intervention plan:

Jacque will be seen in a community setting over the course of 6 months. Occupational therapy intervention will use wellness principles to increase Jacque's coping skills and work habits while empowering him to take a more active role in managing his own well-being. The dimensions of wellness that will be targeted as part of this intervention plan will include occupational and emotional wellness. Although there are eight total dimensions of wellness that can be addressed, and each dimension overlaps and influences the others, particular attention will be paid to occupational and emotional wellness because these areas of wellness will best support Jacque in his pursuit of part-time employment. In this intervention plan, Jacque will have an opportunity to participate in job training and education that will build his confidence and facilitate his ability to obtain a part-time job. This will increase his job satisfaction and create a sense of well-being in the domain of occupational wellness. Additionally, Jacque will learn positive coping strategies such as silent prayer and listening to music when taking breaks from work that will improve his ability to manage his emotions and establish a sense of balance in the domain of emotional wellness.

Figure 17.7 (Continued)

Frame of Reference and/or Practice Model

The Wellness Model was chosen for this intervention plan due to its broad application and its focus on empowering a person to create healthy habits, which promote a sense of well-being (Figure 17.7). Considering intervention will take place in the community, the practitioner will need to create support that will assist Jacque in reaching his goals even after services have ended. The incorporation of healthy habits into Jacque's valued occupations will increase his ability to reach his goals and obtain a sense of balance in each desired area of wellness.

Additionally, the use of a top-down model such as the Wellness Model encourages the practitioner to keep Jacque's ultimate goal in mind throughout the process and ensures that Jacque's valued occupations will be the focus of each session. The use of valued occupations throughout intervention will help to keep Jacque engaged. Furthermore, the use of the Wellness Model Self-Inventory provides an opportunity for Jacque to identify strengths and areas for growth, which become the focus of intervention, thus making the intervention process more person-centered.

The behavioral frame of reference was chosen to supplement the Wellness Practice Model (Figure 17.8). While the Wellness Model's top-down nature is the main approach taken with Jacque's therapeutic process, concepts from the behavioral frame of reference are applicable and useful to ensure that Jacque gets the appropriate support to gain and maintain his skill sets for success in his identified occupations. Concepts such as skill building, reinforcement, and compensatory

Step 1: **Frame of Reference (FOR)**/Practice Model (PM): Behavioral Frame of Reference

Step 2: Words in a Box:

Skill building	Client education	Token economies
Reinforcement	Compensatory strategies	Controlled environment
Behavioral change	Modeling	Behavioral contracts
Splinter skills	Valued occupations	

Step 3: FOR/**PM** Party Paragraph:

The Behavioral Frame of Reference is a guideline for practice used to help clients build the skills necessary for successful occupational performance and eliminating behaviors that are not helpful. Following this guideline, practitioners assist people to build the skills necessary for occupational performance while eliminating behaviors that may interfere with optimal functioning. Two types of deficits can occur, skill and performance deficits. Skill deficits occur when people have not yet learned a skill or if they become impaired and need to re-learn it. Performance deficits take place when people are able to perform the desired skill, but unable to do so consistently or in a situation that calls for it. Practitioners serve as role models who shape behaviors using motivating factors, such as a valued occupation or area of interest, in order to bring about behavioral change and enhance performance skills. Through the use of reinforcements, behaviors can be promoted or extinguished. Methods of reinforcement may include: modeling, token economies, behavioral contracts, splinter skills, relaxation training, systematic desensitization, scaffolding, and fading support. Intervention is typically situated in a simulated and controlled environment where people can practice skills in a safe and predictable manner. Additionally, practitioners are viewed as educators to teach others how to use these strategies upon discontinuation of services.

Step 4: Succinct summary of person's story emphasizing relevant occupational performance issues ᐯ

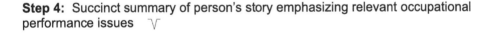

Figure 17.8 MMCR Five-Step Guide to Infusing a Frame of Reference/Practice Model Into a Person's Evaluation Selection and Intervention Plan—Jacque's Behavioral frame of reference.

strategies are all helpful to Jacque given his diagnosis, past difficulties in the community, and assessment results. During individual and group sessions, the occupational therapy practitioner will be modeling behaviors that Jacque can apply when he is accessing community transportation and in the workplace. This approach will also be used to assist Jacque in changing his behavioral response to stress or change, therefore making him successful with pursuing his vocational, social, and independent living goals.

Jacque is a 27-year-old male currently attending a day program for adults with an Intellectual Disability Disorder. During the occupational profile, Jacque expressed an interest in a job detailing cars at a local dealership (top). Jacque has previously attended county-sponsored programs to support his ability to work in the community, but he quickly became overwhelmed with the amount of new information. Jacque has difficulty attending to tasks, particularly if new information is provided, and becomes frustrated when he is unable to follow written instructions provided to complete the task (bottoms). Jacque reports that a job in the community would give him a sense of freedom he does not currently have. Jacque has chosen to participate in services that will support his overall goal of working part-time in a local car dealership detailing cars (middle).

Step 5: Explanation of how the **FOR**/PM will directly influence the specific intervention plan:

Jacque will be seen in a community setting over the course of 6 months. The practitioner will use principles from the behavioral frame of reference to assist Jacque with learning the skills needed for him to take on new roles, routines, and tasks. The practitioner will focus on strengthening Jacque's skills necessary for his desired occupation of detailing cars. There will also be a particular focus on Jacque's performance as he has struggled in previous vocational and community programming, despite having interests as well as abilities that could support success in these endeavors. Positive reinforcement will be essential to help Jacque feel successful as he obtains new skills and will help to extinguish self-harm behaviors that come with his increased frustration. The practitioner will also provide modeling in a variety of intervention sessions in the community, including while on public transportation and in the workplace. In the initial phase of intervention, Jacque will be in a more controlled environment at the day program and progress to new environments as he succeeds. As Jacque progresses through his phases of the intervention plan, he will receive faded support from the staff as he strives towards more independent engagement in occupation.

Figure 17.8 (Continued)

Overview Guide to Intervention Planning

Jacque will be seen in the group home, day program, and community, where he will participate in occupational therapy services for a total of six months. His intervention plan will be divided into three phase (Figure 17.9). All three phases of intervention work toward the same "top", with consideration of his current status per assessment and diagnosis. Adults with IDDs such as Jacque benefit from a client-centered model of care that allows for adaptation and grading of tasks (Johnson et al., 2019). Working toward his top maintains client-centeredness and provides the practitioner with the opportunity to break down the tasks needed for Jacque to succeed over a longer period of time.

Using public transportation in the community in the first phase will provide Jacque with enough time to refine these skills in anticipation of achieving his top or longer-term goal, so he can commute to a future part-time job. Jacque will also be able to practice these skills throughout the duration of the six months such as going to check out different dealerships he may be interested in.

The second phase of intervention will focus on participating in a paid internship through a job training course at his day program. The paid internship will focus on work in the facility's transportation department and introduce him to the work environment in his desired area. The final phase will focus on obtaining a paid internship at a local car dealership and assisting Jacque to acclimate to his new work environment.

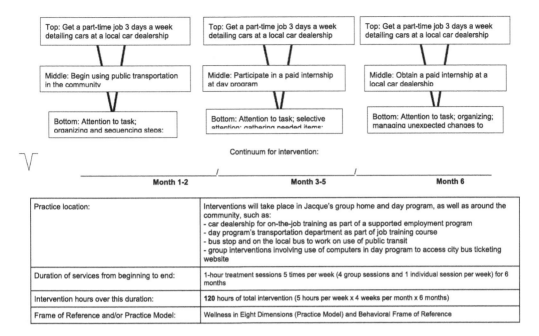

Figure 17.9 MMCR Overview Guide to Intervention Planning—Jacque.

The time frame of six months, with both group and individual sessions, is realistic within the day program setting, as Jacque is undergoing significant transitions during this time in his roles and routines and would benefit from repetition and small, graded steps toward achieving his desired outcome. He benefits from frequent prompting and assistance with basic ADLs and instrumental activities of daily living (IADLs), and therefore achieving his middles during this time frame is practical. The use of different environments during intervention will also support Jacque's understanding of the community outside of his program and group home and will allow him to practice skills in vivo.

Planning Guide to Address Specific Sections of the Overall Intervention Plan

The beginning phase of the overall intervention plan will last two months and will focus on Jacque's ability to use public transportation. The use of public transit not only offers opportunities for Jacque to practice the use of tools such as a simplified bus schedule and visual checklists to support his attention to task and ability to sequence, but it also prepares him for his long-term goal of part-time employment at a local car dealership. In order to obtain and keep a job at a local car dealership, Jacque will need to travel independently to and from his job without assistance from group home staff or the practitioner. Because new learning in adults with IDD typically requires increased time, two months have been allotted for this portion of the intervention plan for increased carryover of new habits and skills. Taking the bus is also something Jacque can continue to practice throughout the course of intervention. Awareness regarding creating a structured routine, social interaction in the community, and of the different features of the bus stop and bus will be targeted as well. This will help prepare Jacque for the experience of getting ready to go to the bus stop, ride the bus, and get off the bus. Figure 17.10 provides a detailed explanation of this phase of intervention.

The middle portion of the intervention plan, covering months three through five, will focus on job-specific training provided by both the occupational therapy practitioner and a job coach. This training will take place through a paid internship offered through Jacque's day program and will

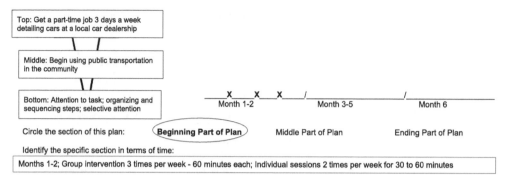

Circle the section of this plan: (Beginning Part of Plan)   Middle Part of Plan   Ending Part of Plan

Identify the specific section in terms of time:

Months 1-2; Group intervention 3 times per week - 60 minutes each; Individual sessions 2 times per week for 30 to 60 minutes

Label and briefly describe the central idea of this specific section of the plan:

The practitioner will focus on specific tasks required for Jacque to use public transportation in order to work towards obtaining a part time job (i.e., locating and reading a bus schedule, knowing when to get on and off the bus in time, understanding the rules of riding a bus). The use of public transportation early on during intervention is beneficial because it provides him with the opportunity to practice these skills and then continue throughout the entirety of the 6 months for more repetition. This phase of intervention will focus on building stronger sequencing, time management, and adaptability skills that will support Jacque being able to more independently ride a bus. New learning will occur through various teaching and learning strategies as well as modeled behaviors by the practitioner in both a group and individual intervention setting.

How does this specific section connect to the overall intervention plan? Describe the ways these intervention ideas are related to ∨ :

This section lays the foundation for empowering Jacque to reach his goal of obtaining a part-time job (top). This step will help him build greater independence while addressing and strengthening some of his attentional needs (bottom) that have been identified at his day program, such as how to read a bus schedule and proper social etiquette in the community. This will also be motivating for Jacque as he mentioned that he would like to go out to eat and shop. The use of public transportation will also provide him with a travel method to a future part-time job. During this beginning phase, Jacque will be working on sequencing, organization, and attention through ADL and IADL tasks at home to facilitate getting to the bus on time and structure his routine to support success in using public transportation to his future part-time job.

Describe the plan for creating **awareness** and/or skill building?

Awareness will be created for Jacque in both group and individual sessions before skill building. Introduction to concepts that support building a routine as well as addressing attention and sequencing will be introduced during treatment as well as the expectations for social interaction behavior in the community. The practitioner may begin by modeling relevant social behavior in the community (i.e., waiting for the bus, taking a seat on the bus) to help create awareness. The practitioner may also take Jacque to the local bus stop to educate him on the different features (i.e., bus stop sign, bus stop numbers, station name, route map, schedule) of the bus stop. Skill building will start to occur with introduction of community living skills in groups, including social etiquette in travel, money/fare management, and reading a simplified bus schedule. Skill building will also occur through the experience of preparing to go to the bus stop, riding the bus, and getting off the bus multiple times during both group and individual sessions with the practitioner in vivo. The setting (bus/bus stop) would be considered new learning and the inclusion of the practitioner offers Jacque support to practice the necessary skills in the new environment.

Select specific methods used to promote change: (therapeutic use of occupations and activities, interventions to support occupations, education, training, advocacy, self-advocacy, group intervention and virtual interventions)

Group: A group setting will provide Jacque a comfortable space to practice and learn skills with peers. Additionally, Jacque will have several opportunities in a group setting to model from both peers and staff. The familiarity of his peers and the practitioner make the group a safe space to practice these new skills and reduce potential stress.
Therapeutic use of occupation and activities: Through the use of both group and individual sessions, Jacque will engage in activities including reading a bus schedule, role playing interactions with the bus driver, making change to pay his bus fare and actually riding the bus route from his home to the local car dealership.
Interventions to support occupations: Activities in both a group and individual setting will help support Jacque in the learning and building skills of attention to task, sequencing of a multiple step process, money familiarity and management, making a routine, ADL management, social skills, and stress/behavior management.
Education and Training: Education on social etiquette, information on bus routes and the bus system, training on how to read a simple bus schedule, and safety education will help Jacque build confidence to succeed in use of public transportation and how to appropriately interact with others in a community setting.

Identify and describe the specific teaching-learning principles to promote change:

Modeling: The practitioner will model how to take a bus and utilize social skills in the community during group and 1:1 sessions, model how to cope with stress that can be associated with frustration or change, and how to ask for assistance in the community.
Education: The practitioner will provide education on the intervention that supports occupations through 1:1 and group intervention. The practitioner will use visual aids, to support the educational process and provide multi-model learning opportunities. The practitioner may also employ the teach-back method to ensure Jacque is able to understand all the steps required for independently taking the bus.
Practice/repetition: The practitioner will provide ample repetitions of the bus taking routine to ensure the skill is learned and a habit is cemented.
Adaptation: The practitioner will provide a simplified bus schedule and adapt a routine checklist for taking the bus that will suit Jacque's unique learning needs and style.

Figure 17.10 MMCR Planning Guide to Address Specific Sections of the Overall Intervention Plan— Beginning portion for Jacque.

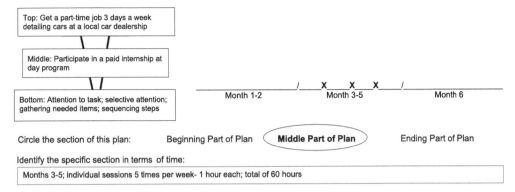

Circle the section of this plan: Beginning Part of Plan   (**Middle Part of Plan**)   Ending Part of Plan

Identify the specific section in terms of time:

Months 3-5; individual sessions 5 times per week- 1 hour each; total of 60 hours

Label and briefly describe the central idea of this specific section of the plan:

In this portion of the plan, Jacque will be learning more about his desired job of detailing cars through a paid internship at his day program in the transportation department. A job coach appointed through the day program's job training course will assist Jacque in preparing for his long-term goal of working in a car dealership, orienting Jacque to the working environment and assisting him to complete tasks related to detailing cars. Support for these tasks will slowly be removed over the course of 3 months to increase Jacque's independence in managing a set workload. The practitioner will engage in task analysis to determine what skills Jacque currently has, as well as ones he may need to acquire or strengthen in order to reach his ultimate goal of working part-time at the dealership. Sample tasks Jacque will learn to complete may include cleaning the exterior of the day program vans, vacuuming the interior van carpeting, and cleaning out stains in the fabric upholstery in the van. The practitioner will help Jacque to identify specific strategies to manage this new information and will assist Jacque in practicing these strategies so that they become habitual. Such strategies may include reviewing visual checklists prior to beginning a task, learning to read and follow step-by-step instructions and using a dry erase marker to check off completed items, and breaking larger tasks down into smaller steps.

How does this specific section connect to the overall intervention plan? Describe the ways these intervention ideas are related to ∨ :

This section of the intervention plan and the specific activities chosen relates to the top in that they directly support Jacque's long-term goal of obtaining part-time employment by teaching him supporting skills that he will eventually use in his desired part-time job. Though Jacque does not have some of the other skills required for part-time work at this stage, his participation in a paid internship through a job training program allows him to work on these skills in a supported environment with the intention of building other habits, such as the use of visual instructions, that will address his areas for growth in attending to tasks (bottom). Participating in a paid internship will also be motivating for Jacque as he will be earning money, which he identified as an interest during the occupational profile, and beginning to learn foundational skills that will be used for a future part-time employment detailing cars (top).

Describe the plan for creating awareness and/or skill building?

This section of the intervention plan will focus on both creating awareness and skill building. The practitioner will work with Jacque to identify everyday tasks that need to be completed within his role as an intern/worker as this will help bring awareness to the tasks he will need to attend to daily. The practitioner may also have Jacque observe other employees at the car dealership so he gains an understanding of what is expected of him. The introduction of visual aids will be incorporated to assist Jacque in attending to and sequencing the steps necessary to complete each task he will be responsible for. With the guidance of the occupational therapy practitioner, Jacque will begin to practice using these strategies on his own over the course of a three-month period, which will allow him time to build on these skills until they start to become habitual.

Select specific methods used to promote change: (therapeutic use of occupations and activities, interventions to support occupations, education, training, advocacy, self-advocacy, group intervention and virtual interventions)

Education: The practitioner will introduce Jacque to the use of visual aids, demonstrating how to use these strategies to complete new tasks. The practitioner, in collaboration with the job coach, will educate Jacque on what is expected of him in his new role as an intern/worker.
Interventions to support occupations: The practitioner will assist Jacque to note the different parts of each task the car detailing employees complete at the dealership and eventually create his own checklists for each task. The practitioner will also encourage Jacque to shadow a current employee to gain a better understanding of how each task is performed.
Therapeutic use of occupations: Jacque will practice the use of these checklists both at the car dealership during the supported employment program and in his group home for chores with assistance from the practitioner to improve carryover of these strategies.

Identify and describe the specific teaching-learning principles to promote change:

Identifying what is to be learned: Through Jacque's participation in a paid internship in the day program's transportation department, the practitioner will guide Jacque in determining what he will need to learn in order to be successful in his future role as part-time employee at the dealership.
Active involvement: By providing Jacque the opportunity to practice the completion of less complex tasks involved in detailing the day program vans, Jacque will gain a better understanding of how to apply the strategies taught by the practitioner to help him successfully complete new tasks without becoming frustrated or losing focus on the work assigned.
Stress with new learning: By managing the stress of new learning, the practitioner will encourage Jacque to practice the use of the new strategies for completing tasks (i.e., visual checklists and visual instructions) during the completion of familiar tasks such as his morning ADLs or his regular chores completed at the group home
Frequent repetition and practice: By practicing the same or similar tasks during his paid internship, Jacque will be able reinforce his sequencing skill until he demonstrates relative mastery, at which point, the practitioner will choose a related but different task to support continued repetition and reinforcement.
Organizing the physical environment: Care will be taken by the practitioner to minimize environmental distractions and create a neat, uncluttered workspace to facilitate Jacque's attention to the task and promote increased retention of new information.

Figure 17.11 MMCR Planning Guide to Address Specific Sections of the Overall Intervention Plan—Middle portion for Jacque.

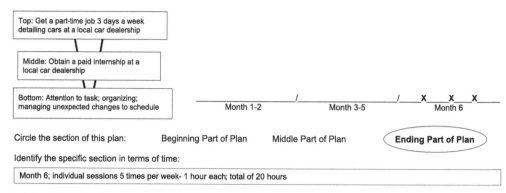

Circle the section of this plan: Beginning Part of Plan   Middle Part of Plan   **Ending Part of Plan**

Identify the specific section in terms of time:

Month 6; individual sessions 5 times per week- 1 hour each; total of 20 hours

Label and briefly describe the central idea of this specific section of the plan:

This portion of the intervention plan will focus on working on site at a car dealership detailing cars. This work will initially occur through a paid internship with assistance from a job coach, with the long-term objective of transitioning Jacque to a part-time position through the dealership. With help from the occupational therapy practitioner and job coach, Jacque will refine his strategies for managing the job's workload and adapting strategies for use in new situations. Though Jacque may now have the necessary skills required for detailing cars, he has not yet learned how to respond to the specific needs and demands of the car dealership. For instance, Jacque may need to follow new protocols for different models of cars or different types of fabric in the interior of a car. Additionally, Jacque will need to learn to work alongside other employees and potentially share portions of a task. If Jacque is to maintain part-time employment at the car dealership, he will need to be able to employ the necessary strategies and coping mechanisms to handle these challenges on his own and without the support of the practitioner. Therefore, intervention will focus on Jacque utilizing skills learned in months 3-5 with gradually decreasing prompts and cues from the practitioner.

How does this specific section connect to the overall intervention plan? Describe the ways these intervention ideas are related to $\bigvee$:

By expanding Jacque's use of such strategies as visual checklists, visual instructions, and written or visual how-to guides, the practitioner will facilitate Jacque's ability to attend to and organize new tasks (bottom) independently while working in a paid internship at the car dealership (middle). Working on his ability to manage unexpected changes during his internship at the car dealership will be skills he will carry over and use in a future part time job (top). His ability to handle increased task complexity at the car dealership will allow him to get and keep a part-time job detailing cars at a local dealership (top).

Describe the plan for creating awareness and/or skill building?

By the beginning of month 6, Jacque has already built the skills required for use of strategies to maintain his attention to familiar and new but closely related tasks. In the ending portion of the treatment plan, the practitioner will assist Jacque in expanding these skills to apply to new situations. By immersing Jacque in a typical schedule at the car dealership and exposing him to novel scenarios (i.e., car cancellations, additional tasks and responsibilities, missing items), the practitioner will encourage Jacque with opportunities to put his new skills to use.

Select specific methods used to promote change:(therapeutic use of occupations and activities, interventions to support occupations, education, training, advocacy, self-advocacy, group intervention and virtual interventions)

Therapeutic use of occupations: Jacque will have the opportunity to practice his desired job of detailing cars and working in a paid internship at the car dealership as part of the occupational therapy intervention, with the practitioner adjusting the complexity and difficulty of Jacque's workload and tasks to a therapeutic level that creates a "just right" challenge.
Interventions to support occupations: The practitioner will be providing cues and feedback, with additional support provided by a job coach, as Jacque works through his assigned workload of tasks at the car dealership to address Jacque's ability to focus, shift, and possibly split his attention between tasks.
Training: In this portion of the treatment plan, the practitioner and job coach will aid Jacque in creating a schedule for each work day using strategies that are similar in structure to the visual checklists and visual instructions Jacque has already learned to use. The implementation of this skill will allow Jacque to effectively manage the increasing demands of his part-time job and support his ability to succeed in this new role.

Identify and describe the specific teaching-learning principles to promote change:

Individual learning progression and timing of new information: To manage Jacque's stress level with new learning, the occupational therapy practitioner and job coach will slowly increase the number of days per week Jacque is working and provide gradually less and less cueing to support the use of the strategies used in months 3-5.
Generalizing to new environments: By practicing new strategies in isolation in months 3-5 and then slowly incorporating these strategies into a gradually increasing workload, the practitioner will provide the opportunity for Jacque to apply skills previously learned to new contexts and environments to support his ability to carry skills over from one context to another.
Trial and error: By having Jacque use his newly learned strategies on the job, the practitioner encourages Jacque to determine when certain strategies will work and when other strategies may be better. In allowing Jacque to try these strategies out in real time, practitioner supports Jacque's ability to problem solve through new situations and decreases the need for support over time.

Figure 17.12 MMCR Planning Guide to Address Specific Sections of the Overall Intervention Plan—Ending portion for Jacque.

occur in the day program's transportation department. Initial job training will occur at the day program to minimize the level of stress that often occurs with new learning considering this is a familiar environment. Jacque's familiarity with his day program and its environments will improve his ability to attend to the new information provided about protocols for detailing cars. This portion of the intervention plan will familiarize Jacque with many of the tasks involved in detailing cars such as selecting cleaning solutions, gathering the necessary tools, and completing cleaning procedures for various vehicles at the day program. Training provided at this stage of intervention will serve to support Jacque in his overall goal of part-time employment at a local car dealership. The use of visual aids and shadowing will support Jacque to attend to tasks, gather necessary equipment/items, and the sequence steps of a task as he begins to learn about his new responsibilities. Figure 17.11 provides a detailed explanation of this phase of intervention.

The ending portion of the intervention plan, occurring over the course of month six, will focus on orienting Jacque to the protocols and procedures specific to the car dealership at which Jacque will eventually work. The job coach and the occupational therapy practitioner will help to arrange a paid internship through a local dealership that will provide Jacque an opportunity to receive on-the-job training that will prepare him for part-time employment. Intervention will occur as part of the paid internship as a means to slowly introduce Jacque to a new working environment and build his confidence and familiarity in this setting. He has already developed the skills necessary for detailing cars and now will learn how to apply them in the desired work environment. As a result, intervention will involve learning his responsibilities, working alongside others, and employing the necessary strategies to manage unexpected changes throughout his shift. At this point, Jacque has also developed the necessary foundational skills to attend to, sequence, and organize tasks. Therefore, intervention will involve less prompting and assistance from the practitioner, allowing Jacque the opportunity to practice his skills in the new environment on his own with the use of his acquired strategies. At the end of month six, the practitioner will re-evaluate Jacque in terms of his job readiness to determine if he requires additional intervention or if services should be terminated. Figure 17.12 provides a detailed explanation of this phase of intervention.

Evaluation Summary Using the POP Acronym

P

Jacque is a 27-year-old male diagnosed with CP, IDD, and major depressive disorder. He identifies as a Black Haitian American male and currently resides in a group home which provides 24-hour supervision, where he has lived for the past four years. Prior to moving to the group home, Jacque spent the first 23 years of his life living with his parents. Jacque had a difficult time in middle and high school, ultimately causing him to fall behind. After completing his high school education at 21, Jacque struggled to find activities he found interesting that also matched his skill level. Jacque's father, Emmanuel, had taught him the value of work early in life, so his mother, Catherine, found a group home and day program in a town two hours from her home and made the decision to move him to the area so that he could receive the support of these programs.

The Wellness Model Self-Inventory (Swarbrick & Yudof, 2017) was utilized to conduct Jacque's occupational profile. This tool helps the individual determine their strengths and areas for improvement within each of the eight dimensions of wellness. During this assessment, Jacque expressed an interest in finding a job. He stated he would like to work in a car dealership detailing cars, but had no previous work experience and was unsure of how to conduct a job search. The COTE scale was used to identify behaviors that impact Jacque's occupational performance, and the Social Profile was used to measure Jacque's social participation during group activities.

Relevant areas to the person's evaluation findings	Strengths	Challenges	Raw Data	Interpretation
Working in car dealership detailing cars (top)	X	X	During the occupational profile, Jacque reported an interest in working at a car dealership to detail cars. While completing the occupational wellness portion of the Wellness Model Self-Inventory, Jacque marked "1" or "sometimes" when responding to these phrases: "I am actively pursuing work and/or training," "I am hopeful in my job search," and "I have considered my options regarding career change…." Jacque reports his father asks him when he is getting a job and that working would "make my dad proud of me" and that it would "feel good to work" and participate in something that "made me feel smart."	**Strengths:** Jacque has expressed an active interest in employment and is able to articulate what area of work interests him most. He has reported that he is hopeful about his job search, demonstrating that he would be motivated enough to engage in a job training program with the right amount of support and training from the practitioner. Jacque's interest in employment due to the influence of his father is a strength and will help keep him motivated as he pursues his desired job of detailing cars. **Challenges:** Jacque has not previously held a job and therefore lacks many of the necessary skills required to work a part-time job. Jacque also does not completely understand the cultural rules and norms surrounding the workplace and will therefore need guidance to navigate this new social situation. His father's desire may potentially place too much pressure on Jacque, overwhelming him and possibly discourage him from seeking or maintaining a job.
Participation in a structured supportive program	X	X	Per occupational profile, Jacque previously attended a county-support vocational training program after graduation from high school but reported it was "too hard" and "made me feel down a lot." Jacque has been attending his current day program and staff reports he likes to attend groups. According to interviews completed with group home staff, Jacque becomes "frustrated" when staff correct him as he completes weekly chores. During the occupational profile, Jacque also reports group home staff sometimes "pissing me off" and that he will punch walls or throw things to "help me feel better." Per the COTE scale, Jacque scored a 0 the reality orientation item (Item A) indicating he was completely aware of person, place, time and situation and considered "typical" per score category definition on the COTE scale	**Strengths:** Jacque is motivated to participate in group activities, as reported by day program staff and by Jacque's own report. His willingness to cooperate with others and engage in a parallel task with the other participants of the group home demonstrates his ability to follow directions and follow through on the task to its completion when the task is at his skill level and he receives the right support. **Challenges:** Though Jacque expresses a desire to return to a structured environment that teaches him to get a job, he has previously had difficulty attending to and managing new information without becoming overwhelmed. Due to his decreased frustration tolerance, Jacque sometimes throws objects or punches walls as a coping mechanism. He will not be able to rely on these coping mechanisms in the workplace due to their disruptive nature. Jacque will continue to develop new strategies for managing new information and effective coping mechanisms for when he feels overwhelmed.
Decreased attention to task (bottom)		X	On the COTE scale, Jacque scored a "3" in the area of concentration and attention (Item P). The 3 indicates that Jacque was on task 75% of the time during the observed group activity. During the Social Profile, Jacque required both visual and verbal cues to attend to the steps for food prep and safety in the kitchen. During the Social Profile group observation, Jacque frequently wandered away from the group area, got distracted by the environment, and required cueing by staff to attend to the gardening task	**Challenges:** Jacque struggles with attending to functional tasks and does require staff assistance to finish many activities. This impacts his ability to fully participate in group activities as well as be safe with more complex ADL and work tasks. Wandering away from a work or task area may also hinder his ability in the workplace as he may leave tasks unfinished which could potentially affect his role as an employee.

Figure 17.13 MMCR Guide to Evaluation Summaries—Jacque.

Community readiness skills	x	X	Day program staff reported that Jacque was previously escorted home by law enforcement due to getting lost, frustrated and yelling at strangers at the bus stop. Jacque reported during the Wellness Model Self-Inventory that he would like to "get my own place" and live on his own "like the guys from high school." Day program staff reported Jacque does not drive but would like to learn to take the local bus transportation so he can go out to eat and shop. Jacque previously had privileges to take the bus but got lost and frustrated and was escorted home by the local sheriff's office after he was seen yelling at others at the bus stop.	**Strengths:** Jacque has an interest in being more independent which will help fosters motivation and receptiveness to participate in intervention to facilitate growth in community readiness skills. He has been able to identify an interest in learning to take the bus which will be a motivating factor. **Challenges:** Jacque has struggled in the past managing his behaviors in the community as well as successfully navigating public transportation. He demonstrates difficulty with frustration tolerance and hesitancy to reach out for help if needed when alone in the community. Jacque has also become overwhelmed when presented with new information which may hinder his ability to navigate the community independently.
Social skills and connections with others	X	X	Staff at the group home stated that Jacque is very friendly with other group home residents but often engages in "one-sided conversations" and often needs to be redirected to a chore or task he is completing. Jacque reports during the social wellness section of the Wellness Model Self-Inventory and the occupational profile that he speaks to his mother via video chat 2 or 3 times per week and speaks to his father on the phone once every two weeks. Jacque gets easily frustrated when he feels staff is "correcting him" too much and will engaging self-injurious behaviors in the form of benign his head	**Strengths:** Jaque's sociability with peers and staff allow him to make his needs known to others and encourages him to connect with persons in his environment. His family connections will provide support during this time of change and his use of video chat, text, and phone calls demonstrate his ability to make meaningful connections with those he values. **Challenges:** Jacque's difficulty with reciprocal conversation may hinder his ability to connect with co-workers and colleagues. His hesitancy to be corrected by staff appears to embarrass him and cause him to show his frustration through behaviors that upset those around him and hinder his relationships with others.
Family involvement in care	X	X	Per a conversation with Jacque's mother Catherine, Jacque's father has always encouraged him to get a job and do well in school. However, Jacque's father Emmanuel has consistently resisted the involvement of county supportive programs such as the day program he currently attends or a supported employment program. After 3 separate involvements with law enforcement officers during his membership to a small local gang, Jacque's mother decided to place his name on the waiting list for Medicare services through the county. Per an interview with Jacque's mother, Jacque's father chooses not to acknowledge the impact of Jacque's Cerebral Palsy and Intellectual Disability Disorder on his daily functioning. Catherine states that Emmanuel would state "Why does he need services? He's fine" whenever the subject of academic or community support programs was raised. Catherine states that Emmanuel tells Jacque that he would be more successful if he just "tried harder."	**Strengths:** Jacque's parents are active participants in his care and show support for his desire to obtain a job. Jacque's mother supports Jacque's ability to engage in his day program and reside in his group home. Jacque's father's focus on other topics beyond Jacque's diagnoses of Intellectual Disability disorder and Cerebral Palsy, such as getting a job, make Jacque feel motivated to pursue employment. **Challenges:** Jacque's delayed involvement in county-sponsored support programs indirectly impacted Jacque's ability to develop skills that would help him to be more independent in the community. As a result, Jacque has limited knowledge of what skills or strategies may work best for him. His father's lack of agreement towards supportive programs may overwhelm Jacque when he has a job coach.
Involvement in church community	x		During the spiritual wellness portion of the Wellness Model Self-Inventory and occupational profile, Jacque reported attending church with his mother once per month. Jacque reports receiving spiritual support and guidance from the members of St. Joseph's congregation during the potluck lunch he attends after mass. Jacque also reports that his *grann* taught him to pray for help when "things are hard" and that "God knows the way, and He will show me, too."	**Strengths:** Jacque's involvement in his church community provides a reliable social support that gives him a sense of connectedness and belonging. He has good relationships with many of the members of the congregation and seeks their advice when he attends church once per month. Jacque has also self-identified a healthy coping mechanism in prayer to help him during difficult times. Though Jacque does not use this coping mechanism consistently, the coping mechanism is already familiar to him and may be able to be generalized to different contexts and new situations.

Figure 17.13 (Continued)

O

Through the occupational profile, Jacque identified his goal as wanting to work part-time detailing cars at a local car dealership. Using the Wellness Model Self-Inventory, Jacque indicated that he has difficulty managing his emotional responses when frustrated. He reported feeling frustrated when a task is too difficult or when he receives constructive criticism from day program and group home staff. Interviews with day program staff revealed that Jacque demonstrated a lack of interest in some of the programming and frequently mentioned wanting to return to supported employment so that he could find a job.

The COTE scale was utilized when observing Jacque in an arts and crafts activity at his day program. The assessment revealed that Jacque often experiences difficulty attending to tasks and processing new information during these groups. He required moderate cueing for group rules and following directions and needed staff's help to organize his materials. He also demonstrated frustration when unable to find needed materials for his craft project. The Social Profile was used during the cooking and gardening groups, and Jacque required staff's assistance in redirecting him back to attend to the task. Jacque also required both visual and verbal cues to support his performance during the activities.

Jacque reports his father asks him about his status of obtaining a job and stated that working would "make my dad proud of me" and that it would "feel good to work" and participate in something that "made me feel smart". Jacque identified wanting to obtain a part-time job detailing cars in a local car dealership to "make a lot of money" and "get a real nice car" of his own. He previously took part in a supported employment program but left due to "feeling down" when he was unable to do something. He then joined a pre-vocational program but reported experiencing frustration when told to do too many things at once.

Jacque will benefit from occupational therapy intervention over the course of six months to assist him in obtaining a part-time job at a local car dealership detailing cars. Intervention will occur five times a week, with each session lasting one hour. Sessions during the first two months of intervention will incorporate both group and individual sessions, and the remainder four months will be individual sessions only. Please see Figure 17.13 to follow how this evaluation summary was developed into the final format.

P

Occupational Therapy Goals

Long-Term Goal: Jacque will improve his attention, ability to sequence, and organize through paid internships in order to obtain a part-time job detailing cars at a local car dealership.

Short-Term Goal 1: Jacque will identify two bus departure times at the stop near his group home in order to use public transportation for a future part-time job detailing cars at a local car dealership with a memory aid and three to four verbal cues for selective attention in two months.

Short-Term Goal 2: Jacque will identify four steps in sequential order for detailing a car in order to be successful in the paid internship at his day program with a visual aid and two to three verbal cues for sequencing in five months.

Short-Term Goal 3: Jacque will demonstrate two positive stress management techniques in order to be successful at his paid internship detailing cars at a local car dealership with one to two verbal cues from his job coach for coping with unexpected changes in the workplace in six months.

Figures 17.14–17.16 demonstrates Jacque's goals for each of the three segments of intervention. Each goal builds on each other so that Jacque can successfully meet his "top" of obtaining a part-time job at the local car dealership where he will be able to detail cars. Due to his past difficulties in vocational programs as well as his cognitive-related challenges, the practitioner will provide six months of intervention to ensure Jacque is comfortable with his job coach as well

1. Jacque   **will**

 (Person's name)

2. identify 2 bus departure times at the stop near   **in order to**
 his group home

 (measurable, comes from bottom occupational performance issues)

3. use public transportation for a future part-time   **with**
 job detailing cars at a local car dealership

 (functional and specific, comes from top or middle occupational performance issue)

4. a memory aid and 3-4 verbal cues for   **in**
 selective attention

 (measurement, how much cuing, prompting or physical assistance)

5. 2 months

 (time frame for achievement)

Figure 17.14 MMCR Guidelines to Formulate a Short-Term Goal—Jacque 1.

1. Jacque   **will**

 (Person's name)

2. identify 4 steps in sequential order for detailing a   **in order to**
 car

 (measurable, comes from bottom occupational performance issues)

3. be successful in the paid internship at his day   **with**
 program

 (functional and specific, comes from top or middle occupational performance issue)

4. a visual aid and 2-3 verbal cues for   **in**
 sequencing

 (measurement, how much cuing, prompting or physical assistance)

5. 5 months

 (time frame for achievement)

Figure 17.15 MMCR Guidelines to Formulate a Short-Term Goal—Jacque 2.

1. Jacque _____ **will**

   (Person's name)

2. demonstrate 2 positive stress management techniques **in order to**

   (measurable, comes from bottom occupational performance issues)

3. be successful at his paid internship detailing cars at a local car dealership **with**

   (functional and specific, comes from top or middle occupational performance issue)

4. 1-2 verbal cues from his job coach for coping with unexpected changes in the workplace **in**

   (measurement, how much cuing, prompting or physical assistance)

5. 6 months

   (time frame for achievement)

Figure 17.16 MMCR Guidelines to Formulate a Short-Term Goal—Jacque 3.

as successful with the transition from a full-time day program to part-time employment. Since each phase is asking Jacque to work on novel tasks, some assistance is expected and acceptable to support Jacque. In addition, Jacque would benefit from visual aids to support the processes of taking the bus and detailing cars as a supplement to the verbal assist he will get from his OT and vocational coach. In the future, as Jacque has multiple opportunities for repetition of tasks in his desired "top" of working a car dealership, it is expected that he may rely less on verbal and visual cueing to be successful.

References

Agency for Health Care Administration. (2021). *Developmental disabilities individual budgeting (iBudget) waiver*. https://ahca.myflorida.com/Medicaid/hcbs_waivers/ibudget.shtml

Agency for Persons with Disabilities. (n.d.) *About us*. https://apd.myflorida.com/about/

American Occupational Therapy Association. (2020). Occupational therapy practice framework: Domain and process (4th ed.). *American Journal of Occupational Therapy*, *74*(Suppl. 2), 7412410010. https://doi.org/10.5014/ajot.2020.74S2001

American Psychological Association. (2014). *Transgender people, gender identity, and gender expression*. www.apa.org/topics/lgbt/transgender

Centers for Medicare & Medicaid Services. (2021). *Home and community-based services 1915*. www.medicaid.gov/medicaid/home-community-based-services/home-community-based-services-authorities/home-community-based-services-1915c/index.html

Donohue, M. (2013). *Social profile: Assessment of social participation in children, adolescents, and adults.* AOTA Press.

GLAAD. (2021). *Media reference guide—transgender.* www.glaad.org/reference/transgender

Johnson, K. R., Blaskowitz, M., & Mahoney, W. J. (2019). Occupational therapy practice with adults with intellectual disability: What more can we do? *The Open Journal of Occupational Therapy, 7*(2). https://doi.org/10.15453/2168-6408.1573

Shotwell, M., & Allison, J. (2020). The comprehensive occupational therapy evaluation. In B. J. Hemphill & C. K. Urish (Eds.), *Assessments in occupational therapy mental health: An integrative approach* (pp. 632–653). Slack Incorporated.

Swarbrick, M. (2006). A wellness approach. *Psychiatric Rehabilitation Journal, 29*(4), 311. https://doi.org/10.2975/29.2006.311.314

Swarbrick, M., & Yudof, J. (2017). Wellness in eight dimensions. *Collaborative Supportive Programs of New Jersey.* https://cspnj.org/wp-content/uploads/2021/09/Wellness-8-Dimensions.pdf

University of South Florida. (2016). *Florida's DD waitlist campaign.* http://ddwaitlist.cbcs.usf.edu/

18 Case Example

Using the MMCR to Guide a Three-Month Intervention Plan in a Homecare Setting

Valerie Hengemuhle, Geraldine Pagaoa-Cruz, Shaniqua Bradley, and Allison C. Inserra

Introducing Jerry

Jerry is a 75-year-old Caucasian male who is a recent widow and a father of three adult children. Jerry was referred to occupational therapy services following the death of Maria, his wife of 50 years who passed away 5 months ago due to a complicated respiratory infection. He plans to continue living in his apartment at the senior complex because he feels most comfortable there.

Medical History

Jerry has a history of diabetes, hypertension, depression, alcoholism and chronic obstructive pulmonary disease (COPD). Per Jerry's report, when walking to the flagpole, sometimes he waits too long to take a rest, and it takes him at least 15 minutes to catch his breath and feel strong enough to walk back to his apartment. Jerry has a history of depression and is prescribed antidepressant medication, but his depression seems to be getting worse since the death of his wife and the stress of living alone. He was previously followed by a psychiatrist; however, he gets his medications renewed by his primary care physician. His primary care physician recommended returning to therapy; however, Jerry has not followed through on seeking weekly therapy sessions, because he reports having no interest in doing so.

Medication List

Jerry has difficulty keeping up with his medication routine, as his wife was the one who reminded him when to take the medications and fill the prescriptions. Jerry reports, "Maria always kept me on track with my medication. She was a nurse, so she was good at that stuff. We would always take our morning medication together with our coffee. Without Maria, sometimes I don't wake up on time and I forget about my medication. I feel very guilty and upset when I forget to raise the flag because if I don't, no one else will." Jerry states, "Daphne says she is going to sign me up to have the medications delivered." See Table 18.1 for Jerry's sample medication list. Please note that although the medications chosen are typical for the diagnoses presented, the medications chosen, dosage and frequency are fictitious and were created to support the case study.

Staff Interview: Siena

Siena, the activities coordinator of the senior complex, recommended Jerry for occupational therapy services as she noticed that he has become very isolated and forgetful lately. Siena discussed how she has been worried about Jerry since his wife's passing. She indicated that Jerry has been consistently late when raising the flag each morning at their complex. Siena stated that he seems

DOI: 10.4324/9781003392408-22

Table 18.1 Jerry's Sample Medication List

Diagnosis	Medication Name	Dosage	Frequency
Diabetes	Metformin ER (white, circular pill)	1000 mg	1×/day with meals
Chronic obstructive pulmonary disease	Advair Diskus (steroid inhalation powder)	250/50 mcg	1 inhalation 2×/day
Chronic obstructive pulmonary disease	Albuterol (inhaler)	2 puffs	Every 4 hours for shortness of breath
Hypertension	Metoprolol succinate (beta blocker; white, oval)	25 mg	1×/day
Hypertension	Amlodipine (calcium channel blocker; white, round)	5 mg	1×/day
Depression	Wellbutrin XL (purple, round antidepressant)	150 mg	1×/day

Source: Whyte et al. (2021).

"more out of breath" and that he sits alone in the lobby for a long time after raising the flag. She indicated that Jerry rarely attends activities and has stopped spending time with his friends at the complex. She also recalls that his carbon monoxide detector went off recently. Siena indicated that Jerry recently participated in a wellness screening and was administered the Montreal Cognitive Assessment (MoCA) by a MoCA-trained and -certified nurse on staff. Jerry scored a 24/30, which is indicative of a mild cognitive decline.

Jerry's Occupational Profile

Using the Interest Checklist to Learn About Jerry and Maria's Story

An in-depth interview was conducted through the lens of the Modified Interest Checklist (Model of Human Occupation Clearinghouse, 2020) in Jerry's home environment, which provided information in regard to his home setup, activities of daily living and instrumental activities of daily living. The Modified Interest Checklist was chosen to help Jerry identify interests that he shared with Maria as well as those he enjoyed alone or with others. This will help the practitioner to create individualized activities that are meaningful to Jerry and potentially reintroduce purposeful activities he enjoyed separate from Maria as he transitions to his new role as widower. See Table 18.2 to review a visual illustration of Jerry's past, present and future interests.

In 1968, Jerry developed an infection in his right leg following an injury while serving in the Vietnam War. The infection resulted in a below-the-knee amputation (BKA) of his right leg. Maria, who had recently immigrated to the United States from the Philippines, was Jerry's nurse at the Veterans Affairs (VA) hospital. Jerry remembers Maria, "She was beautiful." Jerry recalls, "I told her (Maria) how I learned to play the harmonica while I was in the Army. We had a band called 'The Band of Brothers.' She giggled and told me "That's cute" . . . but I knew she liked it." Jerry sighs, "I played that harmonica for her every morning while she was making coffee until she passed."

Jerry and Maria faced criticism and ridicule in the beginning of their relationship because they were from different cultural backgrounds. Jerry said, "They didn't realize how much American culture they have over there. Maria and I loved the same movies. We loved Elvis Presley and dancing. Some of the guys would pull up the ends of their eyes and call her 'China doll' even though

Table 18.2 Synopsis of Jerry's Past, Present and Future Interests Based on the Modified Interest Checklist

Interests Identified From the Profile Using the Interest Checklist	Did You Previously Participate in This Activity? Yes/Sometimes/No	Do You Currently Participate in This Activity? Yes/Sometimes/No	Level of Interest in Participating Again? Strong/Some/None
Playing harmonica	Yes	No	Strong
Salsa dancing	Yes	No	Strong
Gardening	Yes	Sometimes	Strong
Raising the flag	Yes	No	Strong
Child care	Yes	No	Strong
Medication management	No	No	Some
Wood working	Yes	No	Strong
Playing cards	Yes	No	Some
Watching football	Yes	Yes	Strong
Cooking	Sometimes	No	Some
Cleaning	Sometimes	No	None
Managing finances	Yes	Sometimes	Strong

Source: (Adapted with permission from The Board of Trustees of the University of Illinois)

she wasn't Chinese. Even my son, Ethan, came home crying from school one day. The kids asked him if he was black or white and he didn't know what to say. There weren't a lot of Filipinos in our neighborhood back then. That changed a lot in the 70s."

Jerry and Maria shared a love for music and dance: two things that helped him during his rehabilitation following his BKA. When Maria turned 30 years old, Jerry got them salsa dancing lessons as an ode to their first date. One lesson turned into many classes, and eventually, salsa dancing became one of their favorite things to do as a couple and eventually a family. Jerry and Maria's first date was at a "hole in the wall restaurant" in New York City that had salsa dancing. He recalled, "Maria stood up and started to dance and it was apoy," Jerry said with a little smirk. "Apoy" means "fire" in Tagalog, one of the native languages of the Philippines. Jerry stated, "I tried to learn Tagalog (native language), but I only picked up a few words. They were mostly curse words. Maria stopped speaking Tagalog to the kids. She wanted to speak English as clearly and without an accent as she could. Ethan's teacher even said speaking Tagalog was slowing him down at school. Nowadays, I hear they're telling parents to teach languages to kids to make them smarter."

Maria and Jerry are Roman Catholic. Jerry states, "I haven't been to weekly Sunday services since Maria died. We always celebrated the big holidays like Christmas and Easter. We loved listening to Christmas music and dancing together. Maria would want me to go back, I just haven't." See Box 18.1 for a brief explanation of the Roman Catholic religion.

Box 18.1   Brief Explanation of Roman Catholic Religion

Roman Catholicism is one of the three main branches of Christianity. The main pillars of faith and belief are rooted in its scriptures, the Bible. The Bible is believed to be the word of God (Oakley et al., n.d.).

Roman Catholic Holidays

Christmas: The Catholic holiday that celebrates the birth of Jesus Christ, celebrated in December. Customs include holiday songs, attending Mass, hanging lights inside and outside of the house, putting up a tree of decorations, and gift giving (Hillerbrand, 2020).

Easter: The celebration of the resurrection of Jesus Christ on the third day after his crucifixion on the cross. Easter traditions include attending Catholic services in celebration, Easter lamb, and celebrations involving eggs (Hillerbrand, 2021).

Jerry stated his faith helped him while fighting in the Vietnam War. Pointing to his necklace Jerry stated, "My grandmother gave me her crucifix to wear around my neck during the war. I found comfort in knowing I had people praying for me." See Box 18.2 for explanation of Roman Catholic Symbols.

Box 18.2   Roman Catholic Symbols

Rosary beads—The rosary is a physical collection of beads and a crucifix that allows a person to keep count of the number of prayers one says (The Editors of Encyclopaedia Britannica et al., 2020).

Crucifix Is in the shape of a cross, with a representation of Jesus Christ on the cross (The Editors of Encyclopaedia Britannica et al., 2021).

Family Background

For the past 10 years, Jerry has been living in a senior citizen complex. Jerry and Maria raised their family in an urban city on the East Coast of the United States. Jerry's oldest son, Ethan, passed away when he was 18 years old as a result of driving under the influence of alcohol. His middle son, Chris, lives across the country in California. His youngest child is his daughter, Daphne. Daphne, her husband Albert and their six-month-old son, Ethan (named after her brother) live about 60 minutes away from Jerry. Jerry speaks with both Chris and Daphne weekly.

Jerry noted difficulties he faced in his role as a father. Jerry began drinking right after Ethan died in the car accident. Jerry stopped attending Catholic Mass services at this time as well stating, "Faith helped Maria through that time. I couldn't believe in something that took my son away, but . . . drinking helped take that pain away." Jerry said, "My father was addicted to gambling after my mom passed, and I guess I found my vice too." Daphne was only 14 and Chris was 16 at the time. Jerry states, "I wasn't the best father at the time, I was constantly missing big moments in their lives. It was like I had lost all three children, because I had forgotten about the other two."

Both Daphne and Chris moved out once they turned 18. Jerry became increasingly depressed. He "felt like he was turning into his father but couldn't take control over it because the alcohol helped take away the pain of missing Ethan." Jerry attended Alcoholics Anonymous (AA) to get sober and to be a better father, after receiving an ultimatum from Maria. He has been sober for 15 years; however, he reports smoking one pack of Camel cigarettes a day since Maria's passing.

Jerry's Interests and Responsibilities

Jerry has become increasingly withdrawn and socially isolated since his wife's passing, stating, "Daphne says she is worried I will start drinking again because I've been sitting around and feeling sad." Looking away, Jerry states, "Daphne suggested that I start going through 'mom's things' with her, keeping some things and donating others. I just don't want to. It reminds me of the things we did together." Jerry recalls, "Me and Maria spent all of our time together in our garden and while she didn't enjoy it, we would watch the NFL football team, the NY Jets, together on Sundays."

Jerry has the responsibility of raising the American flag every morning and takes this job very seriously and that it "gives him purpose." Jerry reports one of his most valued roles to be that of an Army veteran. Jerry states, "Maria and I would walk and talk about world news or gossip. She would always suggest we take a rest break to chat; she could tell when I was slowing down or out of breath." Jerry reports this activity as an important and necessary part of his day. He is proud of his service to his country and wears his U.S. Army veteran baseball hat every day.

Jerry finds little interest in cooking and eating since Maria's passing. He recently attempted to warm up some premade lechon kawali, crispy pork belly, but he forgot that he had left it in the oven, leaving it burnt and inedible. Jerry's carbon monoxide detector had gone off twice last month because he had forgotten to turn off the gas stove after reheating chicken adobo that Daphne had made for him. Jerry acknowledges that "my memory isn't what it used to be, especially when my blood sugar gets low."

Maria used to make a variety of Filipino dishes that Jerry misses. "She made world class pancit." He reports, "We always celebrated the Filipino tradition of making pancit especially on birthdays, and Maria would make it with the vegetables from our little garden." Jerry pointed to a small garden on their balcony that was full of mostly dead plants. See Box 18.3 for description of these traditional Filipino foods.

Box 18.3   Traditional Filipino Food (a Unique Blend of Spanish, Mexican, Chinese and American Influences)

Adobo: A stew made from a protein, typically chicken or pork, that is marinated or braised in vinegar, bay leaves and pepper. Garlic and onions are also typical ingredients, but there are many variations (Tee, n.d.-c).

Pancit: Pan-fried noodles mixed with typically pork, chicken or shrimp and vegetables such as cabbage, carrots and onion. There are different varieties such as Canton (stir fried egg noodles), Bihon (thin rice vermicelli), Sotanghon (mung bean vermicelli), Palabok (rice noodle dish with rich, shrimp-flavored sauce) and many others. Most celebrations will feature at least one pancit dish. Although it can be served any time, pancit is often prepared for birthdays to symbolize "long life" (Tee, n.d.-a).

Lechon kawali: Traditional dish where pork belly or pork knuckles are boiled for a couple of hours to tenderize, left to air dry for a few hours and then deep-fried in a stainless wok or kawali (Tee, n.d.-b).

Jerry has limited interest in completing several instrumental activities of daily living (IADLs). "Maria was always in charge of the cooking and doing laundry. She made sure my medication was ready. I was in charge of managing the bills, but she reminded me of the due dates." While he is not interested in these IADLs, he does report that he wants to know enough to remain as independent as possible. Daphne or Albert completes his grocery shopping, and Daphne is listed as his "in case of emergency" contact in his smart phone. Daphne has begun to take primary responsibility for the bills; however, once she returns to work from maternity leave, she will have less time to assist Jerry. When Ethan was born, Jerry and Maria were initially going to participate in childcare, and although Jerry still wants to help out, Daphne worries about safety because of Jerry's "forgetfulness." He says, "I think she is worried I will start drinking again or use the baby as a football."

Jerry identifies himself as a husband, father, grandfather and veteran with a strong interest in raising the flag of the United States of America. He knows that his wife is not coming back, and he needs to accept this loss; however, he feels it is too difficult. He describes not having any idea of how to live or do the things he loves without her. "How do you dance, without a dancing partner?" he asked. Jerry had difficulty identifying current interests or goals for therapy. He stated, "I guess I want to be a better grandfather, that is something Maria would have wanted." During the interview, Jerry spoke in a slow voice and was tearful when discussing his wife.

Analysis of Performance Evaluations

Home Assessment: Jerry's Apartment

The practitioner completed a walkthrough of Jerry's home to evaluate potential barriers, safety concerns, opportunities and areas for modification and adaptation. See Figure 18.1 for the layout of Jerry's apartment. In each room of his apartment, the practitioner identified safety issues that

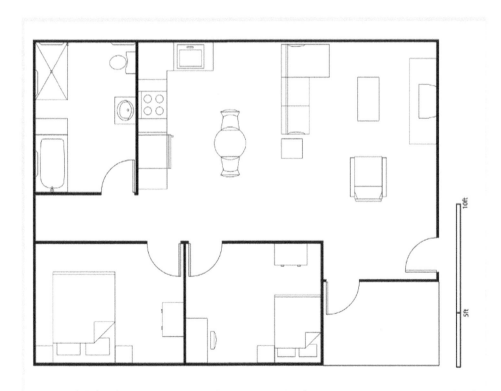

Figure 18.1 Visual rendering of Jerry's apartment.

Source: Used with permission from Noelle Rayment-Cruz (2021).

Table 18.3 Results Based on Jerry's Home Evaluation

Room/Location	Flooring	Features (furniture, appliances, etc.)
Entryway/living room	Low-pile carpeting	L-shaped couch, coffee table, Jerry's recliner, hooks for keys and Army veteran hat, outlet covers.
Kitchen	Hardwood	Gas stove, oven, refrigerator, microwave and coffeemaker, dishwasher, carbon monoxide/smoke detector; fire extinguisher, outlet covers, cabinet locks.
Dining area	Hardwood	Small round table with two armless chairs; unopened mail stacked; outlet covers.
Bathroom	Tile with two bathmats	Walk-in shower with one grab bar on back wall, bathtub, vanity sink; toilet with two handrails; medicine cabinet, closet with a long-handled skin inspection mirror, reacher and long-handled shoe horn, incentive spirometer.
Guest room	Low-pile carpeting	Double-size bed, bedside table, small desk and lamp, rolling chair without mat, small dresser, closet full of Maria's clothes, outlet covers, pack and play.
Master bedroom	Low-pile carpeting	King-sized bed; two bedside tables; tall dresser with "altar" holding a crucifix and Maria's rosary beads; photographs of Jerry's army troop; Jerry and Maria's wedding photo, ashtray, harmonica, outlet covers.
Small balcony	Concrete	Dead potted plants, no chairs, no throw rugs.
Complex facilities	Varies	There is an elevator to access all floors. Jerry's apartment is 50 feet from the elevator. The distance from the lobby elevator to the flag in the courtyard is an additional 50 feet. Staff offices and a community room are located on the first floor. There are benches outside the first-floor elevator, at the front entrance and by the flagpole. There is no bench by the elevator on Jerry's floor. Green exit signs, smoke detectors are located throughout the building. No steps to enter the building.

will be relevant to his intervention plan. These features could facilitate or hinder his performance of his valued occupations (i.e., location of carbon monoxide detector facilitates, ashtrays, flooring, location of commonly used items, kitchen setup, bedroom layout). See Table 18.3 for key features identified during the home evaluation based on each room of Jerry's apartment and building complex.

Six-Minute Walk

Jerry completed the 6-minute walk test in the hallway just outside of his apartment to and from the elevator. He was able to complete the test with five standing rest breaks leaning against the wall. Jerry completed a total of five laps, which is equivalent to 150 meters (492.126 feet). Jerry was noted to have dyspnea on exertion and moderate shortness of breath before taking rest breaks (Steffen et al., 2002).

Vitals/Borg Rating of Perceived Exertion (RPE): See Table 18.4 for the results of Jerry's vitals and the Borg RPE.

Table 18.4 Results of Jerry's Vitals and Borg RPE During the Evaluation

	Rest	*Activity*	*Recovery*
Blood pressure	122/80	150/82	130/80
Heart rate	77 beats per minute	120 beats per minute	90 beats per minute
PO$_2$ saturation	97% on room air	88% on room air; Jerry initiated pursed-lip breathing independently	95% on room air after sitting 120 seconds
Borg RPE	7 (very light activity)	17 (very hard)	12 (between somewhat hard and slight)

Source: Borg, G. (1998). *Borg's perceived exertion and pain scales.* Human Kinetics.

Jerry shows a typical increase of heart rate and blood pressure and decreased in PO$_2$ saturation but with minimal activity. The practitioner can continue to utilize this objective data to monitor Jerry's cardiovascular response to activities throughout the duration of the plan of care.

Explanation of Jerry's Triangle

Review Figure 18.2 to see the details of the MMRC guide to understanding Jerry's individualized "Triangle." The biggest change impacting Jerry has been the death of his wife Maria. Per his profile, we find that Jerry is struggling with many of his day-to-day tasks since her death. Therefore, it was determined that the overall "top" should be his transition to the role of a widower. Jerry's first "middle" ⋁ occupational performance, or overall pressing issue, is developing an individualized,

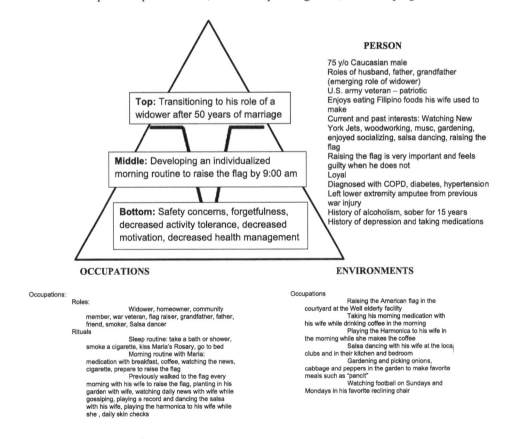

Top: Transitioning to his role of a widower after 50 years of marriage

Middle: Developing an individualized morning routine to raise the flag by 9:00 am

Bottom: Safety concerns, forgetfulness, decreased activity tolerance, decreased motivation, decreased health management

PERSON

75 y/o Caucasian male
Roles of husband, father, grandfather (emerging role of widower)
U.S. army veteran – patriotic
Enjoys eating Filipino foods his wife used to make
Current and past interests: Watching New York Jets, woodworking, musc, gardening, enjoyed socializing, salsa dancing, raising the flag
Raising the flag is very important and feels guilty when he does not
Loyal
Diagnosed with COPD, diabetes, hypertension
Left lower extremity amputee from previous war injury
History of alcoholism, sober for 15 years
History of depression and taking medications

OCCUPATIONS

Occupations:
Roles:
Widower, homeowner, community member, war veteran, flag raiser, grandfather, father, friend, smoker, Salsa dancer
Rituals
Sleep routine: take a bath or shower, smoke a cigarette, kiss Maria's Rosary, go to bed
Morning routine with Maria:
medication with breakfast, coffee, watching the news, cigarette, prepare to raise the flag
Previously walked to the flag every morning with his wife to raise the flag, planting in his garden with wife, watching daily news with wife while gossiping, playing a record and dancing the salsa with his wife, playing the harmonica to his wife while she , daily skin checks

ENVIRONMENTS

Occupations
Raising the American flag in the courtyard at the Well elderly facility
Taking his morning medication with his wife while drinking coffee in the morning
Playing the Harmonica to his wife in the morning while she makes the coffee
Salsa dancing with his wife at the local clubs and in their kitchen and bedroom
Gardening and picking onions, cabbage and peppers in the garden to make favorite meals such as "pancit"
Watching football on Sundays and Mondays in his favorite reclining chair

Figure 18.2 MMCR Guide to Understanding a Person's Story (Triangle)—Jerry.

Location: is 50 feet from his apartment to the elevator, 50 feet from the elevator to the front entrance, and 50 feet to the flagpole from the main entrance; bench is located on the path to the flag; 2nd floor apartment; Jersey City, NJ, USA (urban); CO2 detector in kitchen and in bedroom, coffee maker on counter top near the sink, coffee mugs are in the cabinets above; medication in the medicine cabinet in the bathroom above the sink; ashtray is next to his recliner where he watches TV in the living room; ashtray next to bed; small balcony off the bedroom with planters; adaptive equipment is located in the bathroom closet

Physical: elevator-lives on 2nd floor (50 feet from apartment); left transtibial carbon fiber socket prosthesis; flag, flag pole, pulleys; veteran baseball cap; harmonica; dog tags; grandmother's crucifix; Maria's rosary beads; Maria's clothing and shoes; photos of family; record player with vinyl; apple iPhone 11; alexa radio; various benches; walk in shower stall; gas stove; microwave; camel cigarettes; drip coffee machine; ashtray; recliner; gardening tools; bus/uber; senior home community van; 2 grab bars next to toilet and one in shower; long handled mirror; skin inspection mirror; reacher; long handled shoe horn

Temporal: widower of 5 months; married for 50 years; 75 y/o; served for 4 army terms; retired x 18 years; wakes up at 7am, however forgets to set alarm or sleeps through it; medication with breakfast and dinner; late paying bills; raises the flag at 9am; carbon monoxide detector went off 2x in the past month; living in senior complex for 5 years; raised family in Jersey City, NJ, US for >50 years; Sunday football at 1pm, 4pm, and 8pm EST; daily skin checks (morning and night); smoking in the morning and evening before bed, throughout the day approx. 5-10x, increased smoking since wife's passing; lives 60 min. from daughter and 7 hour plane ride from son; eldest son Ethan died at the age of 18; FaceTimes with his son who lives across the country weekly; sober 15 years; prosthesis 10 years

Social: new grandchild, 6 months old; previously enjoyed spending time with other couples in the complex, not as much since wife died; sees daughter 1x/week; lives around other senior citizens; salsa dancing; senior complex staff (activities coordinator)

Cultural: amputee (prosthesis, skin checks, cleanliness, care); smoker; recovering alcoholic; husband of a Roman Catholic, Filipino wife; rules and regulations as a senior citizen home resident; homeowner; veteran

Figure 18.2 (Continued)

adapted morning routine in order to raise the flag on time. His most valued role, other than that of husband, is the role of veteran. Jerry identified "raising the flag on time each morning" as a specific valued occupation that he is struggling with. Therefore, if he can resume this pressing and valuable occupation without her, that may help to propel him to transition to his widower role (top). The bottoms (safety concerns, forgetfulness, decreased activity tolerance, decreased motivation and decreased health management) were identified after a review of all evaluation results.

Frame of Reference and/or Practice Model

For Jerry, a combination of both the Model of Human Occupation (MOHO) (Taylor, 2017) and the rehabilitation frame of reference were selected to guide his overall evaluation and plan of care. As Jerry has experienced a change in both his volitional subsystem (loss of his wife, the extrinsic and intrinsic motivation of his wife, wanting to be better grandfather) and habituation (routines related to role of a husband, role of a widower) the use of a top-down practice model will utilize

Step 1: Frame of Reference (FOR)/Practice Model (PM):

Rehabilitation Frame of Reference

Step 2: Words in a Box:

underlying impairments unlikely to remediate;   focus on remaining abilities, attain highest level of function,   adaptation,   modification of task, environmental modification;   adaptive tools,   compensation,   potential to learn, motivation to learn,   teaching approach,   learning style,   client strengths, environment,   evaluate environments and social contexts,   energy conservation determine supports and limitations,   work simplifications,   home modification (Cole, M. & Tufano, R., 2008)

Step 3: FOR Party Paragraph:

The Rehabilitation Frame of Reference uses combined and coordinated use of medical, social , educational, and vocational measures to train or retrain the individual to the highest level of function (WHO, 2001). In the Rehabilitation frame of reference the degree to which maximum function or independence can be achieved is dependent on the individual's level of motivation. Underlying impairments are permanent or unlikely to remediate therefore focus is on remaining abilities. Interventions involve retraining and the use of remedial activities to restore function, compensatory techniques as well as assistive devices and environmental adaptations to accommodate loss of function (Ainsworth & de Jonge, 2011).

Step 4: Succinct summary of person's story emphasizing relevant occupational
⋁ performance issues

Jerry has lived and experienced life with his wife, Maria, until her unexpected death 5 months ago. For the past 50 years Jerry's main role has been a husband. While he accepts that his wife has passed, he is having difficulty transitioning into a new role of a widower and participating in occupations previously completed with her.

Prior to the passing of his wife, Jerry's most important roles have been that of a husband and a veteran. While Jerry remains in the home environment that he shared with Maria. Maria is no longer able to assist him in IADL such as medication

Figure 18.3 MMCR Five-Step Guide to Infusing a Frame of Reference/Practice Model Into a Person's Evaluation Selection and Intervention Plan—Jerry's rehabilitation.

his motivations, valued roles and interests to impact his occupational performance (Cole & Tufano, 2008). At the same time, many of Jerry's impairments cannot be remediated. Through the use of the rehabilitation frame of reference, Jerry can learn adaptive strategies to compensate for these impairments while focusing on his remaining abilities and facilitating independence in his valued occupations (Cole & Tufano, 2008). See Figures 18.3 and 18.4 to see how to infuse the rehabilitation frame of reference and the MOHO into Jerry's evaluation and intervention plan.

management, skin integrity checks, meal preparation/ management, safety management and health management. Through this process, Jerry identifies the role of being a grandfather to his grandson, Ethan, as something that is important to him. This self-identified goal of being a better grandfather **(middle)** will help drive him to adapting to his new role as a widower **(top)**. Jerry would like to assist with daily care for his grandson, however, his current state of "forgetfulness" and safety concerns are performance barriers to his daughter allowing him to care for Ethan over extended periods of time.

Based on the occupational profile, Jerry's interests include walking to the flag pole to raise the flag, playing the harmonica to his wife, salsa dancing with his wife to their favorite music, gardening for vegetables for cooking and doing various activities with his wife. Being a veteran of the United States Army was an important role that Jerry held prior to him meeting Maria. Jerry has the responsibility of raising the American Flag every morning and takes this job very seriously as it "gives him purpose". Jerry places a high value on his role as a veteran, wearing his US Army hat and dog tags daily. A valued occupation of his since he and Maria moved into the complex has been raising the flag in his senior complex after having coffee **(middle).**

Recently, capacities related to raising the flag have been compromised by the passing of his wife, including but not limited to, his decreased activity tolerance secondary to COPD **(bottom),** his decreased motivation **(bottom)** and forgetfulness **(bottom).** Jerry demonstrates decreased safety awareness **(bottom)** due to difficulty with concentration and poor health management **(bottom).** Jerry has begun to smoke cigarettes more often than he previously had since the passing of Maria, occasionally forgetting to put them out. which is identified as a safety concern.

Step 5: Explanation of how the FOR/PM will directly influence the specific intervention plan:

Jerry values his previous role as a husband and his current roles as a veteran and grandfather. Guided by the Rehabilitation Frame of Reference, Jerry will engage in various activities to allow him to complete specific valued occupations that support these two roles and help him to transition to his new role of a widower. Through the Rehabilitation Frame of Reference, the intervention will focus on Jerry's remaining abilities and supports to attain the highest level of function in his desired occupations of raising the flag, salsa dancing, gardening and taking care of his grandson.

Jerry is supported by family, friends and senior complex staff. Additional supports are his physical and locational environment including his senior complex building, elevators, seating surfaces (throughout his apartment, building and courtyard), his crucifix, Maria's rosary and his cigarettes. It will be important to include Daphne in family training and incorporate these additional supports, such as, seated rest breaks along the path to the flag throughout his intervention plan.

Figure 18.3 (Continued)

Jerry possesses the cognitive capacities and potential to learn novel strategies, techniques and tools. In order for Jerry to raise the flag outside of his senior complex on time and care for Ethan, he needs to first develop an individualized daily structure without Maria. Additionally, Jerry will need to assess his endurance limitations when performing valued occupations and understand how other, less meaningful, tasks performed in the same day/week could potentially affect overall performance of his valued occupations. For example, will he be too tired from his morning routine to make it down to the building entrance and raise the flag?

Therefore, intervention may initially include compensatory strategies such as creating a morning routine checklist, utilizing a pill sorter as an adaptive tool during morning medication management and hanging various visual reminders (BORG scale, steps for skin inspection, medication lists) in designated areas where he completes his morning routine. These adaptive strategies all compensate for his underlying impairments of decreased memory and health management (bottoms).

As Jerry masters the use of these strategies during his morning routine, intervention will move towards more physically and cognitively challenging occupations. The practitioner will initially provide education and coaching to initiate more complex strategies such as energy conservation, work simplification and basic home modification. For example, Jerry will be trained to move and keep commonly used items in accessible areas around the home. He will be taught how to read his body's interoceptive cues (ex. shortness of breath and fatigue) and implement seated rest breaks or different breathing strategies in real time while performing various tasks such as salsa dancing or gardening. Activity adaptations such as sitting down when gardening or using larger muscles when raising the flag will be incorporated throughout treatment. Intervention will target both selecting the best strategy and implementing perferred strategies independently for Jerry to achieve raising the flag, watching his grandson and performing all tasks related to his new role of widower.

Figure 18.3 (Continued)

Step 1: Frame of Reference (FOR)/Practice Model (PM):

MODEL OF HUMAN OCCUPATION (MOHO)

Step 2: Words in a Box:

Person is an Open-system

3 heterarchical subsystems (Volition, habituation, performance capacities)

Volition + Motivation (interest, values, personal causation)

Habituation (roles, routines + habits),

Performance capacity (objective and subjective; underlying physical and mental components, lived body experiences)

exploration -> skill; competency -> habit; achievement -> role
Environment (physical and social)

Dynamic interaction with environment (input, through-put, output, feedback)

Step 3: FOR/**PM** Party Paragraph:

The Model of Human Occupation (MOHO) is a practice model that conceptualizes the person as an open-system. Human beings are constantly changing and interacting with the environment and have an innate desire to fulfill their need for their occupations to promote well-being. MOHO addressed how occupations are chosen, patterned and what skill set is needed for those chosen occupations to be performed.

This practice model identifies a person as a three heterarchical subsystems: the volitional system (motivations, belief in selfs interests and values), the habituation system (roles and habits which shape and pattern occupational behaviors/routines) and one's performance capacities (foundational skills needed to perform occupations). A person's habits impact how routines are performed, how much time he or she takes and a generalized behavior. The input a person receives is based on his or her dynamic interactions with his or her social and physical environment as well as subjective and objective lived experiences. The objective areas of performance capacity include musculoskeletal, neurological, cardiopulmonary, and mental or cognitive functions. Whereas the subjective areas include the lived body experiences. An environment can be both an opportunity or a barrier to a person and his or her occupational success. All components affect the throughput (volition, habituation and performance capacity) which impacts the output of occupational performance in one's

Figure 18.4 MMCR Five-Step Guide to Infusing a Frame of Reference/Practice Model Into a Person's Evaluation Selection and Intervention Plan—Jerry's MOHO.

most valued roles and occupations.(Taylor, R., 2017).

Step 4: Succinct summary of person's story emphasizing relevant occupational
      ∇   performance issues

Jerry has lived and experienced life with his wife, Maria, until her unexpected death 5 months ago. For the past 50 years Jerry's main role has been a husband. While he accepts that his wife has passed, he is having difficulty transitioning into a new role of a widower and participating in occupations previously completed with her.

Prior to the passing of his wife, Jerry's most important roles have been that of a husband and a veteran. While Jerry remains in the home environment that he shared with Maria. Maria is no longer able to assist him in IADL such as medication management, skin integrity checks, meal preparation/ management, safety management and health management. Through this process, Jerry identifies the role of being a grandfather to his grandson, Ethan, as something that is important to him. This self-identified goal of being a better grandfather **(middle)** will help drive him to adapting to his new role as a widower **(top).** Jerry would like to assist with daily care for his grandson, however, his current state of "forgetfulness" and safety concerns are performance barriers to his daughter allowing him to care for Ethan over extended periods of time.

Based on the occupational profile, Jerry's interests include walking to the flag pole to raise the flag, playing the harmonica to his wife, salsa dancing with his wife to their favorite music, gardening for vegetables for cooking and doing various activities with his wife. Being a veteran of the United States Army was an important role that Jerry held prior to him meeting Maria. Jerry has the responsibility of raising the American Flag every morning and takes this job very seriously as it "gives him purpose". Jerry places a high value on his role as a veteran, wearing his US Army hat and dog tags daily. A valued occupation of his since he and Maria moved into the complex has been raising the flag in his senior complex after having coffee **(middle).**

Recently, capacities related to raising the flag have been compromised by the passing of his wife, including but not limited to, his decreased activity tolerance secondary to COPD **(bottom),** his decreased motivation **(bottom)** and forgetfulness **(bottom).** Jerry demonstrates decreased safety awareness **(bottom)** due to difficulty with concentration and poor health management **(bottom).** Jerry has begun to smoke cigarettes more often than he previously had since the passing of Maria, occasionally forgetting to put them out. which is identified as a safety concern.

Step 5: Explanation of how the FOR/PM will directly influence the specific intervention plan:

Figure 18.4 (Continued)

A change in volition, habituation, performance factors and or the environment can change how one feels about, thinks about and performs occupations. Jerry has experienced change in his volitional subsystem (loss of his wife, the extrinsic and intrinsic motivation of his wife's memory, desire to be better grandfather), habituation (role of a husband to role of a widower, time needed to complete morning routine) and performance factors (forgetfulness, loneliness, decreased activity tolerance etc.) In intervention, we are using the motivation (volitional subsystem) of his valued roles, interests and lived experiences of a veteran and desire to improve his role as a grandfather as a tool for intervention to work towards his top of transitioning to the role of a widower. We will utilize his interests (i.e playing the harmonica, drinking his morning coffee, raising the flag, his wife's memory and playing with his grandson) as the driving volitional force to target and improve his habituation (valued roles, morning routines prior to raising the flag, the act of raising the flag, health management, medication management, etc.) and performance capacities subsystem (decreased activity tolerance, forgetfulness, medication management, safety awareness).

Maria used to wake up in the morning and assist Jerry with most of his daily routines and participate in identified interests with him, Intervention will focus on utilizing valued occupations and identified goals to explore skills needed in order to achieve competency and achievement in his new role as a widower. There is a culture of safety in Jerry's senior complex home which also values independence. Due to the changes in his social and physical environment, the practitioner is asking him to explore and develop independent competencies in activities which were once done with Maria. Due to the temporal nature of this transition, Jerry is hesitant to engage in therapy, thus intervention must utilize the circle of interaction with care to develop rapport and trust through a therapeutic use of self to improve his occupational performance.

Figure 18.4 (Continued)

Overview Guide to Intervention Planning

Jerry will be seen for skilled occupational therapy for one hour, three times a week for three months (36 hours total) in his apartment complex through a home health grant promoting aging in place. See Figure 18.5 for the overview of Jerry's intervention plan over the three months. Jerry relied on Maria for the management of his morning routine, including many of his health management tasks. Without Maria, his routine has become disorganized, resulting in Jerry being late to raise the flag. Therefore, the first middle chosen is developing an individualized morning routine to raise the flag by 9:00 a.m. In this first phase, it will be important to lay the foundation with health management education and training in the use of adaptive strategies to improve personal safety.

As Jerry's individualized morning routine is established, Jerry can focus on his identified goal of raising the flag on time. It will be critical to build on the skills and strategies learned in the first month so that Jerry will not only utilize the different strategies but will begin to select which strategies will work best for him for different tasks.

Finally, Jerry identified a goal as being a "better grandfather." The third middle chosen is to babysit his grandson for a limited time period to allow Daphne to do grocery shopping for Jerry. This is a responsibility that Jerry has only had the opportunity to do with Daphne and/or Maria. His successful achievement of this occupation will further build Jerry's confidence and self-esteem to fulfill his role of grandfather and a widower.

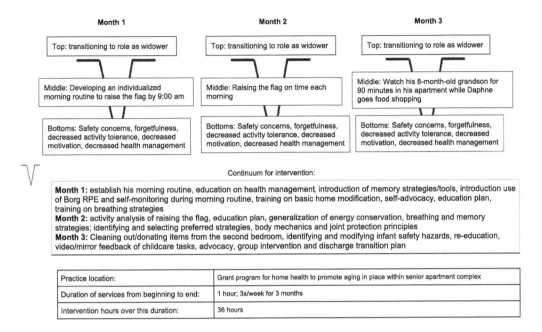

Figure 18.5 MMCR Overview Guide to Intervention Planning—Jerry.

Planning Guide to Address Specific Sections of the Overall Intervention Plan

Explanation of Beginning Intervention Part of Plan Guidesheet

Although Jerry's identified goals are to raise the flag on time and help care for his grandson, intervention needs to begin with setting up his overall routine so that he can successfully and safely engage in those occupations. See Figure 18.6 on how to specifically address the "beginning part" of Jerry's intervention plan.

The practitioner first completes an activity analysis to identify which skills are needed as well as the strengths and barriers to completing Jerry's morning routine. Jerry and the practitioner will begin exploring the task skills needed together, working toward competency in morning habits and routine and creating change to enhance his performance in this occupation. Compensatory strategies for forgetfulness (bottom) and decreased activity tolerance (bottom) will be incorporated in his daily tasks so that he will have the energy and awareness to do them.

During this section of the intervention, the practitioner will implement an education plan to methodically introduce various intervention strategies. First, it is believed that Jerry's forgetfulness is mostly due in part to his identified depression and hypoglycemia (low blood sugar). Considering mild to moderate cognitive deficits related to memory, executive functioning, and attention are associated with depression (Rock et al., 2014), improving medication management during Jerry's morning routine will improve overall ability to recall and learn various new task skills and performance skills. Education will help build a link to an overall healthier lifestyle and how it will positively impact his ability to resume valuable activities such as raising the flag and caring for his grandson. Together Jerry and the practitioner will create visual checklists/reminders (for skin inspection steps, medication types/dosages, etc.) as well as virtual reminders (alarms to wake up).

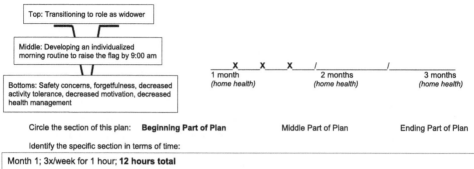

Circle the section of this plan: **Beginning Part of Plan**   Middle Part of Plan   Ending Part of Plan

Identify the specific section in terms of time:

Month 1; 3x/week for 1 hour; **12 hours total**

Label and briefly describe the central idea of this specific section of the plan:

During the first part of skilled services and intervention, focus will be on establishing an individualized morning routine to raise the flag by 9:00 am. Although Jerry is able to raise the flag on some days, he is having difficulty raising the flag consistently and on time because he previously relied on his wife to structure his morning routines. Without her, he now struggles to complete morning tasks effectively, if he remembers to complete them at all. As a result, he often is late too or misses raising the flag. Exploration, competency and achievement in his adapted routine will include various health maintenance tasks such as taking medications, playing harmonica, completing basic ADL/IADL activities and incorporation of strategies so he can both complete these tasks on time and raise the flag on time each day.

How does this specific section connect to the overall intervention plan? Describe the ways these intervention ideas are related to $\vee$:

Frame of Reference and/or Practice Model:	Model of Human Occupation (MOHO) and Rehabilitation Frame of Reference

Without Maria, Jerry does not have any structure in his morning routine and therefore has not been able to consistently raise the flag on time. This connects to the overall plan as Jerry is motivated to raise the flag on time each day due to his valued role of veteran. By having Jerry develop his *own individualized* morning routine (middle), he can create structure for himself. It is critical for Jerry to incorporate adaptive tools and strategies to increase overall safety (bottom) and be successful in his role as a grandfather, veteran and widower (top).

Describe the plan for creating awareness and/or skill building?

The practitioner will conduct an activity analysis of the current morning routine in order to provide adaptive strategies, energy conservation strategies and compensatory techniques to adapt to the new temporal environment and routine. Jerry will learn techniques during his actual morning routine *in the morning* (vs. simulated or practiced later in the day). This helps build his awareness of where the challenges and strengths are in his current routine. It will also reinforce using these strategies in real time while providing teaching and coaching support to facilitate success.

Jerry will be cued to monitor his body for signs of fatigue such as breathlessness and scoring his perceived exertion after physical tasks to build awareness of his cardiovascular endurance. It is expected that he is capable of new learning and adaptation, as it is assumed his current "forgetfulness" may be in part due to his depression and low blood sugar. Mild to moderate cognitive deficits in memory, executive functioning and attention are associated with depression (Rock, P.L et al, 2014). This will prepare him later to implement additional energy conservation techniques, memory strategies and safety awareness as he moves into the next phase (middle part) of intervention.

Select specific methods used to promote change:(therapeutic use of occupations and activities, interventions to support occupations, education, training, advocacy, self-advocacy, group intervention and virtual interventions)

Figure 18.6 MMCR Planning Guide to Address Specific Sections of the Overall Intervention Plan (Beginning)— Jerry.

Jerry will be educated on the use of various and specific compensatory techniques, energy conservation strategies, environmental modification and medication management skills. Methods of change include:

Therapeutic Use of Occupations and Activities
- He will create a morning checklist to include basic ADL, making coffee/breakfast, taking medications, skin inspection, raising the flag, etc. as well as adaptations and changes to routine (i.e he can no longer play harmonica and make coffee at the same time thus transitioning to playing the harmonica seated on the flag bench)
- He will trial various pill box sorters to see which works best for him, if any.
- He will identify and perform all morning tasks and track which morning tasks, if any, are more fatiguing (ex. higher Borg Rating of Perceived Exertion number) and what those symptoms feel like (breathlessness, difficulty speaking, etc.).
- All client centered intervention strategies will utilize meaningful occupations such as listening to the vinyl records, he and Maria enjoyed, playing the harmonica seated on the bench near the flag, phone calls to family
- Jerry will complete all tasks required for his morning routine, trialing adaptive strategies and energy conservation.

Interventions to Support Occupations
- Jerry will perform basic home modifications to support energy conservation, memory strategies and safety
  - keeping medications in visible/meaningful place such as in kitchen by coffee maker,
  - ensuring commonly used items are easily accessible
  - Visual aids will be placed strategically around Jerry's home
  - Morning checklist
    Borg RPE signs in kitchen, bedroom and bathroom
  - Skin inspection reminder/steps and materials visible in bathroom and/or near prosthesis.

Identify and describe the specific teaching-learning principles to promote change:

Modeling and coaching: The practitioner will first demonstrate a range of energy conservation strategies, work simplification techniques, breathing strategies and routine- related tasks. Following the demonstrations, a return demonstration will be completed to demonstrate understanding and carry over.
Trial and error: Jerry will trial strategies and modification through exploration of tasks to develop competencies and achievement in occupations.
Education: An early education plan will begin to establish understanding of his current health status; medication management and what activities may require more effort. The practitioner will educate Jerry and his family on new strategies, medication management and the necessary skills/motions related to routine management with good understanding and carry over. Education will continue to focus on tasks Maria had previously assisted with such as, skin integrity and safety awareness. *Repetition/practice*: Repetition and practice will be implemented during sessions and with a home exercise program. Due to Jerry's decreased motivation, mild forgetfulness, decreased endurance and decreased activity tolerance he may not initially be able to complete multiple repetitions of each breathing exercise, or each adaptive strategy and modification in a generalized manner. However, over time, as Jerry's motivation and self-esteem improves and his endurance improves, the number of repetitions and generalization of task demands will become more habitual to his routine.

Figure 18.6 (Continued)

Explanation of the Middle Part of the Plan Guidesheet

One of Jerry's most valuable roles is that of a veteran; therefore, intervention will focus specifically on his goal of raising the flag as it plays into his volitional subsystem. During the first month, the practitioners will begin to build self-awareness through identifying interoceptive cues in his body and the relation of these cues to different activities in his morning routine. These concepts will be carried over and generalized in various physically demanding tasks which challenge his current cardiovascular abilities in order to focus on the barrier of decreased activity tolerance (bottom). Jerry will learn to proactively recognize these body cues during his daily activities and implement compensatory strategies instead of waiting until he is completely exhausted.

See Figure 18.7 on how to specifically address the "middle part" of Jerry's intervention plan. An activity analysis of raising the flag is performed, and Jerry will complete all aspects of raising the flag through the use of scaffolding activities. Jerry will identify places for breaks and use the Borg RPE to determine when breaks are needed. Utilizing his smart phone to video-chat with his children provides a connection to gossiping with Maria during their walks, so that he can feel connected to his wife while completing this task alone, thus helping him transition to the widower role (top).

The practitioner will encourage Jerry to use previous strategies learned from his long history of COPD, including pursed-lip breathing and incentive spirometer. The education plan will continue to include breathing strategies such as diaphragmatic breathing for deeper and slower breathing. Visual aids such as handouts will be used or displayed in the home to compensate for Jerry's forgetfulness until these strategies are integrated into a routine (habituation) and he demonstrates

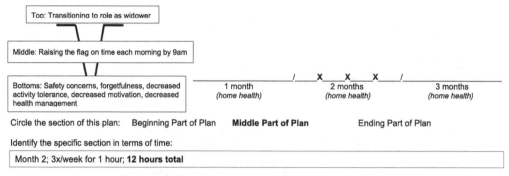

Circle the section of this plan: Beginning Part of Plan   **Middle Part of Plan**   Ending Part of Plan

Identify the specific section in terms of time:

Month 2; 3x/week for 1 hour; **12 hours total**

Label and briefly describe the central idea of this specific section of the plan:

The second month of intervention will continue to address one of Jerry's primary occupations, to raise the flag on time, every morning outside of his senior complex by 9am. At this point, he has established energy conservation techniques, breathing strategies and compensatory strategies for his morning routine which will be carried throughout the remaining interventions. During this time, we will be utilizing his identified interests to further build upon his endurance, activity tolerance (bottoms) and volitional systems needed to wake up and complete the occupation of raising the flag (middle). By the end of this month's intervention Jerry will have developed strategies to honor and stay connected to his wife, by raising the flag on time *alone*; therefore, maintaining his role as a veteran while also transitioning to the widower role (top).

How does this specific section connect to the overall intervention plan? Describe the ways these intervention ideas are related to V :

As Jerry moves into the "middle" phase of the plan, focus moves heavily on his goal of raising the flag (middle). The practitioner and Jerry will identify activities he previously did with Maria, analyze how they were completed and develop strategies to transition doing some of the tasks alone. This connects to Jerry's overall plan as he is spiraling between raising the flag (middle) and his transition to the role of widower (top) through these other tasks.

Describe the plan for creating awareness and/or skill building?

Jerry has been experiencing some forgetfulness thus visual aids for BORG scale and various breathing techniques will be placed strategically around Jerry's home for increased access. Jerry will be asked to utilize BORG scale before, during, after each activity to rate his exertion and begin to recognize those body signs of fatigue quicker. The practitioner will provide objective analysis (ex. 5 minutes of standing activity or 10 minutes of seated task) as well as using visual feedback (i.e., mirror) to raise awareness to the amount of time Jerry can participate in an activity before he starts to demonstrate symptoms. This will help Jerry in planning out activities as part energy conservation throughout the morning, day and week as they impact his ability to raise the flag daily. The practitioner will coach Jerry to use his incentive spirometer, take seated rest breaks and utilize his chosen breathing strategy. Jerry will demonstrate awareness by independently identifying the best strategies and initiating them.

Select specific methods used to promote change:(therapeutic use of occupations and activities, interventions to support occupations, education, training, advocacy, self-advocacy, group intervention and virtual interventions)

Therapeutic Use of Occupations and Activities
- Completing the sequential tasks needed to walk to the flag (selecting appropriate shoes, putting shoes on, taking Army hat and dog tags, locking his door, walking to the elevator, walking to the flag, placing the flag on the line, using the pulley system to raise the flag, saluting the flag.); identifying seating surfaces along the way; the act of raising the flag
- Incorporating interests from Modified Interest Checklist: salsa dancing, throwing a football outside near the flagpole with an old friend of his from the community, repotting plants and herbs on the patio that he used in meals with Maria, playing his harmonica to Ethan and/or during rest break at the flag to honor Maria.
- Home management tasks: simple laundry tasks (matching socks, putting laundry away)

Interventions to Support Occupations
- Jerry will perform basic home modifications to support energy conservation or memory strategies (i.e. identifying and organizing items in accessible places - walking shoes, Army hat, harmonica, veteran tags)
- Including family: inviting Daphne and Ethan to join him in raising the flag, identifying and planning for a place where he can remember Maria on his walk to the flag.
- Incorporate any additional visual aides for new learning
  - Borg RPE and breathing techniques/energy conservation posted for all activities of interest (i.e. salsa dancing, walking to the elevator).
- Family training and education with Daphne

Figure 18.7 MMCR Planning Guide to Address Specific Sections of the Overall Intervention Plan (Middle)—Jerry.

Education
- Continuation of Client Education Plan for medication and health management in order to improve awareness and needed safety awareness to raise the flag
- Identification pin on his ARMY hat that states his name, address and any health concerns,
- Shoes that fit well and compression garments
- Symptom education for diabetes: How much urination is too much urination? Did you drink enough water prior to leaving? Bringing a snack if he feels his insulin levels are low. How to protect his feet and wound care what to look for/signs of foot injury.
- Provide him cognitively appropriate educational materials.
- Family training and education with Daphne

Training
- Jerry will learn more complex body mechanics and energy conservation techniques and how to incorporate them into his daily tasks such as:
  - planning tasks throughout the day/week so that more physically demanding tasks are spread out to improve his overall endurance and activity tolerance
  - delegating very fatiguing tasks (ex. grocery shopping to Daphne)
  - identifying simple meals he can prepare for himself and making a shopping list
  - Using larger muscles to complete tasks

Self-Advocacy
- Jerry will assess his environment to determine areas where resting benches are along his route to the flagpole
- He will advocate to the senior complex staff for an additional bench or seating surface to be added near the elevator

Virtual Interventions
Video call or phone call family while resting on the flag bench to honor the memory of walking with Maria

Identify and describe the specific teaching-learning principles to promote change:

Modeling and coaching: The practitioner will first demonstrate a range of energy conservation strategies, work simplification techniques, breathing strategies with routine-related tasks. Following this demonstration, a return demonstration will be completed to demonstrate understanding and carry over. He will be provided with visual feedback such as self-videos and mirrors for improved understanding, self-reflection and carry over learned strategies.
Trial and error: Jerry will trial the energy conservation strategies, adaptive strategies, techniques and tasks modeled by the practitioner. Trial and error activities will be completed through exploration of tasks, to develop competency and achievement.
Education: The education process will continue in order to improve awareness and needed safety awareness to raise the flag.
The practitioner will provide educational handouts and demonstrations to Jerry and his family. If Daphne cannot be present in person, education can happen virtually.
Repetition/practice: Given the task demands related to raising the flag as well as the emotional and psychosocial barriers it is important that Jerry continues to complete practice activities that are related to his occupation. For example, raising the flag not only requires Jerry to make it to the flag on time, it requires increased upper extremity strength in order to complete the motion and task of raising the flag. Thus, an upper extremity and core exercise program will be developed and used throughout his day to improve activity tolerance, strength and endurance during these tasks demands (i.e lifting his grandson up, throwing a football 10x, resistive exercises using household items) Due to Jerry's identified bottoms he may not initially be able to complete multiple repetitions of each activity. However, over time, as his motivation and self-esteem improve and his endurance improves, he will be able to complete these tasks demands required to raise the flag.

Figure 18.7 (Continued)

increased motivation (bottom) with decreased depressive symptoms. Initially cueing will be given to initiate use of these strategies during various tasks; however, through skilled intervention, Jerry will independently utilize these strategies on his own by the conclusion of month two.

Explanation of the Ending Part of the Plan Guidesheet

In this final section of the intervention practitioners will continue using the motivation of Jerry's valued roles, lived experiences and identified goals as the driving volitional force to improve his role as a grandfather. This will act as a tool for intervention to work toward achievement in his new role of a widower. See Figure 18.8 on how to specifically address the "ending part" of Jerry's intervention plan.

Maria had previously prepared the home with a pack and play, outlet covers, cabinet locks and safe storage of medication to make it "infant proof" before Ethan was born. Since Ethan will now be nine months old, Jerry will continue to develop a safe space for his grandson to sleep, crawl and be changed in his second bedroom, "Maria's closet," so he can safely watch him. The OT practitioner and Daphne will help Jerry clean out some of Maria's belongings and organize items while discussing memories and keepsakes. Other items will be donated to the VA and Catholic Charities, thus utilizing two of his and Maria's preferred groups as a motivator.

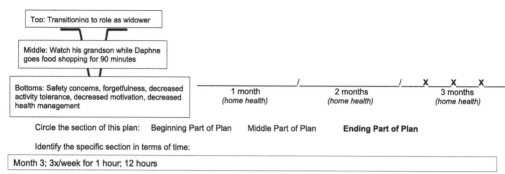

Circle the section of this plan:　Beginning Part of Plan　Middle Part of Plan　**Ending Part of Plan**

Identify the specific section in terms of time:

Month 3; 3x/week for 1 hour; 12 hours

Label and briefly describe the central idea of this specific section of the plan:

During the final stages of the intervention plan, the practitioner and Jerry will begin the process of achieving his identified goal to watch Ethan while Daphne is food shopping in order to feel more confident in his grandfather role. Jerry will continue to be seen 3x/week on Mondays, Wednesdays and Fridays. On Wednesdays, Jerry will be seen in the afternoon, when Daphne would usually go food shopping and around Ethan's nap time. Daphne has been involved in family training for the beginning and middle stages of intervention and will be present for his sessions on Wednesdays. Jerry will complete multiple training sessions with Ethan while Daphne food shops and the practitioner is present. Focus will be on Jerry learning to lift and hold Ethan, change his diapers and feed him utilizing Ethan's own belongings. Jerry will remain in his familiar home environment where he feels comfortable and connected to Maria. It is believed that Jerry will be most successful when intervention is provided in his natural environment, reducing the need for new learning. With improved activity tolerance, health management and daily routine carry over, it is expected that Jerry will be more prepared and motivated to safely watch his grandson. Thus, encouraging improved self-esteem, acceptance and transition into his roles of grandfather and widower.

How does this specific section connect to the overall intervention plan? Describe the ways these intervention ideas are related to ∨ :

In this end phase, Jerry will continue to identify safety concerns in order to make the home more infant friendly. Most recently Jerry has only ever performed hands-on childcare with Daphne present. Thus, training and re-education to perform specific childcare tasks need to occur. Jerry will first identify infant safety hazards in the home environment prior to making necessary adaptations, and he will then continue to transition the space into a safe play space for his grandson Ethan. Jerry will continue to spiral his middle and bottoms by working on activity tolerance/endurance and safety while he prepares his home for his grandson. During this final stage of intervention, Jerry will watch Ethan with the comfort of Daphne still in the home, while she is cooking. Once he has achieved competency and demonstrated confidence and safety, Jerry will watch Ethan for 90 minutes while Daphne is out of the home completing Jerry's food shopping.

Describe the plan for creating awareness and/or skill building?

When Ethan was born, the plan was for Jerry and Maria to assist in childcare. Jerry has previous lived and learned experiences needed to raise and care for children, however those competencies have been challenged (safety, forgetfulness, activity tolerance, etc.). Jerry identifies that Maria would have wanted him to be a good grandfather, and this is important to him. However, Daphne worries about safety. Jerry will begin the exploration process of the skills needed to be a grandfather (identifying and modifying safety hazards, gathering age-appropriate play items, utilizing proper body mechanics, transitioning from sit to stand & floor to stand safely and vice versa, and sustained endurance to lift and sway a baby). Daphne and the OT practitioner will provide coaching and feedback to promote awareness and change. He will develop competencies in the habits and routine needed to watch an infant (preparation of foods, changing a diaper and clothing, identification of emergency numbers) and demonstrate achievement in a grandfather role. The skills and awareness created by targeting this middle will spiral through to the top to facilitate acceptance of his role as a widower.

Select specific methods used to promote change:(therapeutic use of occupations and activities, interventions to support occupations, education, training, advocacy, self-advocacy, group intervention and virtual interventions)

Therapeutic Use of Occupations and Activities
The practitioner will re-educate Jerry on additional techniques to continue to baby proof a home through environmental adaptations and how to incorporate them into his daily tasks such as:
- modifying the rooms in this home for infant safety (i.e., adding changing table, electrical socket covers)
- re-education on child rearing expectation and the culture of raising a child or caring for a child
- identifying and organizing areas for baby food, baby needs that are easily accessible and reachable using the energy conservation strategies and joint protection principles that were previously learned
- watching his grandson in the living room area while his daughter is in the kitchen cooking one her mother's favorite meals

Figure 18.8 MMCR Planning Guide to Address Specific Sections of the Overall Intervention Plan (End)—Jerry.

Interventions to Support Occupations
Jerry will utilize his volitional interests and habits in activities of interest, noting carryover of breathing/endurance strategies; energy conservation and joint protection principles to engage in occupations and achieve middle and tops; examples include:

- making a shopping list for Daphne to cook chicken adobo based on a recipe from Maria's family recipe book
- cleaning out the second bedroom, donating items and choosing which items to save for himself or give to his family
- identify local organization to donate some of Maria's items too
- continuing to childproof the second bedroom and home as a safe space for a child and himself
- identifying safe places and time to smoke cigarettes while watching Ethan, if he must smoke.
- dancing to Maria's favorite music with Ethan to sway him to sleep
- playing his harmonica for Ethan to exercise his respiratory muscles
- visual aids will be placed strategically around Jerry's home

Education
Continue to develop a Client Education Plan for medication and health management that will be spiraled throughout the interventions to achieve to demonstrate an understanding of safety to live independently in this home without Maria:

- identifying emergency numbers and most accessible places to keep them
- infant safety (i.e., choking hazards, smoking safety with a child)

Training

- energy conservation/joint protection strategies and safety for changing a diaper and clothing, making a bottle and managing baby foods
- body mechanics and joint protection principal for lifting and lower an infant
- use of infant tools (highchair, pack and play, bottles, bibs, front infant carrier [Ergo baby])

Self-Advocacy

- Jerry will need to self-advocate for himself to demonstrate to Daphne that he is competent to watch Ethan.

Group Interventions
The practitioner will provide education, group and advocacy opportunities to prepare for discharge planning for Jerry such as.

- education on psychological services following trauma
- joining a grief group or veterans' group
- Alcoholics Anonymous information

Virtual Interventions

- Jerry will watch videos for re-education on changing a diaper, warming up a bottle and/or food.

Jerry will set up his television or virtual devices to have educational shows and songs that Ethan enjoys

---

Identify and describe the specific teaching-learning principles to promote change:

Modeling and coaching: The practitioner will demonstrate a range of energy conservation strategies, work simplification techniques and adaptive strategies needed for changing a diaper, holding an infant and feeding an infant safely. Following this a demonstration/return demonstration will be completed to demonstrate understanding, competency and carry over. He will be provided with visual feedback such as self-videos, mirrors for improved self-reflection and learning. The practitioner will continue to coach Jerry through various activities such as cleaning out the second bedroom to prepare for Ethan. Jerry and the practitioner will identify locations for donations and begin the process of organizing items and donating them.
Trial and error: Jerry will trial various activities to do with Ethan while he is there. Trial and error activities will be completed through exploration of tasks, to develop competency and achievements.
Education: The education process will continue to improve safety awareness needed to care for Ethan independently. It is expected that Jerry will need maximum assistance initially. However, with education, training and demonstration with feedback it is believed Jerry will be able to successfully watch his grandson for ninety minutes. The practitioner will request information from Daphne and educate Jerry on Ethan's needs and routines. While Jerry had previously engaged in child rearing with his own children, the culture around caring for a child may have changed. He will need to be educated on safe areas to smoke with Ethan present and other safety tasks.

Figure 18.8 (Continued)

At this point, Jerry and the practitioner will prepare the home, utilize visual aids and simulate childcare tasks two out of three days per week. However, each Wednesday, intervention will be provided with Daphne and Ethan present in the home so that Jerry can practice this routine and childcare skills with Ethan with the practitioner present. The focus of these sessions will be specifically on holding Ethan, changing his diaper, preparing his bottle/food and feeding him while generalizing previous energy conservation, breathing and home modification strategies. Jerry will have the opportunity to watch Ethan with the support of Daphne and the OT present to provide coaching and feedback.

By the end of the intervention, it is expected that Jerry will still feel connected to his wife; however, he may be more accepting and competent in his role as a widower. In the final session of services, the practitioner and Jerry will attend a group of his choosing within the senior complex community (i.e., a veterans group, a group for widowers, a social group) to develop a transition action plan following discharge.

Evaluation Summary Using the POP Acronym

The following evaluation summary using POP is based on Figure 18.9, which looks at the relevant findings of the evaluation, the strengths/challenges, the raw data and the interpretation of those findings.

Relevant areas to the person's evaluation findings	Strengths	Challenges	Raw Data	Interpretation
Transitioning to role of a widower	X	x	• During the interview, Jerry was observed to speak in a slow voice and was tearful when discussing his wife. • Jerry reported, "Maria was always in charge of the cooking, and doing laundry. She even made sure my medication was ready. I was in charge of managing the bills, but she always reminded me of the due dates." • "How do you dance, without a dancing partner?" • Siena discussed how she has been worried about Jerry since his wife's passing. She indicated that Jerry has been consistently late when raising the flag each morning at their complex. • Jerry stated, "Daphne says she is worried about me sitting around doing nothing all day and feeling sad. She doesn't want me to start drinking again." • Jerry and Maria shared a love for music and dance; two things that helped him during his rehabilitation following his below knee amputation. • "Me and Maria spent all of our time together, planting red, green and chili peppers in the garden, listening to music and dancing in the kitchen." • "Maria and I would walk and talk about world news or gossip. She would always suggest we 'take a rest break to chat', she could always tell when I was slowing down or out of breath." • Per Modified Interest Checklist, Jerry reported that he would like to pursue the following interests in the future: gardening, radio, walking, dancing (salsa), watching football, holiday activities, movies, visiting, checkers, reading, parties, house cleaning, woodworking, television, laundry, exercise, cooking, playing the harmonica and raising the flag.	**Strength**: Jerry continues to identify himself as a husband. While he states he has accepted the death of his wife, he has not transitioned to the role as a widower. This valued role as a husband will act as a strength to engage his volitional subsystem in order to achieve his goals. Jerry had previously used dance and music as a means for rehabilitation; thus, using these interests with the memory of his wife will aid in his motivation during intervention. **Challenge:** Jerry knows that his wife has passed away and he wants to accept this loss, however it is difficult. He relied on Maria for completion of many IADL tasks; therefore, he is now experiencing difficulty in successfully completing these tasks and completing them on time without her. He is experiencing difficulty successfully completing tasks and activities he enjoyed such as raising the flag, playing the harmonica, salsa dancing, socializing with friends and gardening, since many of them involved Maria.
Role of a veteran/ raising the flag	x	x	• "Jerry and Maria met when she was his nurse at the Veterans Affairs (VA) hospital in 1968" • Jerry has the responsibility of raising the American Flag every morning; it "gives him purpose". • "Maria and I would walk and talk about world news or gossip. She would always suggest we 'take a rest break to chat', she could always tell when I was slowing down or out of breath." • He is proud of his service to his country and wears his U.S. Army veteran baseball hat every day. • Siena indicated that Jerry has been consistently late when raising the flag each morning at their complex.	**STRENGTH**-This valued role was one that was already present prior to him meeting his wife, Maria. Additionally, he was previously in a band in the US Army, where he played the harmonica. His volition to raise the flag every day is a strength for Jerry as it is a motivator. Additionally, the use of the harmonica can be used to honor his late wife during his routine of raising the flag as well as a modality to improve his respiratory muscles. **CHALLENGE**-Although Jerry values this occupation, he has a long history of COPD which causes him to be short of breath and have a low activity tolerance. Without Maria, he is having difficulty

Figure 18.9 MMCR Guide to Evaluation Summaries—Jerry.

			• There is a bench in the first-floor lobby and one by the flag. There is no sitting area outside the elevator on his floor. • Jerry played "that harmonica for her every morning while she was making coffee until she passed." • Jerry played harmonica in a band while he was in the Army • Jerry keeps the Harmonica next to his bed	managing his health. He is not always aware of his interoceptive cues regarding his endurance (i.e., shortness of breath/fatigue) and when he needs to implement energy conservation strategies. In addition, since Jerry relied on Maria for the overall structure of his day, he is demonstrating difficulty completing his morning routine and raising the flag on time.
Role of a grandfather	x	x	• "I guess I want to be a better grandfather, that is something Maria would have wanted." • Jerry mentioned that he would still like to help, watching Ethan as Daphne returns to work. • Ethan was named after his late son. • Recently, Jerry has mentioned that Daphne worries about safety (caring for Ethan) because of Jerry's "forgetfulness". He states, " I think she is worried I will start drinking again or use the baby as a football." • All rooms in the house have outlet covers and there is a pack and play in the closet of the second bedroom	**STRENGTH**- Jerry is motivated to fulfill his role of grandfather as it was important to Maria. Jerry has both his two living children as support. **CHALLENGE**-Since Maria's death Jerry has shown difficulty with forgetfulness and safety awareness. If Jerry is unable to safely take care of himself, it will be difficult for him to take care of another person, his grandson Ethan.
Potentially unsafe situations		x	• Jerry's carbon monoxide detector had gone off twice last month because he had forgotten to turn off the gas stove after reheating chicken adobo that Daphne had made for him. • "Daphne says she is worried about me sitting around doing nothing all day and feeling sad. She doesn't want me to start drinking again." • "Sometimes I forget to pick up or refill the medication because Maria always kept me on track with my medication. • "We would always take our morning medication together with our coffee. Without Maria, sometimes I don't wake up on time and I forget about my medication making it difficult to get to the flag on time." • Jerry is currently taking 6 different medications for 4 different diagnoses. They all have different dosages, and they also vary in method. Most are pills, but he also has one inhalant. Also, although most are to be taken 1x/day, the frequency is different for two of medications (Advair Diskus-1 inhalation 2x/day and Albuterol inhaler-every 4 hours)	Jerry's decreased safety awareness is a barrier as his actions put him in potentially dangerous situations (ex. setting his apartment on fire, endangering Ethan when babysitting). He will need to increase his awareness of dangers in the moment, build on anticipating safety hazards/concerns and potentially incorporate strategies to prevent dangerous situations. Although Jerry is implementing a coping strategy, his previous history of alcoholism in times of stress worries Daphne, impacting his ability to watch his grandson. Jerry's decreased independence with his medication routine is a challenge. When Jerry does not complete his medication routine, his blood sugar checks and skin inspection, it affects his abilities negatively. Jerry may benefit from adaptive strategies (medication list, calendar reminders) and adaptive tools (ex. pillbox) to ensure he picks up his medications, takes them on time as well as to complete other health management tasks.
Decreased endurance		x	• Siena stated that he seems "more out of breath" and that she sees him sitting alone in the lobby for a long time after raising the flag. • **Vitals and Borg RPE (see chart in Occupational profile)** |	Rest	Activity	Recovery
---	---	---	---
Blood Pressure	122/80	150/82	130/80		Per subjective report on Borg RPE, Jerry rates his exertion as 17 (very hard) during activity. He has decreased awareness of his interoceptive cues from his body in regard to endurance (ex. shortness of breath, perceived exertion, etc.). Per occupational therapy evaluations, it is also noted that there is increased cardiovascular strain when Jerry is engaged in activities (i.e. increased blood pressure, increased

Figure 18.9 (Continued)

			Heart Rate	77 beats per minute	120 beats per minute	90 beats per minute	heart rate and decreased oxygen saturation). He is below age appropriate norms for the 6 minute walk. This is a challenge because in order for Jerry to perform his valued occupations, he will need to understand his interoceptive cues and be able to respond effectively.
			PO2 Saturation	97% on room air	88% on room air; Jerry initiated pursed lip breathing techniques independently	95% on room air after sitting 120 seconds.	
			Borg RPE	7 (very light activity)	17 (very hard)	12 (between somewhat hard and slight)	
			• 6-minute walk-He was able to complete the test with five standing rest breaks leaning against the wall. Jerry completed a total of 5 laps, which is equivalent to 150 meters (492.126 feet). Noted dyspnea on exertion and shortness of breath.				
Forgetfulness		x	• Jerry's carbon monoxide detector had gone off twice last month because he had forgotten to turn off the gas stove after reheating chicken adobo that Daphne had made for him. • Jerry burnt the lechon kawali he was reheating in the oven because he forgot about it. • He often misses phone calls from friends checking in and forgets to return them. • Jerry is upset that he keeps receiving late notices and fees from the credit card company, and says he often thinks he has paid bills. • Jerry acknowledges that "my memory isn't what it used to be, especially when my blood sugar gets low."				Jerry's forgetfulness is a challenge to him achieving full independence in his valued occupations and day to day tasks. Jerry does have the cognitive ability to learn and will have to rely on this to compensate for his forgetfulness. Jerry will need to consistently manage his health to minimize his overall forgetfulness related to Diabetes and depression. He will also need to explore different compensatory strategies (ex. basic visual aids/checklists, smartphone alarms and virtual assistant technology) to identify which will work best for him and how to implement them throughout the day.
Home and complex layout	x	x	• Jerry lives in a small apartment; one floor, mixed flooring • Jerry's apartment has many handicaps accessible features (walk in shower with grab bar, handrails by toilet) • Jerry has a carbon monoxide/smoke detector and fire extinguisher in his apartment • There are smoke detectors throughout the building. • Jerry lives on the second floor with elevator access • Total distance of 100 feet and an elevator ride from his apartment to flag in the courtyard • There is a bench in the first-floor lobby and one by the flag. There is no sitting area outside the elevator on his floor.				**Strength:** The physical layout of his apartment, elevator access and benches throughout the building are a strength as they support him being able to raise the flag once energy conservation strategies are in place. **Challenge:** Following the passing of his wife, Jerry has been faced with a psychosocial/emotional challenge. Although the familiarity of his housing complex has remained unchanged during this time of transition, he currently remains in the home he once shared with his late wife. This may result in increased feelings of sadness or may make him miss her which can cause a conscious or subconscious emotional response. Although there are many features to assist with energy conservation, there is no sitting area to rest by the elevator on his floor which could pose a challenge to him accessing the first floor or going outside to the flag.

Figure 18.9 (Continued)

P: Jerry is a 75-year-old Caucasian male who is a recent widower and a father of three adult children, two living and one deceased. He also has a six-month-old grandson, Ethan.

Jerry currently resides at his senior citizen complex and plans to continue living independently in his apartment where he feels most comfortable. Jerry's past medical history is significant for a right-sided BKA with a transtibial carbon fiber socket prosthesis. He has a history of COPD, diabetes, hypertension, alcoholism and depression.

He is being referred for skilled occupational therapy evaluation following the death of Maria, his wife of 50 years, who passed away five months ago due to a complicated respiratory infection. He identified his goals as raising the flag before 9:00 a.m. daily and being a better grandfather to Ethan. Upon staff screening via MoCA, Jerry scored 24/30 indicating mild cognitive deficits. Jerry reports that his memory "isn't what it used to be," particularly when his blood sugar is low. Occupational therapy evaluations were completed including a 6-minute walk test, Borg RPE, a home evaluation, vital signs and a Modified Interest Checklist.

O: During the interview, Jerry appears happy when talking about his past with Maria; however, he presents as upset and tearful when speaking about his life without her. Since the passing of his wife, Jerry has had difficulty transitioning to the role of widower. He reports feeling like he is still married and that although he knows she is not coming back, it is difficult to accept. He describes not having any idea of how to live or do the things he loves without her. Jerry has been experiencing difficulty managing his health since his wife passed, as he described Maria's role in reminding him to take his medication, monitor his blood sugar and to rest when becoming out of breath. Based on the home evaluation, his apartment and building complex appear to provide environmental support and are compliant with the Americans with Disabilities Act (ADA). However, he is having difficulty living in the apartment and completing such activities as cooking, doing laundry and paying bills on time. He has been consistently late raising the flag due to the unfamiliarity with incorporating these additional daily activities into this new routine.

Jerry identified a number of interests via the Modified Interest Checklist, including gardening, walking, dancing (salsa), watching football (NY Jets), woodworking, television, playing the harmonica and raising the flag. However, Jerry participated in all of these activities with his late wife Maria and is now having difficulty following his previous activity schedule during the grieving process along with his decreased independence in health management.

With the assistance of his supportive family, Jerry is interested in continuing to fulfill his role as a flag raiser. He describes feeling great pride in being a U.S. Army veteran and reports being proud of his service to his country and the purpose it has brought to his life. Jerry proudly reports wearing a veteran hat wherever he goes. To honor his country, Jerry has consistently raised the American flag at his apartment complex every morning with his wife Maria. He is now struggling to pursue this interest of raising the flag daily due to this recent shift in routines and a cognitive decline. Additionally, the use of the Borg RPE revealed that Jerry rated his exertion at a 17 during activity, which is interpreted as "very hard" (Borg, 1998). This also increases the difficulty of him being able to raise the flag. He was also observed to have poor awareness of his activity tolerance and endurance as evidenced by his lack of taking breaks before becoming short of breath, which may further greatly impact his ability to raise the flag. During administration of the 6-minute walk test, Jerry scored below the norm for his age, indicating that he is at risk for fall, potentially while going to raise the flag or during this activity.

Jerry has recently become a grandfather to Ethan. He values this role deeply and wants to spend more time with his daughter and grandchild. Jerry is planning to assist his daughter, Daphne, with caring for Ethan so she can go food shopping at the store weekly. Daphne has been hesitant to act on this suggestion due to Jerry's forgetfulness and the fact that he tires easily. During the vital sign evaluation, Jerry presented with increased cardiovascular strain with minimal activity as evidenced by his increased blood pressure and heart rate and decreased oxygen saturation. This is of concern, as it may impact his ability to care for his six-month-old grandson, considering Jerry may need to walk to, pick up, carry, hold or play with his grandson. The activity of caring for a six-month-old child may be more challenging if Jerry has difficulty with identifying how to conserve his energy prior to fatiguing or becoming short of breath. Daphne is also worried that he may begin drinking alcohol to deal with the sadness.

See Figure 18.10 to understand how the following goals for Jerry were formulated.

P: Long-Term Goal: Jerry will incorporate health management strategies in and around his home in order to continue raising the flag while adjusting to his role of widower over the next three months.

Short-Term Goal #1: Jerry will implement three memory aids in order to complete his morning routine by 9 a.m. to prepare to raise the flag with minimal assistance in one month.

Short-Term Goal #2: Jerry will implement two energy conservation strategies in order to raise the flag 75% of the time in two months.

Short-Term Goal #3: Jerry will modify three infant hazards in the second bedroom in order to safely watch his grandson for 90 minutes with minimal verbal cues from Daphne in three months.

Short-Term Goal #4: Jerry will tolerate 10 minutes of moderate activity in order to participate in active floor play with Ethan with no more than two rest breaks in three months.

Goal # 1.

1. Jerry   **will**

   (Person's name)

2. implement 3 memory aides   **in order to**

(measurable, comes from bottom occupational performance issues)

3. complete his morning routine by 9AM to prepare to raise the flag   **with**

(functional and specific, comes from top or middle occupational performance issue)

4. minimal assistance from friends at the senior complex   **in**

(measurement, how much cuing, prompting or physical assistance)

5. 1 month.

   (time frame for achievement)

Figure 18.10 MMCR Guidelines to Formulate a Short-Term Goal—Jerry.

Goal # 2.

1. | Jerry | **will** |

(Person's name)

2. | implement 2 energy conservation strategies | **in order to** |

(measurable, comes from bottom occupational performance issues)

3. | raise the flag |

(functional and specific, comes from top or middle occupational performance issue)

4. | 75% of the time | **in** |

(measurement, how much cuing, prompting or physical assistance)

5. | 2 months. |

(time frame for achievement)

Goal # 3.

1. | Jerry | **will** |

(Person's name)

2. | modify 3 infant hazards in the second bedroom | **in order to** |

(measurable, comes from bottom occupational performance issues)

3. | safely watch his grandson for 90 minutes | **with** |

(functional and specific, comes from top or middle occupational performance issue)

1. | minimal verbal cues from Daphne | **in** |

(measurement, how much cuing, prompting or physical assistance)

2. | 3 months. |

(time frame for achievement)

Figure 18.10 (Continued)

Goal # 4.

3. | Jerry | **will**

(Person's name)

4. | tolerate 10 minutes of moderate activity | **in order to**

(measurable, comes from bottom occupational performance issues)

5. | participate in active floor play with Ethan | **with**

(functional and specific, comes from top or middle occupational performance issue)

6. | no more than 2 rest breaks | **in**

(measurement, how much cuing, prompting or physical assistance)

7. | 3 months.

(time frame for achievement)

Figure 18.10 (Continued)

TRY IT: Using the MMCR in an Elementary School Over an Academic Year (10 Months of Intervention): Kody

Katheryne H. Wall, OTR/L, Danielle Minetti, OTR/L, and Shaniqua Bradley, PhD, LCSW
Now that you have a greater understanding of the MMCR, it is time for the final Try It activity. Kody's case example presented here provides the evaluation findings, including the occupational profile and analysis of performance information. Based on this information, complete all of the MMCR clinical reasoning guidesheets to shape your understanding of Kody's story, evaluation priorities, intervention strategy and documentation plan.

TRY IT: Introducing Kody

Kody is an African American 8-year, 3-month-old boy who lives with his uncle Kevin. Kody is beginning third grade in a new school district after moving this past summer. He has a special education classification of Other Health Impaired (OHI), with a formal diagnosis of attention-deficit/hyperactivity disorder (ADHD), which will be explained in further detail within the school record review.

When serving the pediatric population, it is a family-centered approach; therefore, it is important to identify Kody's family and their social history and how it has an impact on Kody.

Family Background

Kody's biological parents are Kenya and David. Kody's adoptive parent is his African American 35-year-old maternal uncle Kevin. Kenya and Kevin were twins. Kevin is the "big brother" as he was born three minutes before Kenya. Kevin and David became best friends in high school. David and Kenya began dating in high school and eventually married and had Kody after graduating college. Shortly after Kody's fifth birthday, David and Kenya died in a tragic car accident at the hands of a drunk driver.

When Kenya and Kevin were younger, they made a pact that when they had children that if something happened to either of them, the other would step in and raise the children. Honoring this pact, Kevin immediately stepped in and went through the process to formally adopt Kody. Though Kevin is now a single parent, he has the support of his parents, "Ma" and "Pa," as well as his other relatives and his church family in raising Kody. In fact, every Sunday, Kevin and Kody go to "Ma and Pa's" house for Sunday dinner, which consists of a big meal where the family gathers to talk, laugh, eat and spend time together. Family is important, and Kevin makes sure that Kody is surrounded by his family as much as possible.

Kevin was recently offered a position at the local university. As a result, Kevin decided to relocate closer to the university, which means Kody will now attend a new school. Currently, Kevin and Kody live in a quiet suburban area in a 3-bedroom, 1.5-bathroom house, with three stairs to enter with a backyard area.

Prior to Kody beginning the new school, Kevin decided that it was time to start talking to Kody about the experiences of the African American male since Kody would now go from attending a school where there were many children that looked like him to a school where he may be one of the only black male children in the school. Kevin tells Kody that racism is real, and he will have people treat him differently simply because he is a black male. He teaches Kody the importance of being respectful to his peers, teachers and those in authority. He tells Kody that he should always make eye contact with his teachers and all adults he will encounter.

Kevin also talks to Kody about being a leader. He tells Kody the importance of doing the right thing and not following after people. He especially tells Kody that since he will now be attending a predominantly white school, that he has to be extra careful and not get into things that he should not. He explains to Kody that just one simple mistake can be disastrous for him as a young black male.

Kevin wants Kody to be aware of what is going on in the world around him and he wants to prepare Kody for some of the interactions that he will experience as a young African American male. Kevin is also worried because Kody has ADHD, which impacts his focus and attention. Though Kody is only 8 years old, Kevin knows that there are many racist people in this world that do not care or see Kody's age and just see another "black face."

Birth, Developmental and Medical Background

Kody was born at 25 weeks and weighed 1 lb 3 oz. He stayed in the hospital for 6 months and underwent 13 surgeries before he was discharged from the hospital. Currently, Kody does not take any medications and does not have any known allergies. He is near-sighted and wears glasses full time.

Educational Background

As a result of the circumstances regarding Kody's birth, he was 6 months to 1 year behind in his skills. He received Early Intervention (EI) services as a result of his development delay (Centers for Disease Control and Prevention, 2019). Preschool and elementary teachers started to call home and share that he "can't pay attention" and "won't sit still." This became the norm every school year; Kody is "constantly on the move" and "can't sit still," and teachers ask, "Have you considered putting him on medication?" Table 18.5 outlines Kody's developmental progression with associated therapies.

Table 18.5 Outline of Kody's History of Services

- **18 months:** Received occupational therapy, speech therapy and physical therapy through early intervention
- **21 months:** Kody began walking and talking
- **3 years old:** Finished Early Intervention and began a specialized preschool program with an Individualized Educational Plan (IEP)
- **6 years old**: Received a formal diagnosis of attention-deficit/hyperactivity disorder (ADHD) from a neuropsychological evaluation

Kody receives the following related services:

Kody's current IEP from his previous school outlines that he attends classes in a mainstream classroom with two teachers (at least one teacher is a certified special education teacher), and he receives additional support services for reading and writing. See Table 18.6 for specific details on Kody's related services as written in his IEP.

Table 18.6 Related Services in Kody's Current IEP

Related Service	Goal	Frequency	Location	Duration	Group Size
Occupational therapy	To improve written communication abilities in the classroom and increase independence with activities of daily living.	2/week	Integrated therapy room	30 minutes	Individual
Physical therapy	To improve safety on stairs and postural control to increase stamina for sitting upright for longer periods of time.	1/week	Therapy room	30 minutes	Group
Speech/ language therapy	To improve his ability to process and utilize language.	1/week	Therapy room	30 minutes	Group

Kody was a delayed reader (did not read with fluency until he was 7 years old) and has a history of writing difficulties (delayed letter formation; difficulties getting thoughts onto paper; illegible writing; difficulties with sizing, spacing and placement of letters on the line). Aside from difficulties with legibility of his numbers and organizing written information on the page, math is an area of strength for Kody. See Table 18.7 for a list of Kody's modifications and accommodations.

Table 18.7 Modifications and Accommodations in Kody's IEP

1. Extra time on assessments and classroom assignments
2. Information broken down into smaller units
3. Use of checklists
4. Allow directions to be repeated as necessary
5. Use of breaks
6. Modify pace of instruction to ensure understanding

Kody's triennial re-evaluation date is approaching. The Individuals with Disabilities Education Act (IDEA) requires that schools conduct a multidisciplinary evaluation at least once every three years to determine whether or not the student continues to be a student with a disability (U.S. Department of Education, 2017). His IEP team that consists of his case manager, his uncle Kevin, current teachers and related service providers are all in agreement that his Child Study Team (CST) evaluations should be updated. Although he knows the evaluation process will be taxing to Kody, Kevin knows the importance of having the most up-to-date information in order to best meet Kody's educational needs at school. See Table 18.8 for evaluations to be completed as part of Kody's triennial re-evaluation.

Table 18.8 Evaluations to Be Completed as Part of Kody's Triennial Re-evaluation

Evaluation	*Purpose*	*Evaluator*
Social assessment	• Student's adaptive social functioning and emotional development • Social and cultural factors that influence the student's emotional development • Relevant family and developmental history	School social worker
Educational evaluation	• Analysis of the student's academic and functional performance • Analysis of the student's learning characteristics	Learning disabilities teacher consultant (LDT-C)
Psychological evaluation	• Analysis of the student's cognitive skills and functional behavioral skills • Appraisal of the student's social and adaptive life skills	School psychologist
Occupational therapy evaluation	• Assessment of the student's fine motor and visual motor skills • Assessment of the student's sensory processing • Assessment of the student's ability to complete self-care tasks • Assessment of the student's need for OT services	Occupational therapist (OT)

Table 18.8 (Continued)

Evaluation	Purpose	Evaluator
Physical therapy evaluation	• An assessment of the student's gross motor skill development • Assessment of the student's need for PT services	Physical therapist (PT)
Speech/language evaluation	• Appraisal of language skills • Appraisal of speech use and production • Assessment of the student's need for speech/language services	Speech and language pathologist (SLP)

Interviews Were Completed With:

1. Mrs. Bott (Kody's main classroom teacher)
2. Mr. Smith (Kody's special education teacher for reading and writing)
3. Kevin (Kody's uncle)

Teacher Interviews

Mrs. Bott has had Kody in her classroom for two months since school started in September. Since then, Mrs. Bott has gotten to know Kody very well. Mrs. Bott describes Kody as "hard working and positive" but "constantly on the go." Mrs. Bott stated that he is observed to frequently fidget in his seat and get distracted by "anything and everything." He is usually seen shifting back and forth in his chair, playing with pencils or erasers and standing up at his desk. Depending on the time of day, he can typically remain seated for up to five minutes at a time before getting out of his seat. After recess and gym class, he can remain seated for up to 10 minutes at a time prior to needing reminders to sit in his chair.

Mrs. Bott reports that math is an area of strength for Kody, and he is currently performing as expected in this subject per testing. However, his performance during math lessons is described as follows: constantly calling out answers, "doodling" on his math worksheets and often dropping his math whiteboard and markers on the floor when trying to hold up his board to show answers to problems. As for science and social studies, Kody does well for the most part; however, if assignments require reading and writing, he has a difficult time keeping up. If he is particularly interested in the topic, he will often call out answers and interrupt other students when speaking. If he is not interested or especially "distracted" he is either seen with his head on his desk, standing up at his seat or trying to spin around in his chair.

Mr. Smith reports that academically, recent class assessments revealed that he is currently reading with fluency on a second-grade level. When completing reading assignments in class, he takes increased time to complete and often has a hard time keeping his place while reading. Mr. Smith provides him with reminders to use his finger to help keep his place, which he benefits from. Mr. Smith provides Kody with significant support with written work. Kody needs assistance to structure his ideas for writing, stay focused while writing and create proper sentence structure. Mr. Smith noted that Kody is "highly creative" but explained that there is often a disconnect between what he can say verbally and what he can directly translate onto paper or type. He often rushes through writing assignments, impacting his overall legibility. When he attempts to type assignments, Mr. Smith stated that he seems to be losing interest, losing motivation and losing confidence while completing these tasks.

Mrs. Bott reported that Kody enjoys all specials and time outside of the classroom (she thinks moving around and changes of scenery help to refocus him). Gym is his favorite special, as he loves to "get up and move," and art is his least favorite, as he has a hard time with using tools like scissors and glue as well as drawing activities. Mrs. Bott shared that during recess aides reported that he has a tendency to seek out high-intensity activities, such as swinging from the monkey bars, playing football and swinging high on the swing set. When playing with other children, he "tries his best" to wait his turn and not "barrel his way through" other students, but this is often an area of difficulty for him.

Mrs. Bott also described his desk and backpack as "total disasters" with papers, school supplies, books, etc., "anywhere and everywhere." When she asks him to take out a worksheet or paper she had given him the day before, he either cannot locate the paper at all, finds it 10 minutes later or takes out the wrong one. This impacts his ability to keep up with work in class. She also said that he appears to be "constantly tripping over his own feet" and seems "pretty clumsy." Despite these areas, Mrs. Bott noted his strengths as being "very kind and social" and indicated that he has positive relationships with other students in class even though he is new to the school and has difficulties waiting his turn and bumping into them. She also noted that he is "always looking out for the other students" and "helps out in class when he can."

Mrs. Bott stated that she would like for Kody to sit still for longer periods of time, not call out answers, be safe around other students (not bump into or push over accidentally) and keep his desk and belongings "more organized." Mr. Smith's main concerns for Kody are primarily his ability to successfully complete reading and writing tasks in the classroom. Specifically, he would like for Kody to keep his place while reading, improve his handwriting, improve his ability to organize his thoughts for writing and determine which method is best for Kody to produce written work (typed, handwritten, etc.).

Parent Interview

Kevin describes a typical day at home with Kody as "long and exhausting," but "never a dull moment." He wakes Kody up for school at 7 a.m. and has his clothes laid out for him the night before. Kevin sets 30 minutes on Kody's basketball buzzer timer so that Kody knows he has 30 minutes to use the shower, get dressed and brush his teeth. Kevin explained that Kody's morning routine was a "constant struggle" for a while before the implementation of the basketball buzzer timer that motivates Kody to "beat the clock" to get ready in the morning. He also knows that Kody benefits from structure and routine, so having all of his clothing laid out and toothpaste/toothbrush ready are critical pieces to Kody completing his morning routine on time.

When Kody gets home from school, Kevin has learned through the years to let him decompress from the day. Kody enjoys playing video games on his Nintendo Switch (loves anything and everything Mario Kart), riding his bike and playing basketball on his portable basketball hoop in the driveway. Kody enjoys playing outside, and because he is still new to the neighborhood, he does not have many children to play outside with. As a result, Kody often ropes Kevin into playing with him outside. Kevin expressed how these are some of their best moments together and Kevin's favorite time of day. When playing, he sees Kody's "clumsy side" come out as Kody often trips and falls "over his own feet" and is constantly on top of Kevin due to his poor spatial awareness. Despite these clumsy moments when playing, he does notice some improvements when Kody goes in the house to sit down and do homework after playing outside.

Kevin recently learned that the university he will now be working for has a clinic that offers a number of different programs and occupational therapy services for children with special education needs such as social skills, swimming, basketball and cooking, to name a few. Kevin wants Kody to be able to regularly participate in some of these activities due to the benefits of socialization and physical activity as well as Kody's love for basketball. When Kody previously attempted an organized sport (baseball last spring), he was "politely asked" to "stop coming" due to his difficulties following directions, paying attention and bumping into other players when out on the field. After this experience Kody stated he "never wants to play baseball again." Kevin is hopeful that this time around, for basketball tryouts, things will be different.

Kevin expressed concern when Kody is completing homework, as he often avoids writing tasks and it takes him a great length of time to complete any homework that requires writing. Reading homework is also tough, as he notices Kody constantly losing his place when reading. He does what he can in order to provide Kody with breaks along the way, but homework is still a "huge struggle." He does not believe assignments are being adequately modified in order to meet Kody's learning needs in class, as this carries over to his difficulty when trying to complete these assignments at home.

Kevin revealed that he has always been a strong advocate for Kody and identifying what his needs are. Since taking Kody in, Kevin finds that every new school year, every new teacher and every new related service provider mean that the process begins again for Kevin to provide information and guide the professionals on how best to work with Kody. Kevin has a history of modifying Kody's assignments himself and giving his teachers and related service providers the strategies that work best for him. Every year Kevin is hopeful that there will be at least one member of the team that will listen to him and take his advice on how to best help Kody. Unfortunately, in the past, that has not always been the case.

The constant need to stand up and speak up for Kody is "extremely taxing" due to the fact that it all falls on him as a single parent. When asked how he copes with the constant stress and need to communicate Kody's needs, he stated that it is his "faith in God" and prayer that helps "get him through." Kevin regularly prays for Kody and prays for strength, guidance and direction to be a good parent to Kody. Kevin also regularly fasts as a method to help him get clarity and focus on what God wants him to do.

Kevin and Kody attend church services every Sunday at 11 a.m. with their family. They are both also actively involved in church. Kevin plays the drums for the choirs, which has sparked a similar interest in Kody. Kody is involved in the Children's Choir, Children's Church Ministry, the Mime Ministry, the Outreach Ministry and the Sight & Sound Ministry. He also serves as one of the flaggers in the Liturgical Dance Ministry. See Table 18.9 for more information on Kody's roles within the church.

Table 18.9 Kody's Roles at Church

Ministry	Purpose	Kody's Role
Children's Choir	Church choir that is made up of children.	Kody plays the drums for the children's choir.
Children's Church	Children's Church is focused on building the children's understanding of the Bible and the importance of a relationship with God. It is held during the same time as the adult services, just in a separate part of the church (Murray, 2020).	Kody is a participant/learner in Children's Church.
Mime	Creative expression of worship in which the individual(s) act out a song through body motions, without using their words. This is done in praise, worship and adoration to God (Maggio, 2017).	Kody serves as a "Junior" or Child Mime.
Outreach	Community service/volunteer ministry that seeks to help the less fortunate (Bast, n.d.).	Kody serves as a "Junior" or child outreach worker/ volunteer.
Sight & Sound	Oversees and manages the Audio & Video (AV) production of worship services.	Kody serves as a "Junior" or child AV team member.
Liturgical Dance	Creative expression of worship in which the individual(s) dance to a song in praise, worship and adoration to God (Britannica, n.d.).	Kody serves as a "flagger" (one who holds, spins and twirls the flags) in the dance ministry.

Evaluation Results From Occupational Therapy

Top Evaluation Results

Kevin completed the Canadian Occupational Performance Measure (COPM) (Law et al., 2019) as part of Kody's triennial evaluation. In this case, Kevin reflected on his perception and satisfaction with Kody's performance in the areas of self-care, leisure and productivity. The following five occupations were deemed as most important for improvement. He has noticed that Kody is frustrated and losing confidence in his schoolwork. Kevin wants for him to succeed academically and complete homework within a reasonable time frame. He also would like to see Kody be "less clumsy" and be able to follow directions better. Kevin wants Kody to feel successful with whatever it is he decides to do with his life. He wants him to develop the necessary life skills he will need to be an independent and successful adult someday.

Kevin reports that Kody can complete all aspects of dressing independently except for tying his shoes. He states that he has "tried and tried" to teach Kody, but he "just does not seem to get it." Kevin would like to see Kody be completely independent in the skill of shoe tying to ease morning routine frustration and improve his safety. Kody successfully uses utensils; however, he will try to eat standing up, put his legs on the chairs next to him while eating or will use the utensils as drumsticks. As a result, he requires constant reminders to "sit nicely" at the table for meals.

Kody's difficulties sitting for mealtimes is carried over into difficulties sitting during church services. Thankfully, Kody's various roles in the church have helped improve his ability to attend church services; however, he can still become "overstimulated" and "distracted" during service.

Kevin expressed concern when Kody is completing homework, as he often avoids writing tasks and it takes him a great length of time to complete any homework that requires writing. Reading homework is also tough, as he notices Kody constantly losing his place when reading. He does what he can in order to provide Kody with breaks along the way, but homework is still a "huge struggle." See Table 18.10 for COPM results.

Table 18.10 Evaluation Results Adapted From the COPM

Occupation	Performance	Satisfaction
Shoe tying	3	3
Completing homework	4	3
Sit for family meals	4	4
Attend church service	5	5
Making the basketball team	4	3

Source: Law, M., Baptiste, S., Carswell, A., McColl, M. A., Polatajko, H., & Pollock, N. (2019). *Canadian occupational performance measure (COPM)* (5th ed. rev.). COPM Inc.

Bottom Evaluation Results

Kody's teachers completed the Sensory Processing Measure, Second Edition (SPM-2) School Form (Ecker et al., 2021) (see Table 18.11). The SPM-2 is a standardized test for children ages 5–12 that measures sensory integration/sensory processing. This test determines a child's sensory functioning specific to the school environment. This test rates six sensory systems (vestibular, proprioceptive, tactile, taste and smell, visual and auditory) as well as praxis and social participation.

Table 18.11 Sensory Processing Measure-2 Child School Form Results

Sections	Raw Score	T Score	Percentile	Interpretation
Vision	16	58	79%	Typical
Hearing	15	57	76%	Typical
Touch	19	67	96%	Moderate difficulties
Taste and Smell	13	58	79%	Typical
Body Awareness	21	78	>99%	Severe difficulties
Balance and Motion	24	78	>99%	Severe difficulties
Sensory Total	108	72	99%	Severe difficulties
Planning and Ideas	28	73	99%	Severe difficulties
Social Participation	22	63	90%	Moderate difficulties

Source: Adapted from Ecker, C., Henry, D. A., Kuhaneck, H., Parham, L. D., & Glennon, T. J. (2021). *Sensory Processing Measure–2nd Edition (SPM-2) Child School Form*. Western Psychological Services.

As per the results of the SPM-2, Kody presents with sensory processing dysfunction, specifically in the areas of Body Awareness (proprioceptive processing), Balance and Motion (vestibular processing) and Planning and Ideas (praxis).

Due to concerns regarding handwriting, typing and coordination, the Bruininks-Oseretsky Test of Motor Proficiency, Second Edition (BOT-2) (Bruininks & Bruininks, 2005) was administered. BOT-2 is a standardized test that measures a wide array of motor skills in individuals aged 4–21 years. A scale score of 11–19 or a standard score of 41–59 is considered average. BOT-2 results revealed that Kody scored below average in the following subtests: fine motor precision, fine motor integration, manual dexterity and upper-limb coordination.

References

Bast, E. C. (n.d.). Simple outreach ministry ideas and tips for getting started. *Faithward.org*. www.faithward.org/simple-outreach-ministry-ideas-and-tips-for-getting-started/#:~:text=What%20is%20outreach%20ministry%3F,or%20a%20five%2Dyear%20plan

Borg, G. (1998). *Borg's perceived exertion and pain scales*. Human Kinetics.

Britannica. (n.d.). Christianity: New liturgical forms and antiliturgical attitudes. *Britannica.com Encyclopedia*. Retrieved October 31, 2022, from www.britannica.com/topic/liturgical-dance

Bruininks, R. H., & Bruininks, B. D. (2005). *Bruininks-Oseretsky test of motor proficiency* (2nd ed.). AGS Publishing.

Centers for Disease Control and Prevention. (2019, December 9). *What is "early intervention"?* www.cdc.gov/ncbddd/actearly/parents/states.html

Cole, M. B., & Tufano, R. (2008). *Applied theories in occupational therapy: A practical approach*. Slack Incorporated.

Ecker, C., Henry, D. A., Kuhaneck, H., Parham, L. D., & Glennon, T. J. (2021). *Sensory processing measure—2nd edition (SPM-2) child school form*. Western Psychological Services.

The Editors of Encyclopaedia Britannica (Ed.). (2020, May 25). Rosary. *Encyclopædia Britannica*. www.britannica.com/topic/rosary/additional-info#contributors

The Editors of Encyclopaedia Britannica (Ed.). (2021, May 5). Cross. *Encyclopædia Britannica*. www.britannica.com/topic/cross-religious-symbol#ref136750.

Hillerbrand, H. J. (2020). Christmas. *Encyclopædia Britannica*. www.britannica.com/topic/Christmas-holiday

Hillerbrand, H. J. (2021). Easter. *Encyclopædia Britannica*. www.britannica.com/topic/Easter-holiday

Law, M., Baptiste, S., Carswell, A., McColl, M. A., Polatajko, H., & Pollock, N. (2019). *Canadian occupational performance measure (COPM)* (5th ed. rev.). COPM Inc.

Maggio, D. (2017). *Gospel mime: Anointed ministry, Afrocentrism, and gender in black gospel performance*. Master's Thesis, University of Pittsburgh. http://d-scholarship.pitt.edu/id/eprint/31664

Model of Human Occupation Clearinghouse. (2020). *Modified interest checklist*. Department of Occupational Therapy, University of Illinois at Chicago. https:\\moho-irm.uic.edu.

Murray, L. (2020). Defining children's ministry. *Children's Ministry Basics*. https://childrensministrybasics.com/2020/08/11/defining-childrens-ministry/

Oakley, F. C., Cunningham, L., Knowles, M. D., Marty, M. E., Frassetto, M., Pelikan, J. J., & John L. McKenzie. (n.d.). Roman catholicism. *Encyclopædia Britannica*. www.britannica.com/topic/Roman-Catholicism

Rock, P. L., Roiser, J. P., Riedel, W. J., & Blackwell, A. D. (2014). Cognitive impairment in depression: A systematic review and meta-analysis. *Psychological Medicine*, *44*(10), 2029–2040. https://doi.org/10.1017/S0033291713002535

Steffen, T. M., Hacker, T. A., & Mollinger, L. (2002). Age- and gender-related test performance in community-dwelling elderly people: Six-minute walk test, Berg balance scale, timed up & go test, and gait speeds. *Physical Therapy*, *82*(2), 128–137. https://doi.org/10.1093/ptj/82.2.128

Taylor, R. R. (2017). *Kielhofner's model of human occupation: Theory and application* (5th ed.). Lippincott Williams and Wilkins.

Tee, S. (n.d.-a). 12 best and unique pancit noodle dishes in the Philippines. *Guide to the Philippines.* https://guidetothephilippines.ph/articles/history-culture/pancit-guide-philippines

Tee, S. (n.d.-b). Lechon in the Philippines: A guide to Filipinos' favorite roasted pig and more. *Guide to the Philippines.* https://guidetothephilippines.ph/articles/ultimate-guides/philippines-lechon-guide#lechon-kawali-and-crispy-pata

Tee, S. (n.d.-c). Philippines' Adobo: A guide to the Iconic Filipino dish. *Guide to the Philippines.* https://guidetothephilippines.ph/articles/ultimate-guides/philippines-adobo-guide

U.S. Department of Education. (2017, May 3). *Sec. 300.304 evaluation procedures.* https://sites.ed.gov/idea/regs/b/d/300.304

Whyte, J., Smith, M., Nazario, B., Bhargava, H., & Pathak, N. (2021, May 5). Drugs & Medications A-Z. *WebMD.* www.webmd.com/drugs/2/index.

MMCR Glossary of Terms

Chapter 1

Analytic processes. Part of the clinical reasoning process and used in conjunction with non-analytic processes; consists of cognitive elements and is based on objective analysis when a practitioner's expertise alone is insufficient, requiring more evidence.

Clinical reasoning. The thinking processes practitioners utilize throughout their therapeutic process to plan, direct, perform, and reflect on client care. Also referred to as professional reasoning in occupational therapy and occurs broadly across all practice settings. Key characteristics of clinical reasoning include critical thinking, problem-solving, therapeutic reasoning, and ethical reasoning.

Conditional reasoning. A type of reasoning that takes on a broader understanding of the person's contexts by considering the social and temporal concerns. This type of reasoning takes into consideration what the best approach for this specific person is and considers current and future outcomes.

Critical thinking. A key characteristic of clinical reasoning based solely on knowledge, evidence, and science rather than intuition or assumptions.

Ethical considerations. A key characteristic of clinical reasoning that emphasizes the practitioner's ability to reason through a dilemma or conflict by collecting the facts of the situation and progress to a morally sound decision.

Interactive reasoning. A type of reasoning that focuses on understanding the illness perspective from the vantage point of the person served. This reasoning emphasizes the interpersonal relationships such as the collaboration between the person and the practitioner.

Narrative reasoning. A type of reasoning that emphasizes the person's story told from their perspective. This helps the practitioner to understand the totality of the story and to assist the person in creating the person's future story.

Non-analytic processes. Part of the clinical reasoning process and used in conjunction with analytic processes; focuses on the affective domain and is more prone to error because those processes are based on subjective analysis, prior knowledge, and the practitioner's expertise.

Problem-solving. A key characteristic of clinical reasoning, problem-solving involves the practitioner utilizing information that is available to them to generate a solution to an existing problem.

Procedural reasoning. A type of reasoning that incorporates more use of science and evidence as the practitioner identifies occupational problems related to disease and disability to implement an intervention plan.

Therapeutic use of self. A key characteristic of clinical reasoning that occurs when the practitioner uses knowledge, personality, and actions to enhance a therapeutic collaboration.

Pragmatic reasoning.   A type of reasoning that considers practitioners' knowledge and experiences when determining an intervention plan within a given practice location. This can include the practitioner's level of experience, organizational policies, time, and available physical resources

Chapter 2

Analysis of performance.   These types of bottom evaluations measure potential client factors and/or performance skills that may facilitate or hinder occupational performance.

Bottom type of evaluations.   In the Matthews Model of Clinical Reasoning, analysis of performance evaluations are categorized as a "bottom" type of evaluation.

Bottom-up approach.   A bottom-up approach emphasizes evaluating analysis of performance measures first to determine how those skills are relevant to a person's valued occupations. The strengths and challenges to a person's client factors and performance skills can be uncovered with numerous bottom-oriented evaluations. Following this line of clinical reasoning, the practitioner begins with understanding the bottom-oriented information and then places it in context of the person's story.

Domain of concern.   This represents our areas of expertise, what makes our profession unique, and details our body of knowledge. It is written in such a way that laypeople are often able to distinguish our areas of expertise and role delineation between professions.

Model.   The way a profession looks at itself, the connection to the other professions, and its relationship with society.

Occupational profile.   This is a type of evaluation used to facilitate a practitioner's understanding of a person's story related to their occupations, activities, interests, and goals. An occupational profile is typically completed in an interview-style format so the practitioner can ask numerous open-ended types of questions with probing, clarifying, and restatements of ideas.

The Occupational Therapy Practice Framework (OTPF):   An example of a document that illustrates our current domain of concern. This document is divided into two parts: domain and process.

Top-down approach.   A top-down approach starts with an occupational profile (top) and provides the practitioner with detailed information about the person's story, interests, occupations, and goals. While this specific information is necessary to learn about the individual person, it does not always emphasize the strengths and challenges of the person's client factors or performance skills. Following this line of clinical reasoning, practitioners begin with the top information and then go down to evaluate a person's client factors or performance skills.

Top type of evaluations.   In the Matthews Model of Clinical Reasoning, occupational profiles are categorized as a "top" type of evaluation.

Chapter 3

The Person section of the triangle.   As part of the MMCR, the practitioner identifies some of the basic, but not limited to, specific information about the individual such as age, education, ethnic identity, cultural identity, diagnosis, gender identity, health considerations, medications and side effects, race, religion, sexual orientation, spirituality, and socioeconomic status.

Reflection-in-action.   This is a process of thinking about what you are doing as you do it. The benefits are that you immediately start to frame the data and begin to identify and transform information into usable pieces. When the triangle guidesheet is completed, the practitioner reflects back on the process and reviews, analyzes, and evaluates to determine what might be missing or further explored.

Chapter 4

Cultural environment.   One of the five facets listed under location, the cultural environment includes the expectations of customs, ideals, values, and thoughts of a social group.

Location.   Viewed as the highest conceptual level of environment, location refers to the sites and places where occupations occur.

Physical environment.   One of the five facets listed under location, the physical environment includes non-human or non-living objects present in various locations that are relevant to a person's life story.

Social environment.   One of the five facets listed under location, the social environment includes people, groups, communities, organizations, and populations that people feel a sense of belonging to, identify with, or have frequent contact with.

Temporal environment.   One of the five facets listed under location, the temporal environment includes understanding a person's story from the perspective of time.

Virtual environment.   One of the five facets listed under location, the virtual environment includes using technology as a means to carry out occupations or communicate with others

Chapter 5

Activities as part of the evaluation process.   Activities represent a general idea held in the minds of a shared culture or society in terms of context, timing, value, and feelings. During the evaluation process, the occupational practitioner uses activities to serve as a starting point in the discussion to understand more about a person's life story.

Occupations as part of the evaluation process.   The practitioner uses the evaluation process to further explore a person's occupations in terms of what they want, need, or are expected to do. The meaning, environmental context, and emotional connection of each occupation places the specific person as central to their story. Using the art of practice, the practitioner begins exploring those most important general activities using open-ended questions, probing, clarifying, and restating pertinent information to understand the person's occupations.

Chapter 6

Bottom.   The bottom is part of a person's occupational performance issues that emphasizes client factors and/or performance skills that may strengthen or hinder the person's top/middle. This information comes from a bottom-oriented or analysis of performance type of evaluation. It is usually selected by the practitioner, in collaboration with the person, to identify what might be getting in the way of a person's goal achievement.

Middle.   The middle is a part of a person's occupational performance issues that represents shorter-term plans, stepping stones, or accomplishments to be achieved. It is specific to the person's story. This information may come from an occupational profile or top-oriented evaluation that facilitates opportunities for practitioners to learn about the person's unique life story, occupations, and environmental facets.

Occupational performance issues.   These are visualized as the center of the triangle using the labels top-middle-bottom to identify the most pressing part of the person's story relative to the person, their environment context, and occupations. In the center of the triangle, there is a square root or letter V–looking symbol ($\sqrt{}$). In the MMCR, this ($\sqrt{}$), or occupational performance issue, symbolizes the first and then subsequent set of life changes that will eventually lead to an intervention plan.

Top.   The top is a part of a person's occupational performance issues that represents a longer-term plan or goal achievement. This information comes from a top-oriented or occupational profile type of evaluation. It is specific to the person's story, identifying the person's longer-term goals and specific interests.

Chapter 7

Characteristics of a frame of reference.   A guideline for action that emphasizes a specific age group or disability, starts with a deficit-driven perspective of the person served, is narrow in scope and content, and intervention moves through stages of dysfunction to function.

Characteristics of a practice model.   A guideline for action that is applicable to all age groups, people (with or without disability), and practice areas so it is broader in scope and content; methods used to conduct evaluations that emphasize occupations and consider the person's unique life story; intervention plans emphasize the interconnectedness of the person, environment, and occupation constructs.

Heuristic.   A decision-making strategy or "rule of thumb" approach. It is the method that experienced practitioners use as a kind of mental shortcut.

MMCR five-step guide to infusing a frame of reference/practice model into a person's evaluation selection and intervention plan:

Step 1: Identify the specific frame of reference(s) and/or practice model(s) to guide the evaluation and intervention process.

Step 2: Words in a box: Create a mental picture by grouping those words, phrases, definitions, evaluations, and intervention ideas together.

Step 3: Create a frame of reference and/or practice model party paragraph: Reflect on these words in a box and begin crafting full paragraphs to link these ideas together into a unifying message.

Step 4: Succinct summary of a person's story emphasizing relevant occupational performance issues: Write a summary of the person's unique story and goals emphasizing the initial top-middle-bottom occupational performance issues.

Step 5: Explanation of how the frame of reference and/or practice model directly influences the specific intervention plan: Reflect on information in steps 1–4 and apply it to guide the person's specific intervention plan.

Chapters 8–12 MMCR Intervention

The beginning part of the intervention plan.   During the beginning part of the intervention plan, the practitioner identifies and creates processes to initiate the change process related to the top-middle-bottom occupational performance issues.

The middle part of the intervention plan.   Once the beginning processes have formed, the middle parts represent the "heavy lifting" of the intervention plan. The middle is the heart of occupation-based practice, emphasizing the top-middle-bottom performance issues. Over the duration of the intervention plan, the practitioner uses the middle part for practice and reinforcement with an increase in task demands.

The end part of the intervention plan.   The end part of the intervention plan, nearing discharge or termination of services, includes specific sections that emphasize preparation to sustain future change. This is influenced by numerous factors such as progress made by the person, relevancy of the intervention approach to the suggested top-middle-bottom, location of services, person's perception of goal achievement, and overall duration of the intervention.

Horizontal line. $\overline{V}$ _____ This horizontal line represents the overall continuum of intervention created specifically for each person served. This line represents a person's total intervention plan from the beginning until the end of services. This line may represent a person who is participating in services within any time frame on any practice area location.

Incorporating activities and occupations to plan intervention.   Using the information gathered about a person's activities and occupations from the evaluation, the practitioner begins formulating a plan incorporating a combination of methods to support occupations that are meaningful to the person and/or central to their well-being.

Methods.   A practitioner carefully selects and uses available methods when implementing occupation-based intervention such as therapeutic use of occupations and activities, interventions to support occupations, education, training, advocacy, self-advocacy, groups, and virtual formats. The type of method(s) selected for intervention depends on multiple factors such as the person's story, environmental context, goals, practice area location, etc.

Peripheral approaches to intervention.   The intervention plan is somewhat related to the person's story, but does not directly address the top-middle-bottom.

Spiral image of intervention that occurs across the entire intervention process from the beginning to the end.   This spiral, incorporating some elements of the top-middle-bottom, continues throughout the entire duration of the intervention plan. By spiraling across, considerable intervention attention is placed on the middle and/or top occupational performance issues in addition to the bottom.

Spiral image of intervention that occurs up and down within each set of occupational performance issues.   During the intervention plan, visualize the top-middle-bottom as a spiral, with the practitioner entering through the middle and addressing all aspects of the occupational performance issues. The practitioner may begin spiraling through the middle, down to the bottom, but also up to the top illustrating the spiral within.

Vertical lines. $\overline{V}$_____/_____/ The vertical lines added throughout the horizontal line delineate and emphasize various sections of the overall intervention plan to make it more manageable. Conceptualizing the overall intervention plan into smaller sections will create a sequential awareness of the change process from the beginning to the end. These vertical lines further assist the practitioner to chunk, or group, relevant methods into smaller sections of the intervention plan while reinforcing top-middle-bottom(s) performance issues during occupational-based practice.

The why factor when creating each section's vertical lines.   The cognitive process behind each vertical line section represents a central idea to describe the intervention emphasis related to the identified top-middle-bottom occupational performance issues. This cognitive process taps into a practitioner's mental skills and knowledge to create rationales for intervention choices and eventual method selection.

Chapter 13

Evaluation summary.   After careful analysis of all evaluations is conducted, this summary provides a snapshot of a person's baseline measure centered on the initial top-middle-bottom(s) occupational performance issues.

Interpretations.   Part of the four basic ingredients of effective documentation, these statements provide a practitioner subjective understanding about the person's behaviors, skills, and/or verbal statements documented within the raw data. This gives meaning to the raw data in terms of the person, their environmental context, and occupations.

Occupational performance issues.   Part of the acronym POP, this next section of the evaluation summary highlights the person's unique life story obtained from the top-oriented (occupational profile) and bottom-oriented (analysis of performance) evaluations. All strengths, challenges, raw data, and interpretations emphasizing the top-middle-bottom occupational performance issues are included in this section of the evaluation summary.

Person.   Part of the acronym POP, this first section of the evaluation summary provides relevant information about the person's situation to see the bigger picture. This will help follow the specific evaluation results described in the evaluation summary. The occupational therapy practitioner strategically selects important background information to understand how the evaluation findings align with the person's story.

Plan.   Part of the acronym POP, this final section of the evaluation summary documents an action plan for change, including both long-term and short-term goals.

Raw data.   Part of the four basic ingredients of effective documentation, these factual or objective statements paint a picture for the reader about a person's behaviors, skills, and/or verbal statements. These objective statements, or the raw data, provide a recollection of what occurred during the evaluation and intervention process without subjective interpretation.

Strengths and challenges.   Part of the four basic ingredients of effective documentation. The practitioners reflect on and document both a person's strengths and challenges related to the top-middle-bottom occupational performance issues.

Chapter 14

Discharge summaries.   These notes are a type of documentation created when the person is nearing the ending section of the continuum for intervention. The practitioner provides a general overview of the progress made toward the selected top-middle-bottom occupational performance issue(s), what may still need to be addressed in the next practice area location, and an action plan of recommendations to continue growth and mastery.

Evaluation summary _____*x*_____ /PN_____ /PN_____ /PN and **discharge summary**

*PN stands for progress note.

Long-term goals.   A long-term goal lays the foundation for a person's short-term goals by establishing an overarching connection to the identified top-middle-bottom occupational performance issue(s). Long-term goals do not need to be measurable, but provide a general description of what the person is trying to accomplish for the duration of the intervention plan.

Progress notes.   These notes are documented opportunities for the practitioner to review each beginning-middle-ending section of the continuum for intervention to determine progress made within each time frame. These notes reflect on the progress toward the top-middle-bottom occupational performance issues initially identified in the evaluation summary and now spiraled across the continuum. As the practitioner has mentally conceptualized how intervention will proceed, progress notes are the "stop and see" measure to track progress made after each beginning-middle-ending intervention section.

Evaluation summary _____*x*_____ /**PN**_____ /**PN**_____ /**PN** and discharge summary

*PN stands for progress note.

Short-term goals.   Following the occupational performance issues highlighted in the long-term goal, there tend to be multiple short-term goals. A short-term goal represents a task that a person intends to accomplish in the near future and is often viewed as the building blocks toward reaching the long-term goals.

Five-step guide to formulating a short-term goal:

1. _____ **will**
(person's name)

2. _____ **in order to**
(measurable, comes from the bottom occupational performance issues)

3. _____ **with**
(functional and specific, comes from the top or middle occupational performance issues)

4. _____**in**
(measurement; how much cuing, prompting, or physical assistance)

5. _____
(time frame for achievement)

The Six MMCR Clinical Reasoning Guidesheets in Sequential Order

Appendix 1: MMCR Guide to Understanding a Person's Story (Triangle):
Appendix 2: MMCR Five Step Guide to Infusing a Frame of Reference/PM into a Person's Evaluation Selection and Intervention Plan:
Appendix 3: MMCR Five Step Guide to Infusing a Frame of Reference/PM into a Person's Evaluation Selection and Intervention Plan:
Appendix 4: MMCR Planning Guide to Address *Specific* Sections of the Overall Intervention Plan:
Appendix 5: MMCR Guide to Evaluations Summaries
Appendix 6: MMCR Guidelines to Formulate a Short-Term Goal

Appendix 1A

MMCR Guide to Understanding a Person's Story
(Triangle)

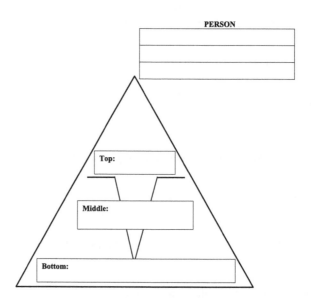

OCCUPATIONS

Occupations: _____

_____

_____

Activities: _____

_____

_____

ENVIRONMENTS

Location: _____

Physical: _____

Temporal: _____

Cultural: _____

Social: _____

Virtual: _____

Appendix 1B

Explanation of MMCR Guide to Understanding a Person's Story (Triangle)

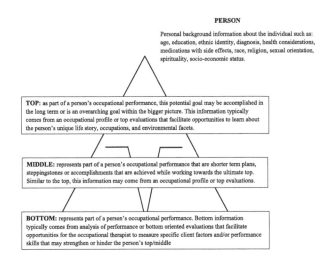

PERSON
Personal background information about the individual such as:
age, education, ethnic identity, diagnosis, health considerations,
medications with side effects, race, religion, sexual orientation,
spirituality, socio-economic status.

TOP: as part of a person's occupational performance, this potential goal may be accomplished in the long term or is an overarching goal within the bigger picture. This information typically comes from an occupational profile or top evaluations that facilitate opportunities to learn about the person's unique life story, occupations, and environmental facets.

MIDDLE: represents part of a person's occupational performance that are shorter term plans, steppingstones or accomplishments that are achieved while working towards the ultimate top. Similar to the top, this information may come from an occupational profile or top evaluations.

BOTTOM: represents part of a person's occupational performance. Bottom information typically comes from analysis of performance or bottom oriented evaluations that facilitate opportunities for the occupational therapist to measure specific client factors and/or performance skills that may strengthen or hinder the person's top/middle

OCCUPATIONS

Occupation:
Personal, subjective, embedded in context, has a beginning and an ending, observed by others, interpreted by a specific person, has an attached emotional connection. Central to a person's well-being in terms of what is desired, needed, or expected.

Activity:
Based on societal norms and expectations, consists of a general idea held in the minds of others, specific context is not relevant, lacks specific ideas to a person's story. Relevant activities will vary depending on the person's story.

ENVIRONMENTS

Location: viewed as the highest conceptual level of environment, location refers to the sites and places where occupations happen

Physical: non-human or non-living objects present in various locations that are relevant to a person's life story

Temporal: understanding a person's story from the perspective of time

Social: people, groups, communities, organizations, and populations that people feel a sense of belonging with, identity with, or have frequent contact with

Cultural: the expectations of customs, ideals, values, and thoughts of a social group

Virtual: using technology as a means to carry out occupations or communicate with others

Appendix 2A

MMCR Five-Step Guide to Infusing a Frame of Reference/Practice Model Into a Person's Evaluation Selection and Intervention Plan

Step 1: Frame of reference (FOR)/practice model (PM):

Step 2: Words in a box:

Step 3: Frame of reference and/or practice model party paragraph:

Step 4: Succinct summary of person's story emphasizing relevant occupational performance issues ∇

Step 5: Explanation of how the frame of reference and/or practice model will directly influence the specific intervention plan:

Appendix 2B

MMCR Five-Step Guide to Infusing a Frame of Reference and/or Practice Model Into a Person's Evaluation Selection and Intervention Plan (Explanation)

Step 1: Frame of reference (FOR)/practice model (PM):

> Write down the potential frame of reference and/or practice model you plan to use. Circle the word FOR or PM, depending on what you select.

Step 2: Words in a box:

> Write down all relevant words, phrases, definitions, evaluations, change processes, and tips relevant to the frame of reference and/or practice model identified in Step 1.

Step 3: Frame of reference and/or practice model party paragraph:

> Incorporating the words and phrases identified in Step 2, create detailed but concise paragraph(s) to provide a general understanding of the frame of reference and/or practice model. You can use the language from the frame of reference and/or practice model, but this party paragraph must make sense to you.

Step 4: Succinct summary of person's story emphasizing relevant occupational performance issues:

> After the evaluation information is analyzed, provide a detailed but concise summary of the person's story emphasizing the top-middle-bottom occupational performance issues.

Step 5: Explanation of how the frame of reference and/or practice model will directly influence the specific intervention plan:

> Reflect on steps 1–4 to understand the person's story and guide the intervention plan. Then integrate this specific information with the frame of reference and/or practice model. When completing this step, use the frame of reference and/or practice model language and explain how it will apply to the specific person.

Appendix 3A

MMCR Overview Guide to Intervention Planning

MMCR Overview Guide to Intervention Planning

V   V   V

Continuum for intervention:

V _____

Practice location:	
Duration of services from beginning to end:	
Intervention hours over this duration:	
Frame of reference and/or practice model:	

Appendix 3B

MMCR Overview Guide to Intervention Planning (Explanation)

The top-middle-bottom occupational performance issue symbols, similar in shape to a square root, provide the practitioner with visual reminders of the initial and/or subsequent issues to be addressed throughout the duration of the intervention plan. This is a dynamic process, as initial tops may move into middles over time, the top may stay consistent throughout the entire intervention plan, or multiple bottoms may be addressed simultaneously.

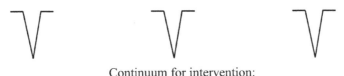

Continuum for intervention:

The continuous horizontal line represents a person's duration of intervention. This line may represent days, weeks, months, or years. The practitioner will draw in vertical lines representing smaller chunks or sections of the intervention process. The top-middle-bottom occupational performance issue symbol is placed at the beginning of the horizontal line to visually cue the practitioner to spiral within AND across the intervention continuum.

Practice location:	Locations matter. Occupational therapy services can be implemented in one central location or across multiple locations. Consider how the facets within these locations (physical, temporal, cultural, social, and virtual) strengthen or challenge intervention plans.
Duration of services from beginning to end:	Identify how long and how often the practitioner has to collaborate with the person seeking services in terms of days, weeks, months, or years.
Intervention hours over this duration:	Consider the amount of intervention time available in terms of hours. This will assist all practitioners to conceptualize the duration of intervention more realistically and consistently.
Frame of reference and/ or practice model:	Is the practitioner following one central guideline for action or a combination of internally consistent guidelines for action? Consider the differences between a frame of reference and a practice model. How will key elements of this guideline(s) for action be used throughout the evaluation and intervention plan?

Appendix 4A

MMCR Planning Guide to Address Specific Sections of the Overall Intervention Plan

$\bigvee$ _____

Circle the section of this plan: Beginning Part of Plan   Middle Part of Plan   Ending Part of Plan

Identify the specific section in terms of time:

| |
| |

Label and briefly describe the central idea of this specific section of the plan:

| |
| |

How does this specific section connect to the overall intervention plan? Describe the ways these intervention ideas are related to $\bigvee$

| |
| |

Describe the plan for creating awareness and/or skill building.

| |
| |

Select specific methods used to promote change (therapeutic use of occupations and activities, interventions to support occupations, education, training, advocacy, self-advocacy, group intervention, and virtual interventions):

| |
| |

Identify and describe the specific teaching-learning principles to promote change:

| |
| |

Appendix 4B

MMCR Planning Guide to Address Specific Sections of the Overall Intervention Plan (Explanation)

$\bigvee$ _____

Circle the section of this plan: Beginning Part of Plan   Middle Part of Plan   Ending Part of Plan

*Use a separate clinical reasoning guidesheet for each beginning-middle-ending part of the plan.

Identify the specific section in terms of time:

> Use the horizontal line to reflect on each specific beginning, middle, or ending section of the continuum for intervention in terms of time for each section (days, weeks, months, years), how many meetings (how many sessions will be offered), and total number of hours.

Label and briefly describe the central idea of this specific section of the plan:

> Describe the part of the change process emphasized in this section of the plan. Is new learning being introduced? Is the person building an awareness of the change process or practicing the development of a skill?

How does this specific section connect to the overall intervention plan? Describe the ways these intervention ideas are related to $\bigvee$:

> All intervention selections with each section must stay aligned with the top-middle-bottom occupational performance issues.

Describe the plan for creating awareness and/or skill building.

> Occupational therapy practitioners are active participants in the change process. Our "doing" incorporates factors such as utilizing relevant teaching-learning principles, selecting relevant methods, and grading activities based on where the person is in the change process.

Select specific methods used to promote change (therapeutic use of occupations and activities, interventions to support occupations, education, training, advocacy, self-advocacy, group intervention, and virtual interventions):

Select relevant methods (therapeutic use of occupations and activities, interventions to support occupations, training, advocacy, self-advocacy, group intervention, virtual interventions) for each section of the beginning-middle-ending part of the intervention plan. Each section of the intervention plan has a different focus and goals, so adjust the methods accordingly. Carefully combining different types of methods will solidify a person's learning process and keep it motivating at the same time.

Identify and describe the specific teaching-learning principles to promote change:

Teaching and learning are at the core of all occupational therapy intervention. We spend a considerable amount of time teaching people new and creative ways to perform meaningful tasks. Become familiar with any new learning before teaching it to others by researching about the topic, interviewing others with similar experiences, watching videos, or practicing the skill directly.

Appendix 5A

MMCR Guide to Evaluation Summaries

Relevant Areas to the Person's Evaluation Findings	Strengths	Challenges	Raw Data	Interpretation

Appendix 5B

MMCR Guide to Evaluation Summaries (Explanation)

Relevant Areas to the Person's Evaluation Findings	Strengths	Challenges	Raw Data	Interpretation
Provide short and concise words, phrases, or statements to identify each relevant area addressed in the evaluation summary.	Place an X next to each relevant area identifying if this is a strength or challenge or considered both. This will help maintain a balance of strengths and limitations throughout the evaluation summary.		Provide all facts and objective information for each area into the person's evaluation findings column. Provide raw data for both the selected occupational profile (top) evaluation and analysis of performance (bottom) evaluation. Consider providing raw data that illustrates both strengths and challenges.	Provide subjective information (within our area of expertise) for each relevant area to the person's evaluation findings column. Provide interpretations aligned with raw data for both the selected occupational profile (top) evaluation and analysis of performance (bottom) evaluations. Consider providing interpretations that emphasize both strengths and challenges.

Appendix 6A

MMCR Guidelines to Formulate a Short-Term Goal

1. [ ] **will**

(Person's name)

2. [ ] **in order to**

(measurable, comes from bottom occupational performance issues)

3. [ ] **with**

(functional and specific, comes from top or middle occupational performance issue)

4. [ ] **in**

(measurement; how much cuing, prompting, or physical assistance)

5. [ ]

(time frame for achievement)

Appendix 6B

MMCR Guidelines to Formulate a Short-Term Goal (Explanation)

1. _____ will

   (person's name)

2. _____ in order to

   (measurable, comes from bottom occupational performance issues)

3. _____ with

   (functional and specific, comes from top or middle occupational performance issue)

4. _____ in

   (measurement; how much cuing, prompting, or physical assistance)

5. _____

   (time frame for achievement)

Quick Explanation Guide:

#1 Use the person's actual name rather than labels such as patient, client, and consumer.

#2 This is a measurable component. Take your bottom from the analysis of performance and adjust the wording so progress is measured. No methods in this section. The wording is less specific to incorporate a variety of intervention options. For example, instead of using the word "pillbox" use "memory aid" instead.

#3 This is the functional component. It comes from your middle or top occupational performance issue. This makes it unique to the person and written so the goal is not interchangeable with other people. This is super-specific. Instead of using the word "grocery store," say "working in the deli department at the community ShopRite."

#4 Think about the physical, verbal, and visual cuing or assistance required for success. All people do not need to be fully independent at the end of intervention.

 # 5 Time frames matter. Do you have one week to accomplish something or a few months?

Note: #2 measurable part, # 4 cueing, and #5 time frames align together.

Index

Note: Page numbers in *italic* indicate a figure and page numbers in **bold** indicate a table on the corresponding page.